Culture and Sexual Risk

Culture and Sexual Risk

Anthropological Perspectives on AIDS

Edited by

Han ten Brummelhuis

University of Amsterdam
The Netherlands

and

Gilbert Herdt

University of Chicago
Illinois, USA

Gordon and Breach Publishers

Australia Austria China France Germany India Japan
Luxembourg Malaysia Netherlands Russia Singapore
Switzerland Thailand United Kingdom United States

RA
644
A25
C846
1995

3 Boulevard Royal
L-2449 Luxembourg

British Library Cataloguing in Publication Data

Culture and Sexual Risk:Anthropological
Perspectives on AIDS
I. Brummelhuis, Han Ten II. Herdt,
Gilbert H.
306.7

ISBN 2-88449-130-9 (hardcover)
      2-88449-131-7 (softcover)

CONTENTS

Acknowledgments vii

Introduction — Anthropology in the Context of AIDS
Han ten Brummelhuis and Gilbert Herdt ix

About the Contributors xxv

Part I CULTURE AND BEYOND: THE WIDER CONTEXT OF SEXUAL RISK

1   Culture, Poverty, and the Dynamics of HIV
    Transmission in Rural Haiti
    Paul Farmer   3

2   Culture, Sex Research and AIDS Prevention in Africa
    Brooke Grundfest Schoepf 29

3   Vulnerability to HIV Infection Among Three Hill
    Tribes in Northern Thailand
    Cornelia Ann Kammerer, Otome Klein Hutheesing,
    Ralana Maneeprasert, and Patricia V. Symonds 53

Part II CONTEXTUALIZING SEXUAL RISK

4   Gender, Age and Class: Discourses on HIV
    Transmission and Control in Uganda
    Christine Obbo 79

5   Sexuality, AIDS and Gender Norms Among
    Brazilian Teenagers
    Vera Paiva 97

6   The Dynamics of Condom Use in Thai Sex Work
    with *Farang* Clients
    Carla van Kerkwijk 115

7   Risky Business? Men Who Buy Heterosexual
    Sex in Spain
    Angie Hart 135

Part III SEXUAL RISK AMONG WESTERN GAY MEN

8 Sexual Negotiations: An Ethnographic Study of
Men Who Have Sex with Men
Benny Henriksson and Sven Axel Månsson 157

9 Social Stress and Risky Sex Among Gay Men:
An Additional Explanation for the Persistence
of Unsafe Sex
John Vincke and Ralph Bolton 183

10 Risk in Context: The Use of Sexual Diary Data
to Analyse Homosexual Risk Behaviour
Anthony P.M. Coxon and N.H. Coxon 205

11 Talking About AIDS: Linguistic Perspectives
on Non-Neutral Discourse
William L. Leap 227

Part IV THE STUDY OF CULTURE AND SEXUAL RISK

12 Disembodied Acts: On the Perverse Use of Sexual
Categories in the Study of High-Risk Behaviour
Michael C. Clatts 241

13 The Social and Cultural Construction of Sexual Risk,
or How to Have (Sex) Research in an Epidemic
Richard G. Parker 257

14 Theory and Method in HIV Prevention:
The Philippine Experience
Michael Lim Tan 271

15 Rethinking Anthropology: The Study of AIDS
Ralph Bolton 285

16 Half-Way There: Anthropology and Intervention-
Oriented AIDS Research in KwaZulu/Natal,
South Africa
E.M. Preston-Whyte 315

Index 339

ACKNOWLEDGMENTS

This volume originated during a University of Amsterdam conference organized as a satellite of the VIIIth International Conference on AIDS in Amsterdam in July 1992. What began as a modest attempt by a few Amsterdam anthropologists, working with AIDS projects in different cultures, to identify colleagues and projects elsewhere, grew precipitously into an energetic meeting with more than 120 participants. All of us were eager to use this opportunity to exchange ideas and experiences within a context free of the now so-frequent concerns of divergent disciplines and competing interests. More than sixty written contributions were presented; some are published here in revised form.

In preparing this book we acknowledge especially Richard Parker's advice and help. Iman Boot organized the greatest part of the process of revising and rewriting. Ian Priestnall, Sue Williams, and Alan Grusd helped in correcting and improving the language.

Special thanks to those who made the conference, 'Culture, Sexual Behavior and AIDS,' possible. Financial support was provided by the Koninklijke Akademie voor Wetenschappen in Amsterdam; the faculty of Social-Cultural and Political Sciences, University of Amsterdam; the FUOS (Funds for Development Cooperation), University of Amsterdam; the Centre for Asian Studies, University of Amsterdam; and the Amsterdam Universiteits Fonds.

The work of many volunteers was crucial to the success of the conference. We wish to acknowledge especially: Paul Grifhorst, Mirjam Schieveld, Carmencita Boekhoudt, Marietta Blokhuis, Inge van Oeveren, Lia Sciortino, Anneloes van Staa, Beate Wesdorp, Rudie van de Berg, Trudie Gerrits, Maria Piscaer, and Jetske Bijdendijk, whose help was invaluable.

INTRODUCTION

Anthropology in the Context of AIDS

Han ten Brummelhuis and Gilbert Herdt

What has anthropology to offer those who work in the area of AIDS/ STDs? Stated simply: The study of culture. For many professionals working on AIDS prevention, culture enters and then inflates itself as a 'barrier' they confront. Thus, 'culture' serves as the 'explanation' for failures to effectively fight the epidemic (see, e.g., Schoepf in this volume). Theoretically, for the anthropologist, culture defines much of the world in which people situate themselves and live. If we do not enter and attempt to understand this world, our efforts to convince, change or console others will be ineffective, even harmful. This theme of the priority of culture is central to all the contributions in this volume. And it is explored and documented here in many case studies from all over the world.

The chapters in this book highlight a series of issues with which social scientists involved in AIDS prevention research are confronted. These ethnographic studies illustrate how a particular culture and, indeed, a special context within it, defines the 'risks' of sexual HIV transmission. We use the term 'risks' in the plural to acknowledge the multiple pathways of infection that may result in HIV/AIDS. Moreover, some authors describe and analyse attempts to develop strategies of intervention that are tailored to the 'risk' requirements of a given group or cultural setting.

Anthropologists comprise the majority of the authors in this volume, which reflects how aspects of the AIDS crisis challenge anthropological theory, method, and practice. Several of the chapters argue that, so far, anthropology has had little reason to assume an attitude of self-confidence about its dynamic contribution to solving the AIDS crisis. At the same time, there are valid reasons why anthropologists, as well as non-anthropologists, should expect a substantial contribution from a discipline whose object of study is 'culture.'

The significance of the issues raised here is not, however, limited to the circle of professional anthropologists. Hence, we see how other disciplines are also confronted with the cultural side of AIDS but respond to this dimension in divergent ways. In the presence of scholars from other fields, working from the perspectives of their own disciplines, we find AIDS investigators who also met 'culture' and did not treat it merely as an awkward barrier to eliminate, but rather as the medium in which to work (see, for instance, the chapters by trained psychologists Paiva and Vincke). More generally, understanding and cooperation among the various disciplines challenged by the AIDS crisis are essential for contributions to have their desired effects in research, prevention, and education.

CHANGING ANTHROPOLOGY?

Anthropology does not have a clear-cut set of tools that have only to be applied in order to create solutions. On the contrary, AIDS has had the cumulative effect of opening a crisis in our discipline. As stated above, HIV/AIDS challenges the discipline to rethink some of the core elements of culture theory, method, and practice (see Bolton's, indeed, sometimes painful remarks). How continuing involvement with the AIDS crisis tends to influence and change anthropology can be illustrated threefold.

First, behavioural change is crucial for AIDS prevention, and anthropologists increasingly see themselves in the role of agents who attempt to change, re-interpret, or re-invent culture (especially Bolton; Schoepf; and Preston-Whyte in this volume; also Herdt 1992). Such a role is far removed from the old rhetorical position of functional anthropology, which advised, 'do not change the culture you are studying' (cf. Herdt and Stoller 1990). Such a role is even infamous for some — especially in light of the large-scale surreptitious involvement of anthropologists with counter-insurgency in the early 1970s. Several chapters of this volume express the ambiguities of this new activist or interventionist anthropological role (Preston-Whyte; Bolton). Such activism has led to experimenting with old and new solutions to the dilemma: 'observe but don't change the culture.' Noteworthy are the adaptation of group methods from social psychology (Schoepf); the rediscovery of Socialist models of mass education (Paiva); and the use of role playing and staged drama (Preston-Whyte; Tan). These solutions to the dilemma come amid growing doubts about the adequacy of classical fieldwork methods (Parker et al. 1991). It is not only time pressure that forces teamwork, but also a need to create a balanced perspective between, for instance, male and female, and outsider and insider points of view. In all such ways AIDS is changing the practice of anthropology.

In what sense is this AIDS-initiated practice different from the old and familiar 'applied' anthropology? What is new is how anthropologists assume increasing responsibility for the application of their knowledge, and then participate in the application of this in a culturally sensitive way. Thus, it is not just a report to be presented to decision-making officials within a government body, international agency, or NGO that matters. Given the pressure to not do just a study and look on, it should hardly surprise us to see anthropologists construct their research as a new kind of dialogue (Preston-Whyte, in this volume). In other words, we want to continually test our interpretations with our 'informants,' men and women who seek new ways to learn and teach about sexual risk.

Second, more than the other social sciences involved in AIDS research, anthropology rests upon a method that can be called intensively subjective; subjectivity constitutes its method and object (Mead 1977). Anthropology lives in the tension between subjective experience and objective reality; it always has to deal with both, in its sensitivity to local context and individual meaning. Our instrument is not an objectified procedure or a neutral tool but, instead, a trained, disciplined, and experienced subject. This human instrument, and thus our knowledge, is necessarily situated in and shaped by an individual researcher's history and experience. Anthropological research on AIDS has brought this subjective anchor of fieldwork to the fore.

Let us highlight at least the forms of 'commitment' among anthropologists studying AIDS. These tend to constitute different research paradigms — one exemplified by Western gay and lesbian anthropologists, another by Third World anthropologists. By 'commitment' we mean the lived experience and embodied knowledge of the social actor, who is a practising scientist combining theory and practice in the field. One of the merits of the present volume is how these elements are represented. To take into account and reflect about such 'constitutive' differences more systematically represents a modest step towards the destruction of the old myth of the self-sufficient and solipsistic anthropological researcher (see Lindenbaum 1992). More than any other 'social problem' AIDS seems to create cooperation — perhaps more accurately, mutual challenge and control of perspective — both between and within segments of anthropology.

Third, anthropology in its traditional form deals almost exclusively with local culture and the ways of people. More recently, anthropologists have come to realize how extremely difficult it has become to identify villages or locations in the world that have not been affected by the encroachment of the 'modern world system.' AIDS has thus imposed upon anthropology its totalism and global effects, shattering our prior particularistic conceptions of culture and society. AIDS articulates a tension between global patterns and frequencies of interaction and the local perspective that nourishes anthropology. For a generation now, anthropologists have emphasized the importance of taking into account this wider context (cf. Wolf 1980). AIDS has truly accelerated and completed this trend.

The AIDS crisis is 'global' in several senses. It is a multicultural problem which has to be combatted on a worldwide scale (see Mann et al. 1992). This collection reflects the fact that AIDS, apart from its Western pattern of distribution, is bringing moral, personal, and socio-economic crises to an increasing number of societies in the Third World. And, simultaneously, AIDS has become global in the sense that, even if no alarming HIV seroprevalence or AIDS figures are known, there is no reason to assume that any region or country will be spared. Further, AIDS entails sexual risk to populations of many kinds of sexual actors; and most of these actors are represented among the contributors to this book.

MODES OF COMMITMENT

As Ralph Bolton suggests in his essay (chapter 15), a larger number of anthropologists working on AIDS are gay or lesbian, with their involvement dating back almost a decade. These fieldworkers developed a discourse, criteria for research, research methods, and ethical guidelines. They helped to move issues such as sex and sexual identity from the periphery of the discipline to the agenda of 'normal' science. However pessimistic and skeptical these scholars were, or became (see also Clatts in this volume), regarding the effects of anthropologists' efforts to contribute solutions to HIV prevention, nevertheless they helped transform 'AIDS and Anthropology' into a recognized field, with its own research problems, networks, and informal research agendas (see Bolton and Singer 1992; Feldman 1990; Bolton and Kempler 1992; Herdt and Lindenbaum 1992). In the beginning, only a few Third World specialists in the United States (Schoepf, Farmer, among others) from outside the gay perspective joined them. Since the late 1980s, however, an increasing number of area specialists have realized how AIDS is changing their countries more than they could have imagined. This first occurred to specialists of sub-Saharan Africa; then to Latin Americanists; and finally to Asianists.

It is obvious that AIDS work is committing scholars in a probably not unique but — given the dominant atmosphere of the late 1980s and early 1990s — unexpected way. Commitment is also expected or required by those affected daily by the 'war' against the epidemic, those people with whom anthropologists in most cases have to cooperate. But, as stated above, there are important differences and varieties of commitment, especially between the gay/lesbian anthropologists and the Third World anthropologists. Here we do not want to question sincerity and honesty: Rather, we wish to recognize the differences between two kinds of cultural commitment — the social formations of gays and those of the Third World — observed at our conference and reflected in these papers. Bolton's chapter especially challenges many readers to reflect on the specifically 'gay' form of commitment in contrast to the work of those in the Third World.

Gay men — anthropologists in North America and Europe — who became involved with AIDS were themselves 'natives.' Their professional involvement was part and parcel of their personal, sexual, and social identity; therefore, the feelings and beliefs that made up their commitment differed from Western scholars working in or about areas in the so-called developing world. Gay anthropologists had to live and cope with AIDS in their personal lives. For them there was no temporary escape, no middle course between involvement and denial (see Levine 1992). They were assaulted by AIDS as a community; many of their friends, lovers, and colleagues were lost to the epidemic; and thus they were led to total involvement in the effort to stop the epidemic. Their motive was so evident that no one could reasonably question their commitment to the research effort.

The situation is distinct, more compound and less 'pure,' in the case of Western anthropologists working on AIDS in the Third World. They cannot escape the doubts inherent in all Western commitment to, and intervention with, the Third World (cf. the heritages of colonialism, orientalism, third worldism; see Schoepf and Preston-Whyte in this volume). Thus, a foreigner-anthropologist becomes engaged with AIDS research, and suspicion arises immediately that he or she is only interested in bringing home 'data' for use in a thesis or article. In other words, the anthropologist is suspected of valuing career and academy more than the suffering of people. This poses a problem of ethics with which the colonial and post-colonial discourses of the field seldom dealt and which can no longer be avoided (see Farmer 1992).

Area-specialist ethnographers deal with 'others,' with a 'they–problem.' Their commitment is not necessarily personal, although it might be. In most cases they are dependent upon academic funding, with a greater chance of becoming 'sponsor-spoiled.' Where Bolton (in this volume) criticizes colleagues and incites them to step out of their offices and 'do something' about AIDS, they still have to wait for a budget. After they have the budget, they often have to work their plans out in a process of bargaining and compromising with doctors, policy-makers, bureaucrats, and indigenous co-researchers. This process rarely strengthens the original anthropological commitment.

Moreover, these different modes of commitment belong to the wider social reality of differences between AIDS in the Western world and in the Latin American, African, and Asian continents. The wealth and power of the First and Third Worlds constitute a material difference between a 'Northern' and 'Southern' pattern of AIDS infection epidemiology (see Obbo, chapter 4) which goes far beyond the disparity of the present historical period. As in medical and epidemiological research more broadly, the amount of money and energy spent on AIDS in Western countries is many times greater than elsewhere. The gap can be noticed in this volume too; generally speaking, the contributions by gay-identified scholars on populations of gay and bisexual males demonstrate an enlarged division of labour in their focused demarcation of research areas and in the connections between theory and intervention. Their research agenda illustrates a somewhat more sophisticated, dedicated or specialized type that is explained only in part by the longer period of time involved in AIDS research on gays. It is remarkable but understandable, then, that the approach and framework of studies such as those presented in Part III of this book — 'Sexual Risk Among Western Gay Men' — are extremely rare in the Third World. However, this situation is also changing.

The work of gay anthropologists, their models and research questions have to be critiqued, rethought and translated before their lessons may be applied to Third World contexts. Of course, for anthropology such translation is expected, since culture theory thrives on posing a counterforce to the universalizing models of international agencies and organizations. Let us spell out some of the specific characteristics of what might now be labelled as a social geography of perspectives reflected in the chapters of this volume.

'NORTHERN' AND 'SOUTHERN' AIDS

In Third World countries affected by AIDS, heterosexual intercourse has been identified as the main mode of HIV transmission. There is a great dissimilarity in cultural contexts of sexual behaviour leading to infection. Compare, for example, Brazil, Uganda, and Thailand: These nations were slow to realize the inadequacy of their identification of the threat with respect to specific risk practices. Their policies had to change; they had to learn painfully that AIDS prevention was an issue for the majority of the population, not just a fringe or margin (Farmer 1992). In numerous Third World countries, AIDS has remodelled astonishingly swiftly and profoundly the public discourse about, for example, sexuality, STDs, condom use, and prostitution. For those familiar with AIDS in Western nations, it is amazing how encompassing and intruding the mobilisation against AIDS has been among developing countries, at least those less hampered by tradition, religious taboo, human rights, or state attempts to deny the AIDS stigma. As a consequence, AIDS in such places is on the national political agenda, and it is not an exclusive concern of minorities or action groups.

Who among us will doubt that sexual tolerance and a sex-positive attitude is a requirement for effective safe sex behaviour? The example of Thailand is particularly instructive in this way (cf. Hanenberg et al. 1993). Yet, we are not so sure that these attitudes are valid to all Third World countries in the same manner. We think not, even if we do not agree with all of their spokesmen ('condoms create promiscuity'). For instance, Obbo has expressed skepticism about the adequacy of the 'open' Danish approach as applied to African societies. Anthropologists have to acknowledge that in many cultures, a sudden introduction of sexual openness might have adverse effects, and even damage long-term efforts to make culturally appropriate interventions. Initiating sex-positive attitudes or practices in an environment where sexuality was hitherto repressed will provoke, and anthropologists must anticipate such, unintended consequences.

Westerners, including social scientists, often understand only with the greatest difficulty how other cultures suppress the expression of sexual feelings on many occasions and in many contexts. Conversely, in certain non-Western contexts, taboos on sexual behaviour provide unexpectedly elaborate ways of dealing with the sexual. For instance, that no kissing is permitted in public places or porno-videos are not made available in shops does not indicate *per se* an atmosphere of general sexual repression; one should not simply conclude from such cases that individuals and communities are not ripe to discuss in detail safe sex behaviour. Defining the proper context for such discussion of sexuality is extremely important when designing interventions. One has to take into account the difference between 'sexuality' as something private and 'sexuality' to be addressed in public (Mead 1961; Herdt and Stoller 1990). It is necessary to spell out for certain societies the distinctions between prudery, sex-positivity, openness and repression in specific — public and private — cultural contexts (Parker, in this volume). Actually, the Western case might be extreme and atypical, due to its high tolerance for sex in public discourse, compared to the face of its elaborate ideologies and practices of repression (Foucault 1980).

GLOBAL AND LOCAL DIALECTICS

The epidemic has its global as well as local manifestations, as we have noted. Research input and funding are, however, very much directed globally by such agencies as the World Health Organization and the United States Centers for Disease Control. Not surprisingly — who can object? — these agencies look for universal answers to policy guidelines. Indeed, as Berridge (1992) has noted, historically this has long been the case in epidemiology and the treatment of disease. Anthropologists emphasize the local context; and doing this within generalizing and global frameworks creates particular potential for policy conflict. An obvious solution would be to work with the 'indigenous' social scientists, anthropologists, or interventionists, and so on, who normally belong to a middle class that is Western educated and increasingly global in orientation (see also Obbo, in this volume).

However, cooperation between foreign and local social scientists may fail, as a result of competing personal and institutional interests. These circumstances may counteract the anthropological commitment which authors such as Bolton and Clatts demand. However, this is the nature of the contested world in which we live; we are forced to spell out the impediments to a culturally sensitive approach (see Herdt and Lindenbaum 1992; Vance 1991; Lindenbaum 1992).

Local scholars are dependent on foreign cooperation for all kinds of input and human resources, not all of them exclusively related to funding. Local interests are defined and organized politically to make claims on foreign funds. All those involved have to adopt a kind of interface or common denominator discourse — a global or universal idiom heavily dominated by the medical discourse, and insensitive or even inimical to anthropological concerns within the local culture (see Farmer, in this volume). In some places, a new middle class, built on the emerging resource base, benefits from representing the 'natives' to the outside world (see Parker, in this volume). Such groups develop their social profile and identity in response to their involvement in global networks; and such Third World researchers tend to live in a 'global village' in which local voices of particular people are muted (Obbo, in this volume).

Here, a dialectic that tends to corrupt anthropological commitment presents itself. First, it may be difficult to find a local social scientist who shares the commitment of anthropology, and if one is found, he or she tends to study the 'other' — for instance, tribal groups or ethnic minorities — within his own society. Second, our social scientific 'counterparts' tend to view their own culture preferably from a universalizing perspective, according to which anthropology's interest in the particular is easily felt as denigratory of their own culture. Situations can arise in which, for instance, Thai HIV-counsellors follow translated 'American' models to the letter, while a rare foreigner searches for the 'Buddhist' model in consoling people living with HIV/AIDS. An illustration regarding the use of research methods is given by Michael Tan (in this volume), whose Philippine experience seems typical. He signals the local preference for a rigid type of Western social science insensitive to the specifics of local culture. Inevitably, these remarks lead to a question repeatedly addressed at the Amsterdam conference: 'What is an apt form of cooperation between Western anthropologists and "native" researchers?'

Western anthropologists themselves can pose a barrier too. Recently, Maxine Ankrah commented — at the Kampala conference in December 1992 — on the incongruence between the solutions proposed for 'Africa' and African cultures. She noted that most scientists perceived and interpreted the epidemic from the perspective of other cultures and other continents, making no exception for anthropologists. She even criticized the dependence on the expertise of anthropologists who are trained in, or imported almost exclusively from, industrialized countries, because they tend to view the

'African experience' of AIDS from the perspectives of their own cultures. This should remind us that there is no ready-made, 'context-free tool' for cultural specificity, as so desired by epidemiologists: One cannot guarantee cultural sensitivity in advance (Lindenbaum 1992). Ankrah certainly does not want to suggest that the foreigner-anthropologist should stand back and let the Africans 'solve their own problems.' Rather, she seeks a precise qualification of the potential role and contribution of a foreigner-anthropologist. Here we have found a common concern.

The potential advantages of cooperation between foreign and local researchers go far beyond the fact of having easier access to foreign funding. A strong argument emerges for the benefits of teamwork. AIDS is requiring us to abandon the models of the lonely researcher, able to make his own way, to create his own world (Bolton, in this volume). We must develop new models of cooperation wherein the anthropological project itself is conducted by teams (see chapter 3 by Kammerer, Hutheesing, Maneeprasert, and Symonds). Such teams should be balanced for gendered perspectives, but also for a foreign and 'native' point of view (Schoepf). Not only can an international project provide extra opportunities for training in theory, method, and prevention, it can more easily generate fresh perspectives. Teams can help shield local workers from harassment by their own bureaucracies — concerning problems about allocation of funds, researching sexual, or illegal behaviour. They benefit the research effort in personal ways too, by new possibilities for locating settings that cope better with feelings of stress, despair or burn out. And, finally, such teams have a greater chance to find a proper balance between pure research and prevention efforts in every country. If such a trend is not the 'wave of the future,' it is at least a significant tide that anthropology may now harness.

Although culture is the key focus, this book starts with papers that show how AIDS impacts countries in the Third World beyond a cultural perspective. The chapters by Farmer, Schoepf, and Kammerer et al. represent three continents, but have in common a concern with the wider socio-economic and political context of the HIV/AIDS epidemic in Haiti, sub-Saharan Africa and the mountains of Northern Thailand. They remind us that culture study must address what Farmer calls 'social analysis,' or what is 'political economy' in Schoepf's paper, and a 'materialist approach' in the contribution by Kammerer et al. They all attempt to situate AIDS perceptions within ramifying situations of economic and political relations.

While these approaches echo the political activism of the past, there is an important difference. The wider context is not invoked to make claims for change more encompassing and totalizing, resulting in postponement or delay. The papers attempt to show the wider connections, without giving up the attempt to analyse and identify those elements of culture, behaviours, and relations that can be changed immediately and will contribute to saving lives. Although the chapters reflect the tension between the need for immediate action and analysis of the wider context, they are not limited to the dilemma between blind activism and summons to revolutionary change. They assume that political economy rarely determines people's behaviour completely; in most circumstances there is space left for empowerment of individuals and communities.

Haiti (Farmer) is one of the first locations in the Third World that became part of the international AIDS epidemic and it has played a role in the Western construction of the epidemic. Thailand (Kammerer et al.) is one of the latest examples of a country whose image in the international media became largely identified with HIV/AIDS. It is evident that the social and political contexts in both cases differ widely, and again differ from the one described by Schoepf for Africa.

By employing the perspective of vulnerability Kammerer et al. suggest that there is no need to wait for so-called 'reliable' data about actual infections for doing relevant anthropological work. One could add that several of their 'theoretical' points have been confirmed by epidemiological data about the spread of HIV infection among the mountain people since their first writing.

Part II, Contextualizing Sexual Risk, contains four papers that are ethnographic in the strict sense. Gender is more or less important to all of them, and these perceptive descriptions of situations of sexual risk open new understanding of these cultural spaces. Christine Obbo's chapter documents a deep cultural entrenchment of AIDS — its representation in political and cultural discourse. She has shown a society's adaptation to AIDS, and not just individual reaction and response.

Paiva and van Kerkwijk report on two countries — Brazil and Thailand — that have much in common: A strong local tradition; a powerful and often wealthy middle class; incorporation in global networks; and cultural forms of sexuality that challenge Western categories. For this reason, Paiva's attempt to find a balance between a sex-positive approach and existing sentiments of shame and taboo in her work with Brazilian teenagers is particularly stimulating. Her attempt of 'eroticization' of prevention reflects that Brazilian culture — like Thai culture — has its own undercurrent of sex positivity which in the recent past was suppressed partly by Western-influenced middle classes.

While van Kerkwijk's study is located in Thailand and illuminates its epidemic, she shows that interactions between Western male tourists and Thai girls cannot be understood in terms of Western or Thai culture. These interactions are from a specific subculture of sex tourism which has played a role in the introduction of the virus into Asian countries. The importance of chapter 6 is in drawing attention to the dynamics of sexual interactions in the specific places and locations where representatives of different cultures interact, e.g., border areas, especially at places where large economic differences and ethnic distinctions go together.

Hart's chapter 7, set in Europe, contains rare analyses that deal with male customers of female prostitutes. She spells out how clients create their own ideology of risk by adapting cultural notions at the individual level. She further demonstrates forcefully the problems that remain unsolved when an analysis of risk in terms of groups is given up and replaced by analysis of risk behaviours.

As elaborated above, the third part of this book, consisting of papers about Western gay men written by gay social scientists, contrasts in a relevant way with the other papers in the volume. We can add that each paper contains incentives and suggestions for more focused research in Third World countries. In this section non-anthropologists dominate. It is no surprise that all that chapters go beyond the boundaries of classical anthropological method, drawing on techniques from other disciplines. Although Henriksson and Månsson use the common method of participant observation, the way they bring this method to sex research certainly transgresses boundaries.

Chapter 9 by Vincke and Bolton has a format that reflects its origin in a different discipline. It also demonstrates how anthropological reasoning can contribute to other disciplines. Notice how the authors move away from a strict individual conceptualization and focus on the social support for safe sex behaviour. They account for the cultural patterning and variation of such social support. This chapter can also remind anthropologists that culture never socializes an individual totally; there is an 'anti-social' core to sexuality. Much criticism of individualizing and socializing approaches is supported by good arguments. However, this cannot do away with an unalienable psychological dynamic.

Coxon and Coxon (chapter 10) provide another example of promising cooperation between social-scientific sub-disciplines. They developed a diary method which draws on sociologists' greater familiarity with a quantifying approach. As they suggest in the concluding part of their paper, this method challenges its use in other cultural contexts. They demonstrate also that quantification is able to derive insights from diary data that are difficult or impossible to gain from interpretation alone.

William Leap's concentration on the language used in discourse about AIDS presents a model for linguistic analysis, in chapter 11, although he works as an anthropologist. How people talk about AIDS as rule-governed speech events provides the backdrop for an approach which draws on text-centered methods of linguistic research. The challenge is to adapt such an approach for other cultures, to spell out the connections between language, experience, and culture.

Part IV — The Study of Culture and Sexual Risk — addresses issues that immediately concern the anthropological discipline and its relationship to AIDS. No doubt the dominating piece is Bolton's paper (chapter 15), much as it dominated the conference from which this volume derives. The author chooses a format close to the original oral presentation. Bolton does not conceal his dissatisfaction with anthropology's commitment to AIDS research in Western countries. His catalogue of issues deserves to be rethought carefully in the context of HIV/AIDS in the Third World. For a few issues, this has been done in the first part of this introduction. Others are explicitly reflected in the contribution of Preston-Whyte, whose point of departure is Bolton's keynote paper as presented at the original conference.

Preceding these two concluding chapters are three papers that reflect critically on ongoing anthropological AIDS research. Clatts (chapter 12) points to what escapes categories derived from an anthropological framework. He demonstrates the necessity to work with concepts that are sensitive to local perceptions instead of looking for decontextualized categories suitable for a social control approach. Like the chapters in the first section, Clatts reminds us again that the context which is relevant for HIV/AIDS is not to conceive exclusively in cultural terms. Particularly in a Third World context, a micro-approach that forgets about economic inequality and poverty becomes extremely naive.

Parker's critical assessment of the state of sex research in relation to HIV/AIDS, in chapter 13, reveals that sex research is largely limited to the developed world. His discussion of research priorities exposes the strained relations between epidemiology and ethnography, although he explicitly points to the necessity of ethnographic insight guiding epidemiological research.

In several respects, Michael Tan's contribution (chapter 14) complements Parker's. His description of the use of Western social science techniques in AIDS research in the Philippines can be generalized to fit several other developing countries, where a local social science tradition has been established since World War II. Dependence on research instruments designed in the West, often in combination with an uncritical belief in their universal applicability, results in a 'pick-up sticks' approach that is not only insensitive toward the local culture but even imposes Western assumptions. Tan, finally, illustrates what also has been exemplified by Schoepf and Paiva, that possibly there is no country outside the West where the dominant discourse of sexuality is not deeply influenced by forms of Western discourse (here Spanish Catholicism).

REFERENCES

Berridge, V. 1992. AIDS: History and Contemporary History. In: *The Time of AIDS: Social Analysis, Theory, and Method*, edited by G. Herdt and S. Lindenbaum. Newbury Park, CA: Sage Publications.

Bolton, R., and E. Kempler, eds. 1992. The Anthropology of AIDS: Syllabi and Other Teaching Materials. Washington, DC: American Anthropological Association, AIDS and Anthropology Task Force.

Bolton, R., and M. Singer, eds. 1992. *Rethinking AIDS Prevention: Cultural Approaches*. Philadelphia: Gordon and Breach Science Publishers.

Farmer, P. 1992. *AIDS and Accusation: Haiti and the Geography of Blame*. Berkeley: University of California Press.

Feldman, D., ed. 1990 *Culture and AIDS*. New York: Praeger Press.

Foucault, M. 1980. Trans. R. Hurley. *The History of Sexuality*. New York: Pantheon Books.

Hanenberg, R., P. Benjarattanaporn, and P. Mugrditchian. 1993. The Use of Sexually Transmitted Disease (STD) Statistics to Evaluate Thailand's HIV Prevention Program. Paper presented at the IXth International Conference on AIDS, Berlin, June 6–11, 1993.

Herdt, G. 1992. Introduction. In: *The Time of AIDS: Social Analysis, Theory, and Method*, edited by G. Herdt and S. Lindenbaum. Newbury Park, CA: Sage Publications.

Herdt, G., and R. Stoller. 1990. *Intimate Communications: Erotics and the Study of Culture*. New York: Columbia University Press.

Herdt, G., and S. Lindenbaum, eds. 1992. *The Time of AIDS: Social Analysis, Theory, and Method*. Newbury Park, CA: Sage Publications.

Levine, M.P. 1992. The Life and Death of Gay Clones. In: *Gay Culture in America*, edited by G. Herdt. Boston: Beacon Press.

Lindenbaum, S. 1992. Knowledge and Action in the Shadow of AIDS. In: *The Time of AIDS: Social Analysis, Theory, and Method*, edited by G. Herdt and S. Lindenbaum. Newbury Park, CA: Sage Publications.

Mann, J.M., D.J.M. Tarantola, and T.W. Netter, eds. 1992. *AIDS in the World*. Cambridge: Harvard University Press.

Mead, M. 1961. Cultural Determinants of Sexual Behavior. In: *Sex and Internal Secretions*, edited by W.C. Young. Baltimore: Williams and Wilkins.

Mead, M. 1977. *Letters From the Field 1925–1975*. New York: Harper Colophone Books.

Parker, R.G., G. Herdt, and M. Carballo. 1991. Sexual Culture, HIV Transmission, and AIDS Research. *Journal of Sex Research* 28:77–98.

Vance, C.S. 1991. Anthropology Rediscovers Sexuality: A Theoretical Comment. *Social Science and Medicine* 33:875–884.

Wolf, E.R. 1980. *Europe and the People Without History*. Berkeley: University of California Press.

ABOUT THE CONTRIBUTORS

Ralph Bolton is Professor of Anthropology at Pomona College, Claremont, California. His current research focuses on sexual behaviour and HIV prevention among gay men in Europe and the United States. A specialist in human sexuality and medical anthropology, he has edited two volumes on AIDS, both published by Gordon and Breach: *The AIDS Pandemic* (1989) and *Rethinking AIDS Prevention: Cultural Approaches* (1992, with M. Singer).

Han ten Brummelhuis, as a Thai specialist with an interest in medical anthropology, has followed the Thai AIDS epidemic from its beginning in 1987. He became involved in several projects dealing with cultural and social aspects of AIDS in Thailand. Recently he studied Thai marriage and family, Thai communities in Europe, and the Buddhist potential for HIV/AIDS care.

Michael C. Clatts is associated with the National Development and Research Institutes, Inc., New York.

Anthony P.M. Coxon is Research Professor in Sociology, University of Essex; Emeritus Professor of Sociological Research Methods, University of Wales; and principal investigator, Project Sigma, University of Essex.

N.H. Coxon is research assistant, Project Sigma, University of Essex.

Paul Farmer, author of *AIDS and Accusation* (1992), is Assistant Professor at the Harvard Medical School and an infectious disease fellow at Boston's Brigham and Women's Hospital. He conducts his research and medical practice in rural Haiti, where he specializes in community-based efforts to improve the health of the poor.

Angie Hart is a lecturer in Social Studies at LSU, a college of the University of Southampton, England. Her research is concerned with sexuality, gender studies, and the social aspects of health (especially HIV/AIDS) in European contexts. She is currently writing *Buying Power: Prostitution in Spain*, a book based on her D.Phil. research.

Benny Henriksson is a social researcher at the Department of Social Work at the University of Göteborg. He has done research in general youth issues, homosexuality, and HIV prevention.

Gilbert Herdt is Director of the Center for Culture and Mental Health Research, and Professor of the Committee on Human Development, University of Chicago. His most recent books are *Children of Horizons: How Gay and Lesbian Youth Are Forging a New Way Out of the Closet* (with Andrew Boxer) and *Third Sex, Third Gender: Beyond Sexual Dimorphism in History and Culture.*

Otome Klein Hutheesing, author of *Emerging Sexual Inequality Among the Lisu of Northern Thailand,* has taught at Bernard Baruch College in New York and Universiti Sains Malaysia in Penang.

Cornelia Ann Kammerer is a Resident Scholar in the Women's Studies Program at Brandeis University who has done fieldwork on religion, kinship, gender, and social change among Akha highlanders in Thailand.

William L. Leap is a Professor in the Department of Anthropology at the American University, Washington, DC. A linguist by training, he has published on American Indian languages, Indian varieties of English, and on language and AIDS. He is currently exploring conversation, narration, and negotiation in gay men's English.

Ralana Maneeprasert has done fieldwork among Akha and Hmong in Thailand in her capacity as a Social Science Researcher at the Tribal Research Institute, Chiang Mai. Her central interests are women, children, and health, particularly nutrition.

Sven Axel Månsson is Professor and Chair of the Department of Social Work at the University of Göteborg. He has done extensive research in sociology, mainly in areas concerning prostitution and HIV prevention.

Christine Obbo is a Ugandan social cultural anthropologist currently working as an independent research consultant on HIV/AIDS and gender issues in Africa. She is carrying out research on changes in family obligations and entitlements, and writing a book on women and HIV/AIDS and the historical/cultural construction of disease and death in Uganda. Currently, she is an associate of the Centre of

African Studies at the School of Oriental and African Studies, University of London.

Vera Paiva is Professor of Social Psychology at the University of São Paolo, Brazil. She serves on the steering committee of the Interdisciplinary Group for AIDS Prevention (NEPAIDS/USP).

Richard G. Parker is Professor of Medical Anthropology and Human Sexuality in the Institute of Social Medicine at the State University of Rio de Janeiro and a Director of AVIA, the Brazilian Interdisciplinary AIDS association.

Eleanor M. Preston-Whyte is Deputy Vice-Chancellor for Research and Development and Professor of Anthropology at the University of Natal. For her Ph.D. she examined the position of African women migrants in the Durban region. Her research interests have for some years included issues of family and domestic structure, gender interaction, sexuality, and the empowerment of women; more recently, she has been actively involved in developing AIDS intervention strategies.

Brooke Grundfest Schoepf is a medical and economic anthropologist with twenty years of teaching and research experience in Africa. From 1985 to 1990, she led Project CONNAISSIDA in Zaïre. Since 1991, she has worked as an AIDS prevention consultant for international, bilateral, and non-governmental agencies.

Patricia V. Symonds, currently a Visiting Assistant Professor in Brown University's Department of Anthropology in Providence, Rhode Island, is a medical anthropologist who has done fieldwork among Hmong in the United States and Thailand.

Michael Lim Tan is Executive Director of the Health Action Information Network (HAIN), Quezon City, and Assistant Professor at the University of the Philippines. He is a medical anthropologist.

Carla van Kerkwijk graduated in 1991 in Anthropology at the University of Amsterdam. For her MA, she did fieldwork among female sex workers in Bangkok.

John Vincke, Ph.D., is a sociologist and research associate at the AIDS Reference Center, University Hospital, University of Ghent in Flanders, Belgium.

Part I

Culture and Beyond:
The Wider Context
of Sexual Risk

Chapter ONE

Culture, Poverty, and the Dynamics of HIV Transmission in Rural Haiti

Paul Farmer

Over the course of the past ten years, important work regarding HIV transmission has been conducted in urban Haiti. There has been a dearth, however, of studies conducted in *rural* Haiti. This is significant, because Haiti, a country of well over six million inhabitants, is generally considered to be a substantially rural nation.[1] As the ties that link rural and urban Haiti are economically and affectively strong, a brief review of studies from urban Haiti is a useful prolegomenon to a consideration of HIV transmission in rural areas. Together, insights from studies in both places enhance our understanding of HIV infection not just in Haiti, but in many settings where poverty seems to favour rapid sexual spread of HIV.

Table 1. HIV Seroprevalence Among Healthy
Adults in Haiti (1986–1987)

Category	N	Mean age (years)	Percent HIV-positive
Urban Haiti (Port-au-Prince area)			
Hotel workers	25	45	12.0
Factory workers	84	30	5.0
Pregnant women (1986)	1240	29	8.4
Mothers of sick infants	502	29	12.0
Other adults:			
High SES	54	35	0.0
Low SES	190	33	13.0
Medical workers	57	40	0.0
TOTAL	2152	37	9.0
Rural Haiti (outside Port-au-Prince)			
Mothers of sick infants	97	25	3.0
Pregnant women	117	27	3.0
Blood donors	245	32	4.0
Other adults (rural village)	191	29	1.0
TOTAL	650	30	3.0

Source: Pape and Johnson (1988).

HIV IN HAITI

HIV was probably introduced to Haiti in recent years: careful review of clinical records and pathologic specimens has revealed no confirmed case of AIDS until 1979, when Dr. Bernard Liautaud diagnosed Kaposi's sarcoma in two previously well young adults. As of December 1990, the latest date for which official data are available, Haiti had reported 3086 cases of AIDS to the Pan-American Health Organization. Most clinicians feel that the actual number of cases is several times this figure, which would make Haiti one of the world's 20 most affected nations. In the years since its arrival, HIV infection has become as common as other, more well-established sexually transmitted diseases such as syphilis (Liautaud et al. 1992).

How has HIV infection become so widespread, at least in urban Haiti, in such a short period of time? In the early 1980s, the epidemic seemed to have an epicentre in the city of Carrefour, a centre of prostitution bordering the south side of Port-au-Prince. Haitian researchers documented a high prevalence, among the first Haitians with AIDS, of 'accepted risk factors,' i.e., the risk factors for AIDS identified by the US Centers for Disease Control (CDC). Of all of these factors, bisexual activity was by far the most significant, according to studies conducted in urban Haiti in the early 1980s; a significant percentage of the homosexual contact had been with North Americans.[2] Another recognized risk factor was also important at the time: the rate of transfusion-associated transmission was then higher in Haiti than in the United States.

With the passage of time, however, it has become increasingly clear that HIV infection has become a predominantly heterosexually transmitted disease. By 1986, heterosexual transmission — or, in the language of the day, 'no risk factor' — was demonstrated or strongly suspected in approximately 70 per cent of Haitian AIDS cases. Additional evidence for heterosexual transmission of HIV are the high rates (over 50 per cent) of infection among prostitutes in the Port-au-Prince area, the ever decreasing male:female ratio among Haitians with AIDS, and the growing number of paediatric AIDS cases (for reviews of this research, see Desvarieux and Pape 1991; Farmer 1990a; Pape and Johnson 1988).

How far has HIV spread in Haiti? During 1986 and 1987, sera from several cohorts of healthy adults were analysed for antibodies to HIV (see Table 1). In a group of individuals working in hotels catering to tourists, HIV seroprevalence was a sobering 12 per cent. In a group of 502 mothers of poor children hospitalized with diarrhoea and among 190 urban adults with a comparable socio-economic background, the seroprevalence rates were 12 per cent and 13 per cent, respectively. Among urban factory workers, 5 per cent were found to have antibodies to HIV. In both series, rates were comparable for men and women, which suggested to many observers that the high attack rate in Haitian men would slowly give way to a pattern like that seen in parts of Central Africa, where men and women are equally affected.

Overall, researchers of the Haitian Study Group on Kaposi's Sarcoma and Opportunistic Infections (GHESKIO) found that approximately 9 per cent of 912 healthy urban adults (medical workers, college graduates, factory or hotel workers, mothers of sick infants, and other adults) were seropositive to HIV. Sadly, studies in other urban settings have confirmed those of the GHESKIO team.[3] More recent studies, also conducted in Port-au-Prince by Pape and co-workers (Desvarieux and Pape 1991:275), would seem to confirm this trend.

In summary, then, large numbers of urban Haitians have been exposed to HIV, and it is now clear that, in urban settings, HIV infection is most often a heterosexually transmitted disease. But what of rural regions? Based on small studies conducted in 1986–87, Pape and Johnson (1988) report that, 'in rural areas,' the seroprevalence rate averaged 3 per cent. The seroprevalence rate in 97 mothers of children hospitalized with dehydration was 3 per cent; 4 per cent of 245 unscreened rural blood donors had antibodies to HIV. In an area even more distant from urban centres, 1 per cent of 191 adults who came for immunizations were seropositive.

Unfortunately, we know little about the individuals bled for these studies: Just how rural were they? What was the nature of their ties to Port-au-Prince and other high-prevalence regions? How did the seropositive individuals come to be at risk for HIV? How did they differ from seronegative controls? How rapidly is HIV making inroads into the rural population? By what mechanisms does poverty serve to heighten risk of exposure to HIV? What, in short, are the dynamics of HIV transmission in rural Haiti?

We will address these questions by considering the means by which large-scale social forces become manifest in the lives of particular individuals. We argue that it is necessary to move beyond the concept of 'risk groups' to a consideration of the interplay between human agency and the powerful forces that constrain social life, especially those activities which promote or retard HIV transmission. In Haiti, the most powerful of these forces, we believe, have been the deepening poverty and political dislocations that have together conspired to hasten the spread of HIV.

AIDS IN A HAITIAN VILLAGE

The setting for the research described here is the Peligre basin of Haiti's central plateau, home to several hundred thousand, mostly rural, people. Although all parts of Haiti are poor, the Peligre basin region may be especially so: in 1956, thousands of families living in this region were flooded out by a large hydroelectric dam. The displaced persons were all peasant farmers, and they received little or no compensation for their lost land.

The hilltop village of Do Kay was founded by refugees from the rising water. Although initially a dusty squatter settlement of less than 200 persons, Do Kay has grown rapidly in the past decade and now counts over 1,000 inhabitants. In spite of the hostile conditions

— Do Kay is stony and steep — most families continue to rely to some extent on agricultural efforts. Many more are involved in a series of development projects designed to improve the health status of the area's inhabitants. Since 1984, for example, a series of outreach initiatives have complemented the efforts of a growing team of clinicians based in Do Kay. The most significant efforts were those undertaken under the aegis of Proje Veye Sante, the 'health surveillance project.' Proje Veye Sante is conducted in large part by village-based community health workers from over a dozen nearby communities and provides preventive and primary care to more than 30,000 rural people. AIDS surveillance began well before the epidemic was manifest in the region, and it is thus possible to date the index case of AIDS to 1986, when a young school teacher fell ill with recurrent superficial mycoses, chronic diarrhoea, and pulmonary tuberculosis. Seropositive for HIV, he died a year later (see Farmer 1990b, 1992).

Although the schoolteacher was from another part of the central plateau, it was not long before natives of Do Kay were diagnosed with the syndrome. Below are brief case histories of the first three villagers known to have died of AIDS. None had a history of transfusion with blood or blood products; none had a history of homosexual contact or other 'risk factors' as designated by the CDC. We believe, however, that they share an important, if poorly understood, risk factor: poverty.

Anita

Anita Joseph was born in approximately 1966 to a family that had lost its land to the Péligre dam. One of six children, Anita briefly attended school until her mother, weakened by the malnutrition then rampant in the Kay area, died of tuberculosis. Anita was then 13. Her father became depressed and abusive, and she resolved to run away: 'I'd had it with his yelling ... when I saw how poor I was, and how hungry, and saw that it would never get any better, I had to go to the city. Back then I was so skinny — I was saving my life, I thought, by getting out of here.' Shortly thereafter, Anita left for Port-au-Prince with less than three dollars and no clear plan. She worked briefly as a *restavèk*, or live-in maid, for $10 per month, but lost this position when her employer was herself fired from a factory job.

Cast into the street, Anita eventually found a relative who took her in. The kinswoman, who lived in a notorious slum north of the capital, introduced her to Vincent, a young man who worked unloading luggage at the airport. Anita was not yet fifteen when she entered her first and only sexual union: 'What could I do, really?' she sighed in recounting the story much later. 'He had a good job. My aunt thought I should go with him.' Vincent, who had at least one other sexual partner at the time, became ill less than two years after they began sharing a room. The young man was cared for by Anita throughout his illness and died after repeated infections, including tuberculosis. Not long after his death, Anita herself fell ill with tuberculosis. Upon returning to Do Kay in 1987, she quickly responded to appropriate therapy. When she relapsed some months later, an HIV test was performed and the true cause of her immunosuppression was revealed. Following a slow but ineluctable decline, Anita died in February 1988.

Dieudonné

Dieudonné Gracia, born in Do Kay in 1963, was also the child of two 'water refugees.' One of seven children, he attended primary school in his home village and, briefly, secondary school in a nearby town. It was there, at the age of 19, that he had his first sexual contact, with a young woman from a nearby town. Dieudonné remarked that she had had 'two, maybe three partners' before they met, and was sure that one of them was a truck driver from a city in central Haiti. When the destruction of Haiti's swine population further immiserated his family, Dieudonné was forced to drop out of school, and also to drop out of his relationship with the young woman. He returned to Do Kay to work with his father, a carpenter. In 1983, however, the young man decided to 'to try my luck in Port-au-Prince.' Through a friend from Do Kay, Dieudonné found a position as a domestic for a well-to-do family in a suburb of the capital.

While in the city, Dieudonné's sexual experience broadened considerably: he had five partners, all of them women approximately the same age as he, in little more than two years. Asked about the brevity of these liaisons, Dieudonné explained that 'a couple of them let go of me because they saw that I couldn't do anything for them. They saw that I couldn't give them anything for any children.' He worked in Port-au-Prince until 1985, when he became ill and was dismissed. Shortly thereafter, Dieudonné returned to Do Kay, and began seeing his former lover. She soon became pregnant and moved to Do Kay as the young man's *plase*, a term designating a partner in a more stable conjugal union. It was during this interlude that Dieudonné was seen at the Kay clinic for a number of problems that suggested im-

munodeficiency: herpes zoster and genital herpes, recurrent diarrhoea, and weight loss. In the months following the birth of her baby,
the young mother fell ill with a febrile illness, thought by her
physician to be malaria, and quickly succumbed. Less than a year
later, Dieudonné, much reduced by chronic diarrhoea, was diagnosed with tuberculosis. Following an initial response to anti-tuber-
culous agents, Dieudonné relapsed. He died of AIDS in October
1988.

Acephie

Acephie Joseph was born in 1965 on a small knoll protruding into the
reservoir that had drowned her parents' land. Acephie attended
primary school somewhat irregularly; by the age of 19, she had not
yet graduated and decided that it was time for her to help generate
income for her family, which was sinking deeper and deeper into
poverty. Hunger was a near-daily occurrence for the Joseph family;
the times were as bad as those right after the flooding of the valley.
Acephie began to help her mother, a market woman, by carrying
produce to a local market on Friday mornings. It was there that she
met a soldier, formerly stationed in Port-au-Prince, who began to
make overtures to the striking young woman from Do Kay. Although
the soldier had a wife and children, and was known, in fact, to have
more than one regular partner, Acephie did not spurn him: 'What
would you have me do? I could tell that the old people were uncomfortable, worried — but they didn't say no. They didn't tell me to stay
away from him. I wish they had, but how could they have known?...
I looked around and saw how poor we all were, how the old people
were finished.... It was a way out, that's how I saw it.' Shortly
thereafter, the soldier fell ill and was diagnosed in the Kay clinic with
AIDS. A few months after they parted, he was dead.

Shaken, Acephie went to a nearby town and began a course in
what she euphemistically termed a 'cooking school,' which prepared
poor girls for work as servants. In 1987, 22 years old, Acephie went to
Port-au-Prince, where she found a $30-per-month job as a
housekeeper for a middle-class Haitian woman working for the US
embassy. Also at this time, Acephie began seeing a man, also from
Kay, who chauffeured a small bus between the central plateau and
Port-au-Prince. Acephie worked in the city until late in 1989, when
she discovered that she was pregnant. This displeased both her
partner and her employer. *Sans* job and *sans* boyfriend, Acephie
returned to Do Kay in her third trimester. Following the birth of her

daughter, Acephie was sapped by repeated opportunistic infections, each one caught in time by the staff of the clinic in Kay. Throughout 1991, however, she continued to lose weight; by January 1992, she weighed less than 90 pounds, and her intermittent fevers were unresponsive to broad-spectrum antibiotics. Acephie died in April 1992. Her daughter, the first 'AIDS orphan' in Do Kay, is now in the care of Acephie's mother. The baby is also ill. A few months after Acephie's death, her father hung himself.

Sadly, however, this is not simply the story of Acephie and her family. The soldier's wife, who is much thinner than last year, has already had a case of herpes zoster. Two of her children are also HIV-positive. This woman, who is well known to the clinic staff, is no longer a widow. Once again, she is the partner of a military man. And her late husband had at least two other partners, both of them poor peasant women, in the central plateau. One is HIV-positive and has two sickly children. The father of Acephie's child, apparently in good health, is still plying the roads from Mirebalais to Port-au-Prince. His serostatus is unknown.

When compared to age-matched North Americans with AIDS, Anita, Dieudonné, and Acephie have sparse sexual histories. Anita had only one partner; Dieudonné had six; Acephie had two. Although Pape's and co-workers (see Pape and Johnson 1988) case-control study suggested that urban men, at least, had larger numbers of partners than did our patients, research conducted in Anita's neighbourhood in Port-au-Prince suggests that her case is not as unique as it would seem:

> The high seropositivity rate (8 per cent) found in pregnant women 14 to 19 years of age suggests that women [in Cité Soleil] appear to acquire HIV infection soon after becoming sexually active.... Moreover, this age group is the only one in which a higher seropositivity rate is *not* associated with a greater number of sexual partners. Women with only one sexual partner in the year prior to pregnancy actually have a slightly higher prevalence rate (although not significantly so) than the others. This suggests that they were infected by their first and only partner. (Desvarieux and Pape 1991:275)

The stories of Anita, Dieudonné, and Acephie are ones in which are revealed the push-and-pull forces of contemporary Haiti. In each case, young adults were driven to Port-au-Prince by the lure of an escape from the harshest poverty; once in the city, each worked as a domestic; none managed to find the financial security so elusive in the countryside. The women were straightforward about the non-voluntary aspect of their sexual unions: in their opinions, they had been driven into unfavourable unions by poverty.

Over the past several years, the medical staff of the Kay clinic has diagnosed dozens more cases of AIDS and other forms of HIV infection in people presenting to the clinic with a broad range of complaints. With surprisingly few exceptions, however, those so diagnosed shared a number of risk factors, as a modest case-control study would suggest. The study was conducted by interviewing the first 17 women diagnosed, by clinic staff, with AIDS or AIDS-related complex (ARC) who were residents of Kay or its two neighbouring villages. Their responses to questions posed during the course of a series of open-ended interviews (conducted in Haitian Creole by a medical anthropologist) were compared with those of 17 age-matched, seronegative controls. In both groups, ages ranged from 17 to 37, with a mean of about 25 years.

None of these 34 women had a history of prostitution; none had used illicit drugs; only one, a member of the control group, had a history of transfusion. None of the women in either group had more than 6 sexual partners. In fact, four of the afflicted women had had only one sexual partner. Although women in the study group had on average more sexual partners than controls, the difference is not striking. Similarly, there was no clear difference between the study and control group vis-à-vis number of intramuscular injections received or years of education (see Table 2).

The chief risk factors in this small cohort seemed to involve not number of partners, but rather the professions of these partners. Fully 14 of the women with AIDS/ARC had histories of sexual contact with soldiers or truck drivers. Two of these women reported having only two sexual partners: one a soldier, one a truck driver. Of those women diagnosed with AIDS or ARC, none had a history of sexual contact exclusively with peasants (although one had as sole partner a construction worker from Do Kay). Among the control group, only one woman had as a regular partner a truck driver; none reported contact with soldiers, and most had only had sexual relations with peasants from the region. Histories of extended residence in Port-au-Prince and work as a domestic were also strongly associated with a diagnosis of AIDS or ARC.

Conjugal unions with non-peasants — salaried soldiers and truck drivers who are paid on a daily basis — reflect these women's quest for some measure of economic security. In this manner, truck drivers

Table 2. Case-Control Study of AIDS in Rural Haitian Women

Patient characteristics	AIDS/ARC (N = 17)	Control (N = 17)
Number of sexual partners	2.7	2.2
Partner of truck driver	9	1
Partner of soldier	7	0
Partner of peasant only	0	15
Port-au-Prince residence	14	4
Worked as servant	11	0
Years of education	4.8	4
Received blood transfusion	0	1
Used illicit drugs	0	0
Received > 10 IM injections	11	13

and soldiers have served as a 'bridge' to the rural population, just as North American tourists seemed to have served as a bridge to the urban Haitian population. But just as North Americans are no longer important in the transmission of HIV in Haiti, truck drivers and soldiers will soon no longer be necessary components of the rural epidemic. Once introduced into a sexually active population, HIV will work its way into those with no history of residence in the city, no history of contact with soldiers or truck drivers, no history of work as domestics. Nevertheless, these risk factors — all of which reflect a desperate attempt to escape rural poverty — are emblematic of the lot of the rural Haitian poor, and perhaps especially of poor women.

HIV IN A HAITIAN VILLAGE

Extended residence in Port-au-Prince, work as a servant, and sexual contact with non-peasants — although these risk factors were far different from those described for North Americans with AIDS, they embraced the majority of our male and female patients afflicted with AIDS. The majority of the residents of the area served by Proje Veye Sante share none of these attributes: did this suggest that few would prove to be infected with HIV? Although a good deal of ethnographic research into the nature of AIDS has already been conducted in the region, no research had addressed the question of HIV prevalence among asymptomatic adults.

Troubled by this lacuna, the staff of the clinic and of Proje Veye Sante established the Groupe d'Étude du SIDA dans la Classe Paysanne (GESCAP). GESCAP has a mandate to inaugurate research that attempts to expose the mechanisms by which poverty puts young adults, and especially young women, at risk of HIV infection. With community approval, GESCAP is attempting to illuminate case histories with serologic surveys, an expanded case-control study, and cluster studies such as those that revealed the means by which a single HIV-positive soldier came to infect, as was the case with Acephie's partners, at least eight natives of the region.

After considerable discussion, the members of GESCAP decided to undertake a study of all asymptomatic adults living in Cange. 'Adults' were held to include all members of the community who might plausibly be sexually active (15 years and older); 'asymptomatic' was held to mean free of any suggestion of immunodeficiency. For reasons discussed below, patients with active tuberculosis were excluded from this study. Another exclusion criterion was status as the regular sexual partner of a person with known HIV infection.

Given that the staff of the clinic and of Proje Veye Sante are accountable to the communities served, rather than to funding organizations or to research institutions, and given the poverty and non-HIV-related sickness in the region, it is not surprising that research is not seen as a high priority. In order to meet our obligations to the community, all serologic studies became part of a 'dossier preventif.' This instrument included a series of laboratory examinations (such as haematocrit and rapid plasma reagin (RPR)), a chest radiograph, and a physical examination. Any abnormal findings were to be pursued aggressively; free dental care was also offered as part of the programme. This proposal was presented to members of the community in four different public meetings, engendering considerable enthusiasm for the undertaking.

Of the first 100 villagers enrolling in the programme, 99 were seronegative for HIV.[4] The young woman with HIV infection — Alourdes — had a history of extended residence in Port-au-Prince and also, in 1985, of regular sexual contact with a salaried employee of the national electric company; this man, who had several sexual partners during his tenure in central Haiti, was rumoured to have died of AIDS, although we have not been able to confirm this. Alourdes was also found to have been, in 1986, the partner of a young man from her home village, a construction worker. He later developed tuberculosis, which was initially attributed to respiratory contact with his wife, who had pulmonary tuberculosis. Both were later found to be infected with HIV; neither had ever had sexual contact outside of the Kay region. The discovery of HIV infection in Alourdes, known to have risk factors as defined in the case-control study, illuminated the routes of exposure of the couple with HIV-related tuberculosis.

Although initially not part of the CDC diagnostic criteria for AIDS, most Haitian physicians regard tuberculosis as an early opportunistic infection in patients with HIV. As early as 1983, in fact, tuberculosis was recognized to be the most common infection among Haitians with the newly described syndrome, AIDS. Table 3 gives a summary of the available studies of this concurrence. Recent data from urban Haiti suggest that a majority of those hospitalized for tuberculosis are seropositive for HIV.

Data from the Hôpital Albert Schweitzer, described by many as rural, would seem to confirm this as a *nation-wide* pattern. It is important to note, however, that this hospital is a large referral institution serving a highly mobile and far-flung population. Our own study of HIV seroprevalence among peasants with tuberculosis was conducted from a clinic serving a smaller, less mobile community of rural peasants. It is a relief but no surprise that only 5 per cent of 60 ambulatory patients were HIV-infected (Farmer et al. 1991). If tuberculosis was the leading cause of death among rural Haitian adults before the advent of HIV, it makes little sense to assume that a large percentage of TB cases in the same population are now 'attributable to HIV.' It is nonetheless interesting to note that the rate of seropositivity in ambulatory patients with tuberculosis appears to be at least three times greater than the seroprevalence of HIV among asymptomatic adults.

GESCAP will continue the clinical and epidemiological research now underway; this work is grounded in ethnographic research inaugurated in 1983. Such discrete studies suggest, but do not fully define, the nature of the large-scale forces mentioned above. In the following discussion, we summarize the factors that we believe to be most significant in the ultimate rate of progression of HIV. We hope this discussion will serve as a model for other parts of Latin America, and also parts of Asia and Africa, where rural areas are currently

Table 3. HIV Seroprevalence Among Haitians with Tuberculosis

Site, year of study	N	HIV positive	Study authors
Central Plateau, 1990	60	5%	Farmer et al. (1991)
Deschapelles, 1989	274	24%	Long et al. (1991)
Port-au-Prince, 1987	>200	31%	Johnson and Pape (1989)
Port-au-Prince, 1990	100	57%	Desvarieux and Pape (1991)

low-prevalence regions. It is a cautionary tale that argues for aggressive preventive measures:

> If a disaster is to be prevented in rural Haiti, vigorous and effective prevention campaigns must be initiated at once. And although such efforts must begin, the prospects of stopping the steady march of HIV are slim. AIDS is far more likely to join a host of other sexually transmitted diseases — including gonorrhoea, syphilis, genital herpes, chlamydia, hepatitis B, lymphogranuloma venereum, and even cervical cancer — that have already become entrenched among the poor. (Farmer 1992:262)

Only massive and co-ordinated efforts may yet avert the ongoing disaster that has befallen Haiti, Puerto Rico, inner-city North America, and many nations in sub-Saharan Africa.

DISCUSSION: THE DYNAMICS OF HIV TRANSMISSION IN RURAL HAITI

Wherever HIV infection is a sexually transmitted disease, social forces necessarily determine its distribution. Cultural, political, and economic factors, while each inevitably important, cannot be of *equal* significance in all settings. In Haiti, we have identified a number of differentially weighted, synergistic factors promoting HIV transmission:

Population Pressures

Haiti, which covers 27,700 square kilometres, is one of the most crowded societies in the hemisphere. In 1980, only 8,000 square kilometres were cultivated, giving an effective population density of

626 persons per square kilometre. Unfortunately, Haiti's topsoil is now prey to runaway forces that further compound the overcrowding: 'The land suffers from deforestation, soil erosion and exhaustion; the country is periodically ravaged by hurricanes which cause enormous damage' (Feilden et al. 1981:6). As the land becomes more exhausted, more and more peasants abandon agriculture for the lure of wage-labour in cities and towns. Indeed, one of the most striking recent demographic changes has been the rapid growth of Port-au-Prince. More than 20 per cent of the Haitian population now lives in the capital, a city of more than 1 million inhabitants. Although this is not impressive by Caribbean standards (more than 30 per cent of Puerto Ricans live in San Juan), Port-au-Prince has grown rapidly in recent years: 'The urban population was 12.2 per cent of the total in 1950, 20.4 per cent in 1971 and an estimated 27.5 per cent in 1980' (Feilden et al. 1981:4). Haitian demographers estimate that, by the year 2000, urban dwellers will constitute 37 per cent of the total population.

As is the case with so many Third World countries, internal migration has played the significant role in the growth of the capital. Locher (1984:329) estimates that 'between 1950 and 1971 rural-urban migration accounted for 59 per cent of Haitian urban growth, while natural population increase accounted for only 8 per cent.' As Neptune-Anglade (1986:150) has noted, the growth of Port-au-Prince is substantially the result of a 'feminine rural exodus,' leaving the city approximately 60 per cent female. The most common form of employment among younger women of rural origin — women like Anita and Acephie — is that of servant.[5] Regardless of gender, these migrants maintain strong ties with their regions of origin. In these respects, the three index cases of AIDS from Kay are illustrative of the trends documented by demographers and others who speak of Port-au-Prince as 'a city of peasants.'

Economic Pressures

Rural Haiti, always poor, has become palpably poorer in recent decades. A per capita annual income of $315 in 1983 masked the fact that it hovered around $100 in the countryside.[6] Accompanying population growth and a loss of arable land to erosion and alkalinization has been an inevitable growth in landlessness. All of these factors have had, inevitably, a devastating effect on agricultural production. For example, Girault (1984:177) typifies the decade preceding 1984 as marked chiefly 'by the slow-down of agricultural production and by a decrease in productivity.' This decline has been further compounded by striking rural-urban disparities vis-à-vis every imaginable service. In 1984, Girault (1984:178) was able to complain that 'Port-au-Prince with 17–18 per cent of the national population consumes as much as 30 per cent of all the food produced in the country and a larger share of imported food.' Government statistics reveal that the 'Port-au-Prince agglomeration' consumed, in 1979, 93 per cent of all electricity produced in the country. As Trouillot (1986:201) notes, the city 'houses 20 per cent of the national population, but consumes 80 per cent of all State expenditures.'

In short, current economic conditions push people out of the countryside and into the city or, if possible, out if the country altogether. The Haitian people have long since left behind a peasant standard of living. Whereas Haiti was once a nation with an extremely high percentage of landholders, late-twentieth-century Haiti is increasingly a country of unemployed and landless paupers. When in 1992 the Population Crisis Committee published their 'international index of human suffering' based on a variety of measures of human welfare, Haiti had the dubious distinction of heading the list of all countries in this hemisphere. Of 141 countries studied, in only three were living conditions felt to be worse than in Haiti — and all three of these countries are consumed by civil wars.

Sexuality in Rural Haiti

There have been a number of studies of conjugal unions in rural Haiti, and most have underlined the classic division between those who are *marye* (joined by civil or religious marriage) and those who are *plase*, joined in a conjugal union that incurs significant and enduring obligations to both partners. *Plasaj* (from French, *plaçage*) has generally been considered to be the most common form of conjugal union in rural Haiti, outnumbering marriages by two or three to one. Early studies usually considered *plasaj* to be polygamous, with one man having more than one *plase* partner. In fact, this is often no longer the case, as Moral (1961:173) suggests: 'It is "plaçage honnête" — that is, monogamy — that best characterizes matrimonial status in today's rural society.' The reason for this shift toward monogamy, he believes, is the same one that leads many rural people to avoid marriage in the first place: formal unions are costly. 'If the considerable growth of *plaçage* is to be explained in part by economic factors,' continues Moral, 'the form that *plaçage* now takes is greatly influenced by the poverty spreading throughout the countryside.'

Allman's (1980) review suggests that contemporary sexual unions are considerably more complex than the bipolar model mentioned above. In a survey in which women who had sexual relations for a minimum of three months were considered to be 'in union,' interviews revealed an emic typology with five major categories: three of these — *rinmin*, *fiyanse*, and *viv avèk* — did not usually involve cohabitation and engendered only slight economic support; two others — *plase* and *marye* — were deemed much stronger unions, generally involving cohabitation as well as economic support. Finally, there are a number of sexual practices that have often been loosely termed 'prostitution,' a largely urban phenomenon and much understudied (but see Laguerre 1982). It is clear, however, that unemployed women from rural areas may become involved in occasional and often clandestine sex work when other options are exhausted. For example, the commonly heard terms *ti degaje* and *woulman* both imply, in these contexts, sexual 'survival strategies'. There are few avenues of escape for those caught in the web of urban migration, greater than 60 per cent unemployment, and extreme poverty.[7]

To those working in rural clinics, *plasaj* is often implicated in the rapid spread or persistence of sexually transmitted diseases (STDs) such as gonorrhoea. Treatment of one or two members of the network is of course inadequate, as even women who have but one sexual partner are indirectly in regular sexual contact with the other *plase* partner(s) of their mate. As regards HIV, *plasaj* may be considered a pre-existing socio-cultural institution that serves to speed the spread of HIV and constitutes in and of itself a risk, particularly for monogamous women. 'For most women,' notes the United Nations Development Program (1992:2), 'the major risk factor for HIV infection is being married.'

The unremitting immiseration of Haiti has had a palpable effect on long-standing patterns of sexual union. Stable unions such as marriage and *plasaj* are undermined by the economic pressures to which women with dependents are particularly vulnerable. In the wake of these pressures, new patterns have emerged: 'serial monogamy' might describe the monogamous but weak unions that lead to one child but last little longer than a year or so. After such unions have dissolved, the woman finds herself with a new dependent and even more in need of a reliable partner. Equally dangerous is the quest for a union with a financially 'secure' partner. In rural Haiti, men of this description once included a substantial fraction of all peasant landholders. In recent decades, however, financial security has become elusive for all but a handful of truck drivers, the representatives of the state (viz. soldiers and petty officials), and landholders (*grandon*). As noted, truck drivers and soldiers are clearly groups with above average rates of HIV infection.

Sexism

The Haitian economy counts a higher proportion of economically active women — most of them traders — than any other developing society, with the exception of Lesotho (see Mintz 1964; Neptune-Anglade 1986; Nicholls 1985). It is less surprising, then, that the *machismo* that has so marked other Latin American societies is less pronounced in Haiti (see Murray 1986). Even the head of Duvalier's dreaded paramilitary force was a woman. But sexism is clearly a force in political, economic, and domestic life, and it would be difficult to argue with Neptune-Anglade (1986:155) when she states that, in all regards, rural women 'endure a discrimination and a pauperization that is worse than that affecting [rural] men.'

'The ability of young women to protect themselves from [HIV] infection becomes a direct function of power relations between men and women' (UNDP 1992:6). Sexism has thus weakened women's ability to negotiate safe sexual encounters. Preliminary ethnographic research in the Kay area would lead us to doubt the authority of many women to demand that *plase* partners (or husbands) use condoms. A growing literature documents similar patterns throughout the developing world and in the inner cities of the United States.[8] All of these considerations lead us to agree with those calling for preventive efforts that are 'women-centred.' 'In societies where the female has a weaker hand,' note Desvarieux and Pape (1991:277), 'effective methods of prevention have a better chance of working if the woman does not have to rely on either the consent or the willingness of her partner.'

Other Cultural Considerations

Other cultural practices, such as the widespread and unregulated use of syringes by 'folk' practitioners unschooled in aseptic techniques, received a fair amount of attention as possible sources of HIV transmission. But far more frequently invoked were 'voodoo practices,' which played a peculiarly central role in speculations about the nature of the Haitian epidemic. None of these leads, when investigated, panned out. In urban Haiti, the GHESKIO did not even consider these hypotheses to be worthy of serious investigation. In our small-scale but in-depth study of AIDS in the central plateau, we did not find any strong implication of non-sexual transmission of HIV (Farmer 1992). Similarly, the 'Collaborative Study Group of AIDS in Haitian-Americans' initiated the first and (so far) only controlled study of risk factors for AIDS among Haitians living in the United States. Compiling data from several North American research centres, the investigators reached the following conclusion: 'Folklore rituals have been suggested as potential risk factors for HTLV-III/LAV transmission in Haiti. Our data do not support this hypothesis' (Collaborative Study Group of AIDS in Haitian-Americans 1987:638). Such hypotheses reflect less an accurate reading of existing data and more a series of North American 'folk theories' about Haitians.[9]

There have been few anthropological studies of Haitian understandings of AIDS, and most of these have been conducted in Montreal, New York, or Miami. To our knowledge, the only such study conducted in rural Haiti demonstrated that such understandings were in fact changing, at first quite rapidly. Over time, however, a stable illness representation of *sida*, as AIDS is termed, seemed to evolve. In the Kay region, serial interviews with the same group of villagers permitted the delineation of a complex model of illness causation, one linked fairly closely to understandings of tuberculosis. Sorcery was often, but not always, invoked in discussions about *sida*, which nonetheless came to be seen as a fatal illness that could be transmitted by sexual contact (see Farmer 1990b). Local understandings of *sida* were not demonstrated to affect disease distribution, but may hamper preventive efforts if not taken into account when designing interventions. Far more disabling, however, has been the current political situation.

Political Disruption

It is unfortunate indeed that HIV arrived in Haiti shortly before a period of massive and prolonged social upheaval. Political unrest has clearly undermined preventive efforts and may have helped, through other mechanisms, to spread HIV. Although many commentators observed that political struggles served to divert the public's interest away from AIDS, this was clearly not the case in the Kay region. On the contrary, periods of increased strife were associated with increased public discourse about the new sickness (Farmer 1990b, 1992). Unfortunately, the same political disruptions that may have stimulated commentary about AIDS also served to paralyse co-ordinated efforts to prevent HIV transmission. For example, although AIDS prevention has been identified as one of the top priorities of the Haitian Ministry of Health, the office charged with co-ordinating preventive efforts has been hamstrung by six *coups d'état*, which have led, inevitably, to personnel changes — if not worse. At the time that GESCAP was founded, in 1991, there had been no comprehensive efforts to prevent HIV transmission in rural Haiti. Even in Port-au-Prince, what has been accomplished thus far has been marred, all too often, by culturally inappropriate messages, or by those designed for a small fraction of the population (e.g., Haitians who are francophone, literate, and television-owning). These messages are especially unhelpful in rural areas, where well-funded 'social marketing' schemes have had little cultural currency.

Political upheaval did not just hobble coordinated response to the epidemic. It has had far more direct effects. One of the most epidemiologically significant events of recent years may prove to be the *coup d'état* of September 1991. As noted, a number of surveys of asymptomatic adults living in Cité Soleil, an urban slum on the northern border of the capital, revealed seroprevalence rates of approximately 10 per cent. Following the *coup*, these areas were targeted by the army for brutal repression. A number of journalists and health-care professionals estimated that fully half of the adult residents of this slum fled to rural areas following the army's lethal incursions. It takes little imagination to see that such flux substantially changes the equations describing HIV transmission dynamics in rural areas sheltering the refugees. Similar patterns have been noted elsewhere:

> Women living in areas plagued by civil unrest or war way be in a situation of higher risk. In many countries, relatively high percentages of male military and police personnel are infected and their unprotected (voluntary or forced) sexual encounters with local women provide an avenue for transmission. Patterns of female infection have been correlated with the movements of members of the military in parts of Central and Eastern Africa. (de Bruyn 1992:253)

Concurrent Disease

The progression of HIV disease depends on host variables such as age, sex, and nutritional status; T-cell number and function; and intercurrent disease. Concurrent illness may alter the progression of HIV disease in at least three different ways: (1) any serious illness, including opportunistic infections, may hasten the development of AIDS among the HIV-infected; (2) various diseases are able to heighten an individual's 'net state of immunosuppression,' rendering him or her increasingly vulnerable to infection; and (3) certain infections seem to increase the risk of *acquiring* HIV. We will consider here only the latter.

STDs have been cited as 'AIDS co-factors' in a number of studies, especially those conducted in tropical and sub-tropical regions. STDs have been held to be particularly important in the heterosexual spread of HIV, as the retrovirus is less efficiently transmitted from women to men than vice versa. Thus vaginal and cervical diseases, even those as ostensibly minor as trichomoniasis, may increase the risk of HIV transmission through 'microwounds' and even through mere inflammation (as lymphocytes are, after all, the target cells of HIV).[10] Although important data about STDs are now being collected in Port-au-Prince (e.g., Liautaud et al. 1992), there are as yet no careful studies being conducted in rural areas.[11] But there is little data to suggest that villagers are more sexually active than their urban counterparts; there are even less data that suggest that rural Haitians are more sexually active than age-matched controls from North America. What is clear is that a majority of STDs go untreated, which certainly suggests that sores, other lesions, and inflammation will persist far longer in rural Haiti than in most areas of the world.

Other diseases — including leprosy, yaws, endemic syphilis, and various viruses — have been suggested as possible co-factors in 'tropical' AIDS, but their roles have not been clarified. It seems safe to add, however, that serious co-infections do enhance the net state of immunosuppression. Similarly, malnutrition clearly hastens the advent of AIDS among the infected, although this dynamic may lessen the risk of transmission: the Haitian variant of 'slim disease' is now popularly associated with AIDS, and frank cachexia is likely to drive away potential sexual partners.[12]

Access to Medical Services

Finally, in seeking to understand the Haitian AIDS epidemic, it is necessary to underline the contribution, or lack thereof, of a non-functioning public health system. Medical care in Haiti is something of an obstacle course, one in which innumerable barriers are placed before poor people seeking care. Failure to have an STD treated means persistence of important co-factors; failure to have pulmonary tuberculosis treated means rapid progression of HIV disease and death, to say nothing of its impact on HIV-negative individuals. Contaminated blood transfusions alternate with no transfusions at all. Condoms are often not available even to those who want them. The cost of pharmaceuticals, always prohibitive, has skyrocketed in recent years. Antivirals are in essence unavailable: in February 1990, 'local radio stations announced ... that for the first time, the drug AZT is available in Haiti. It might as well have been on Mars. A bottle of 100 capsules costs $343 — more than most Haitians make in a year' (Lief 1990:36).

CONCLUSIONS

It is clear from the above studies that a number of social forces are indeed shaping the HIV epidemic in rural Haiti. But what, more precisely, are these forces and how may each of them be weighted? This is a perennial problem, but one too rarely addressed by medical anthropology, which has often been asked to elucidate the 'cultural component' of particular sub-epidemics. We contend that by combining social analysis with ethnographically informed epidemiology, we have identified the most significant factors determining the rate of HIV transmission in rural Haiti. These factors are differentially weighted, of course, but each demonstrably plays a role:

1. Deepening poverty
2. Sexism
3. Traditional patterns of sexual union
4. Emergent patterns of sexual union
5. Prevalence of and lack of access to treatment for STDs
6. Lack of timely response by public-health authorities
7. Lack of culturally appropriate prevention tools
8. Political upheaval

Many of these factors are a far cry from the ones that anthropologists were exhorted to explore — for example, ritual scarification, animal sacrifice, sexual behaviour in 'exotic subcultures' — during the first decade of AIDS. But the forces underpinning the spread of HIV to rural Haiti are as economic and political as they are cultural, and poverty seems to underlie all of them. Although many working elsewhere would agree that poverty is the strongest enhancer of risk for exposure to HIV, once again this subject was neglected at the VIIIth International Conference on AIDS. Of the epidemiology-track posters presented in Amsterdam, only three used 'poverty' as a key word; two of these were socio-culturally naïve and did not seem to involve the collaboration of anthropologists.

In order to move beyond the stifling notion of 'risk group,' anthropologists would do well to remember that they are trained in *social analysis*. While cultural considerations — such as racism or the nearly universal stigma attached to AIDS — may very well be of overriding significance in settings in the Northern hemisphere, we would argue that they are often less so wherever poverty and economic inequity serve as the most virulent co-factors in the spread of this disease.

ACKNOWLEDGMENTS

The research upon which this chapter is based was made possible by a collaboration between two community-based organizations: Zanmi Lasante and Partners in Health. I would like to thank all the members of GESCAP, a study group funded by the World AIDS Foundation, for their contribution to the research and, more importantly, to the care of those with HIV disease: thanks especially to Patrick Samedi and Maxi Raymonville. I am also grateful to Jim Yong Kim, Roger Grande, Brèdy Pierre-Louis, Paul Grifhorst, Mirjam van Ewijk, Tom White, Arthur Kleinman, Ophelia Dahl, and Didi Bertrand for their editorial (or otherwise inspirational) comments.

NOTES

1. In their consideration of unequal exchange and the urban informal sector, Portes and Walton (1982:74) designate Haiti as the most rural of all Latin American nations: in 1950, the nation was held to be 88 per cent rural; in 1960, 85 per cent; in 1970, 81 per cent.

2. In a key paper published in 1984, Guerin and co-workers from Haiti, North America, and Canada stated that, '17 per cent of our patients had sexual contact with [North] American tourists' (Guérin et al. 1984:256).

3. In Cité Soleil, a slum on the northern fringes of Port-au-Prince, 8.4 per cent of 1240 healthy women receiving prenatal care in 1986 were seropositive for HIV (Halsey et al. 1987). In 1987, 9.9 per cent of 2009 'sexually active women' in Cité Soleil were HIV-positive; in 1989, 10.5 per cent of 1074 such women were found to have been exposed to HIV (Brutus 1989a). In Gonaives, the third-largest Haitian city, 9 per cent of

1795 patients reporting to a clinic that serves a predominantly low-income clientele were found to be seropositive in 1988 (Brutus 1989b).

4. One young woman, the regular sexual partner of a truck driver, was also found to be seropositive. She died suddenly during the course of the study, less than a week after a negative physical examination. Although the cause of death is unclear — she had explosive, watery diarrhoea and presented in shock — she is not considered in this cohort.

5. 'Note that, in the cities, the [economically] active 10–14 year-old girls are essentially all domestics.... These 'restavèks' find themselves at the very bottom of the social hierarchy' (Neptune-Anglade 1986:209).

6. See Farmer (1988) for a review of these and other data concerning the Haitian economy.

7. This is of course a cursory discussion of a very complex — and changing — subject. See the studies by Lowenthal (1984), Murray (1976), Neptune-Anglade (1986), and Vieux (1989) for a more complete discussion of sexual unions in Haiti.

8. For a helpful review of these issues as regards women in developing countries, see Maria de Bruyn: 'Even if they dare suggest avoiding risky sexual acts or using condoms, they often encounter male refusal, are accused of adultery or promiscuity (the desire to use condoms being interpreted as evidence of extramarital affairs), are suspected of already being infected with HIV or are said to accuse their partners of infidelity' (de Bruyn 1992:256). A recent issue of *Culture, Medicine and Psychiatry* examines sex and risk among poor women living in the inner cities of the United States (Farmer et al. 1993).

9. On American 'folk models' of Haitians, see Lawless (1992) and, as regards AIDS, Farmer (1992a).

10. Poor, young women may be especially at risk of genital trauma: 'Non-consensual, hurried or frequent intercourse may inhibit mucous production and the relaxation of vaginal musculature, both of which would increase the likelihood of genital trauma. A lack of control over the circumstances in which the intercourse occurs may increase the frequency of intercourse and lower the age at which sexual activity begins. A lack of access to acceptable health services may leave infections and lesions untreated. Malnutrition not only inhibits the production of mucus but also slows the healing process and depresses the immune system' (UNDP 1992:3–4).

11. We do know that, in one study of 100 women presenting to our women's health clinic in 1991, fully 25 per cent of them had trichomoniasis. GESCAP thanks Dr. Anna Contomitros for conducting this study, which included Pap smears.

12. Data from GHESKIO (e.g., Deschamps et al. 1992) suggest, however, that those ill with HIV disease continue to have sex.

REFERENCES

Allman, J. 1980. Sexual unions in rural Haiti. *International Journal of Sociology of the Family* 10:15–39.

Brutus, J.R. 1989a. Seroprevalence de HIV parmi les femmes enceintes à Cité Soleil, Haiti. Paper presented at the Fifth International Conference on AIDS. Montreal, Canada, 5–7 June.

Brutus, J.R. 1989b. Problèmes d'éthique liés au dépistage du virus HIV-1. Paper presented at the Congrès des Médécins Francophones d'Amérique. Fort-de-France, Martinique, 12–16 June.

Bruyn, M. de. 1992. Women and AIDS in Developing Countries. *Social Science and Medicine* 34(3):249–262.

Collaborative Study Group of AIDS in Haitian-Americans 1987. Risk Factors for AIDS Among Haitians Residing in the United States: Evidence of Heterosexual Transmission. *Journal of the American Medical Association* 257(5):635–639.

Desvarieux, M., and J.W. Pape. 1991. HIV and AIDS in Haiti: Recent developments. *AIDS Care* 3(3):271–279.

Deschamps, M., J.W. Pape, M.E. Beaulieu, K. Thermil, and W. Johnson Jr. 1992. HIV Seroconversion Related to Heterosexual Activity in Discordant Haitian Couples. Abstract Number C1087, VIIIth International Conference on AIDS/IIIrd STD World Congress. Amsterdam, 19–24 July.

Farmer, P. 1988. Blood, Sweat, and Baseballs: Haiti in the West Atlantic system. *Dialectical Anthropology* 13:83–99.

Farmer, P. 1990a. The Exotic and the Mundane: Human Immunodeficiency Virus in Haiti. *Human Nature* 1(4):415–446.

Farmer, P. 1990b. Sending sickness: Sorcery, Politics, and Changing Concepts of AIDS in Rural Haiti. *Medical Anthropology Quarterly* 4(1):6–27.

Farmer, P. 1992. *AIDS and Accusation: Haiti and the Geography of Blame.* Berkeley: University of California Press.

Farmer, P., S. Robin, S. Ramilus, and Jim Yong Kim. 1991. Tuberculosis, poverty, and 'compliance': Lessons from rural Haiti. *Seminars in Respiratory Infections* 6(4):254–260.

Farmer, P., M. Raymonville, S. Robin, S. Ramilus, and Jim Yong Kim. 1992. The Dynamics of HIV Transmission in Rural Haiti. Abstract Number C4608. VIIIth International Conference on AIDS/IIIrd STD World Congress. Amsterdam, 19–24 July.

Farmer, P., S. Lindenbaum, and M.-J. Del Vecchio Good. 1993. Women, Poverty and AIDS: An Introduction, *Culture, Medicine and Psychiatry* 17(4):387–397.

Feilden, R., J. Allman, J. Montague, and J. Rohde. 1981. Health, Population and Nutrition in Haiti: A Report Prepared for the World Bank. Boston: Management Sciences for Health.

Girault, C. 1984. Commerce in the Haitian economy. In: *Haiti — Today and Tomorrow: An Interdisciplinary Study*, edited by C. Foster, and A. Valdman. Lanham, MD: University Press of America.

Guérin, J., R. Malebranche, R. Elie, A. Laroche, G. Pierre, E. Arnoux, T. Spira, J. Dupuy, T. Seemayer, and C. Péan-Guichard. 1984. Acquired Immune Deficiency Syndrome: Specific aspects of the disease in Haiti. *Annals of the New York Academy of Sciences* 437:254–261.

Halsey N., R. Boulos, J. Brutus, et al. 1987. HIV Antibody Prevalence In Pregnant Haitian Women. Abstracts of the Third International Conference on AIDS, Washington, DC, June 1987.

Johnson, W., and J. Pape. 1989. AIDS in Haiti. In: *Treatment*, edited by J. Levy. New York: Marcel Dekker.

Laguerre, M. 1982. *Urban Life in the Caribbean*. Cambridge, MA: Schenkman.

Lawless, R. 1992. *Haiti's Bad Press*. Rochester, VT: Schenkman.

Liautaud, B., B., L. Mellon, J. Denizé-Vieux, R. Grand-Pierre, M. Mevs, C. Nolté, and J.W. Pape. 1992. Preliminary data on STDs in Haiti. Abstract Number C4302. VIIIth International Conference on AIDS/IIIrd STD World Congress. Amsterdam, 19–24 July.

Lief, L. 1990. Where Democracy Isn't About to Break Out. *U.S. News and World Report* 12 February 1990: 34–36.

Locher, U. 1984. Migration in Haiti. In: *Haiti — Today and Tomorrow: An Interdisciplinary Study*, edited by C. Foster, and A. Valdman. Lanham, MD: University Press of America.

Long, R., M. Sarcini, J. Manfreda, G. Carré, E. Phillipe, E. Hershfield, L. Sekla, and W. Stackiw. 1991. Impact of Human Immunodeficiency Virus Type 1 on tuberculosis in rural Haiti. *American Review of Respiratory Diseases* 143:69–73.

Lowenthal, I. 1984. Labor, Sexuality and the Conjugal Contract in Rural Haiti. In: *Haiti — Today and Tomorrow: An Interdisciplinary Study*, edited by C. Foster, and A. Valdman. Lanham, MD: University Press of America.

Mintz, S. 1964. The Employment of Capital by Market Women in Haiti. In: *Capital, Saving and Credit in Peasant Societies*, edited by R. Firth, and B. Yamey. Chicago: Aldine.

Moral, P. 1961. *Le Paysan Haïtien*. Port-au-Prince: Les Editions Fardins.

Murray, S. 1986. A Note on Haitian Tolerance of Homosexuality. In: *Male Homosexuality in Central and South America*, edited by S. Murray. Gai Saber Monograph 5.

Neptune-Anglade, M. 1986. *L'Autre Moitié du Développement: A Propos du Travail des Femmes en Haiti*. Pétion-Ville, Haiti: Éditions des Alizés.

Nicholls, D. 1985. *Haiti in Caribbean Context: Ethnicity, Economy and Revolt*. New York: St. Martin's Press.

Pape, J., and W. Johnson. 1988. Epidemiology of AIDS in the Caribbean. *Baillière's Clinical Tropical Medicine and Communicable Diseases* 3(1):31–42.

Portes, A., and J. Walton. 1982. *Labor, Class, and the International System.* New York: Academic Press.

Trouillot, M.R. 1986. *Les Racines Historiques de l'État Duvaliérien.* Port-au-Prince: Imprimérie Henri Déschamps.

United Nations Development Program (UNDP). 1992. *Young Women: Silence, Susceptibility and the HIV Epidemic.* New York: UNDP.

Vieux, S.H. 1989. *Le Plaçage: Droit Coutumier et Famille en Haïti.* Paris: Éditions Publisud.

Chapter TWO

Culture, Sex Research and AIDS Prevention in Africa

Brooke Grundfest Schoepf

AIDS is the leading cause of death among sexually active youth and adults in a number of African countries. As elsewhere in the Third World, the majority become infected through sexual relations unprotected by condoms. Considered 'normal and natural,' heterosexual penetrative sex with ejaculation is invested with cosmological significance, strongly valued by many as the essence of life, crucial to the health, beauty, and survival of individual, family, and community. Thus freighted with extraordinary symbolic power, AIDS may be more damaging to society than other fatal afflictions often attributed to sorcery — a potent metaphor for human relations gone awry (Schoepf 1990a).[1]

These significations contribute to denial of risk, to stigmatization of the afflicted and their families, and to withdrawal of social support. The meanings with which AIDS is invested, the social contexts of transmission, and cultural constructions of contagion and disease create constraints to understanding and acting upon information about prevention. The heavy cultural and emotional load does not render prevention or compassionate care for the sick and survivors impossible, however. Rather, it renders urgent the search for both effective culture change and self-sustainable development, both in support of sexual risk reduction and of resources for affected families and communities. Because the semiology of AIDS is as important as its biochemistry, applied research needs to be grounded in theory, in broad participative experience, and in an extensive Africanist literature informed by Afrocentric views 'from below.'[2]

GENDER, CRISIS, AND AIDS

Globally, AIDS is a disease of development and 'under-' or 'uneven' development. It has struck with severity in nations with economies in crisis. Africa's present crisis has its roots in distorted production structures inherited from colonialism, heavy debt burdens, exports of a limited number of tropical products on unfavourable world markets, and rapid class formation propelled by privileged access to the state. Research in Zaïre linking macrolevel political economy to microlevel socio-cultural analysis shows how poverty and hopelessness born of prolonged crisis and increasing disparities in wealth contributed to a burgeoning HIV epidemic (Schoepf 1988, 1990b; Schoepf et al. 1988; Rukarangira and Schoepf 1991). Together with institutionalized male dominance, they led in the 1970s to increases in multiple partner relations and widening sexual networks (Schoepf 1978, 1981).

AIDS places gender relations, the status of women and women's knowledge at the centre of analysis. While the majority of Zaïrean women make major contributions to household incomes, most are in positions of social, economic and emotional dependency (Schoepf and Walu 1991; Walu 1991, 1992). With high levels of background infection, gendered differences in power, earning capacity, and ideology combine with biological factors to make young females especially susceptible. Structural Adjustment Programs (SAPs) have exacerbated the poverty of poor urban and rural women particularly (Newbury and Schoepf 1989; Schoepf et al. 1991b). Reduced public health budgets and user fees for services make it unlikely that the poor majority will obtain adequate care. Few men and even fewer women are adequately treated for sexually transmitted infections.

AIDS spread initially in cities and towns crowded with unemployed, where few women hold well-paid formal sector jobs. The informal economy is over-crowded, and earnings in both sectors are generally very low. Inflated food prices and user fees for health care add to women's burdens. The crisis has fostered risky situations and forced numerous women to use sex with multiple partners to provide for themselves and family members. Adolescents from poor families are especially vulnerable to offers of gifts. Some exchange sex for food, clothes, or grades in school. Fear of AIDS prompts older men to seek out youngsters whom they reason are unlikely to be infected. HIV is spreading most rapidly among adolescent women.

Most women, including faithful wives, are unable to negotiate safer sex practices with partners whom they know or suspect have multiple partners. When men refuse to use condoms, women without independent incomes cannot refuse risky sex. Powerlessness in the face of a dreaded disease leads many women to deny their risk. In the presence of HIV, what was once a survival strategy for poor women leads to AIDS and death (Schoepf 1988; Schoepf et al. 1988). These findings are confirmed by studies in neighbouring countries, and recent literature indicates their relevance in other areas of the world where HIV is transmitted heterosexually (Kisekka 1990; Bassett and Mhloyi 1991; Obbo 1993a, and in this volume; Kammerer et al., in this volume; studies reviewed in de Bruyn 1992; Schoepf 1992a, 1993a).

Women informants agree on the need to prevent abuse of power by men in sexual relations. This requires a major change in existing culture, beginning with social and legal legitimation of women's right to say 'No,' and the economic independence to do so. This basic human right is violated not only in Zaïre, but in many other societies. It is essential to cultural survival in the time of AIDS. Another major change envisioned by informants is increased communication between stable partners and lovers about sex, not only to allow realistic risk assessment and condom use, but also to enhance the quality of sexual relations. Desirable as the latter strategy is, however, it takes second place in the eyes of some women to augmenting their economic and social power to refuse sex.

Research in Zaïre suggests that in the cities today, male dominance sometimes leaves fewer opportunities for negotiation than were available to women in rural communities a generation ago. Nevertheless, teaching empowerment techniques in women's groups enables some to discover ways to protect themselves and children. Moreover, while the main efforts to promote risk reduction and change in sexual relations must focus on men, women, too, need to make personal risk assessments and to accept condoms in risky relationships.

Given the context of gender, age, and class inequality, and the rapid spread of HIV, this contribution examines four interrelated issues. The first is the nature of premises and methodologies driving sex research in Africa. The second is the nature of interdisciplinary collaboration between anthropologists and biomedical researchers. Linking both are questions about the uses made of the concept of culture. Finally, there are epistemological questions about 'the nature of cultural knowledge and the nature of knowledge of cultural knowledge' (Fabian 1990b:18). Although the illustrative examples come from Africa, the concepts and problems are general ones, related to anthropology's post-colonial encounter with its 'object' on a global scale. They are relevant to other areas of the world where AIDS affects poor and relatively powerless people.

SEX RESEARCH IN AFROCENTRIC PERSPECTIVES

Lindenbaum (1991) writes that, with the publication of Malinowski's work on sex in the Trobriand Islands, anthropology acquired an early, perhaps undeserved, reputation for free inquiry into tabooed subjects. She locates renewed interest in the cultural construction of sexuality in research driven by feminist concerns published in the 1970s. In the US, legitimacy for this interest was not easily won in the biomedical arena, as I can attest from experience teaching courses on sexuality in two major universities. The legitimacy of sex research is still strongly contested in the wider American society. The religious right has impeded both national and local KAP surveys.[3]

In Zaïre, too, sex research is an arena of cultural politics on national and international levels (Schoepf 1991a, 1992c, 1992d, 1993c). Contests over meaning are power struggles of 'race,' class, gender, and age. AIDS has set in motion discourses about sex grown from 500 years of unequal relations between Africa and the West — since, in fact, trade in human beings by Christians required ideological justification. Western discourse about 'African sexuality,' with its stigmatizing myths of super-potent men and wild, lascivious women, has been reinvented in both biomedical and popular accounts of AIDS in Africa.[4] Not unpredictably, stigma provoked defensive reactions among African governments, intellectuals, and peoples.

History aids in understanding the strength of this refusal. Missionary ideology invested the colonial terrain with sexual prudery (Richards 1956; Schoepf 1980, 1981; Yates 1982). Women who aspired to Christian respectability were taught to suppress their feelings and their expression of pleasure.[5] Whereas African cultures in the region had endowed sex with both sacred ritual power and danger of pollution, the missionary view stressed pollution. Female sexuality was exclusively for reproduction, and otherwise deemed 'dirty.' Although men were excused by dint of their 'natural, animal' needs, they were warned that 'too much sex' would sap their vitality. As in Europe, parents and teachers were enjoined to prevent children and adolescents from masturbation and non-penetrative sex in order to protect their charges' health. Same-sex relationships were driven underground. Missionary intervention created new sexual guilts that resulted in illness and — ironically, in view of strong missionary opposition — expanded the reach of African healers (Central African examples in Janzen 1978; Corin 1979; Taylor 1992).

One means of colonial domination involved scrutiny of intimate relations. Discourse about bodies was also a set of metaphors about the body politic (Douglas 1966). The missionaries' cultural engineering project combined with the interests of elder African males as well as those of employers in controlling women's labour in agricultural production and reproduction of the labour force, and with those of the colonial state in maintaining order. In the process, free women's roles were reinvented, their autonomy undermined, and their status depressed. Colonial discourses converged in moral texts of missionary medicine (Seidel 1993; Vaughan 1991). As in the West, women were blamed for spreading sexually transmitted diseases and for sterility.

Sexuality has been reinvented in various ways, with patent anachronisms sanctified as 'tradition.' Constructing an 'archaeology of sexuality' is now extremely difficult. In Central Africa Christianity is now a hegemonic discourse, with Islam a minor theme. Even people with little formal schooling value badges of 'middle class respectability.' Governments in the region are frequently led by men educated in mission schools. Some have refused to legalize contraception or to authorize condom promotion to the general population, particularly to youth at risk; girls who become pregnant may be expelled from school, which leaves many with no resort but risky illegal abortion — or sex work to support their children.

Repression notwithstanding, some cultures in Eastern Zaïre have resisted sexual alienation.[6] For example, in the 1970s villages in Southeastern Shaba retained the *chisungu*, the girls' fertility celebration witnessed among the neighbouring Bemba by Audrey Richards in 1931 (Richards 1956). Women's sexual pleasure was cultivated along with the duty of wives to please husbands and to produce descendants. 'Sexual archaeology' is of more than antiquarian inter-

est. Since communication about sex and fertility is central to prevention, silencing ideologies that narrow the space for sex-positive
prevention strategies are an obstacle to HIV prevention. Throughout
the world, the power of fundamentalist religious leaders constitutes
one of the most intractable cultural constraints.

The legitimacy of sex research in Africa labours under another, not
unrelated, cloud (Schoepf 1983; Ahlberg 1991). In the 1970s agencies
concerned about high rates of population growth funded demographic surveys and ethnographies of sex and fertility. Some of these
afforded research opportunities to young African social scientists,
including some who are now distinguished contributors to AIDS
research. While many African governments have adopted population policies, few have proceeded to effective implementation. The
association of sex research with 'population control' renders it
suspect to many of those who believe that this concern is a smoke
screen for withholding health resources and for lack of effective
development policies. AIDS was seen as a pretext to gain acceptance
for contraception when other means had failed. Rumours about the
dangers of condoms for women, ubiquitous in Central and East
Africa, are fuelled by this broad cultural resistance, as well as by
some religious leaders. Women are warned of potential infection,
permanent sterility, and death should a condom break and remain in
the vagina. Men who refuse to diminish their pleasure by 'taking a
shower in a raincoat' use these imaginary dangers as justification.

This example shows how converging elements of macrolevel cultural politics are bolstered by microlevel gender relations. Some men
use the threat of insemination as a means to control women's
sexuality. The subtext of the often-heard statement that 'condoms
lead to immorality,' is the reasoning that a woman who fears pregnancy is more likely to remain faithful than one who uses contraception.[7] One consequence was that prior to the spread of HIV, sexually
active single women would risk pregnancy and illegal abortion,
rather than seem to be prepared for sex, for fear that they would be
considered 'prostitutes.'[8]

Male-oriented discourses on issues of sexuality appeal to
'tradition' for support. Already present in debates about sex education and population policy among African leaders, these debates
have dogged responses to HIV/AIDS. They reinforce the need for
integrated approaches to reproductive health, gender, and development, rather than to vertical, single-disease programmes.

Biomedical researchers stepped into this complex arena less than
fully prepared. When heterosexual transmission of HIV was dis-

covered in Africa, biomedical researchers regarded it as a new epidemiological paradigm (Quinn et al. 1986). Anthropologists were asked to answer a set of questions about African difference:

Why is AIDS in Africa transmitted differently from in the West?
Why are as many African women as men infected with HIV?
Why does African sexuality result in heterosexual infection?

Ethnographic literature was searched for data on African cultural traditions related to exotic sexual practices, blood and sorcery; the results included examples of a genre Pellow (1990) terms 'ethnopornography.' Survey research was funded to locate individual risk behaviours in 'knowledge, attitudes and practices' (KAP). Partner numbers were reported — without comparative empirical data — to be significantly higher than in the West. Some accounts featured the terms 'promiscuity' and 'prostitution.' The subtext (indeed, sometimes the text) was about a special 'African sexuality.' Both variability and change were lost in an opaque 'ethnographic present' (Schoepf 1992d).

Two decades of socio-medical research on disease in African contexts were ignored in favour of an approach to epidemiology and public health that focused on individual behaviours divorced from social contexts, and stripped them of their origins in power, gender and class relations. The narrow biomedical approach ignored the work of both African and Africanist scholars in women's studies showing how the social positions and ideologies of researchers condition knowledge-gathering. Instead, by treating sex research as a value-neutral process, KAP studies neglected opportunities to learn how women's experiences differ from those of men. Translated into policies, these epistemological blinders resulted in predictable failures of prevention campaigns. Ignoring epistemic adequacy for political convenience has cost millions of lives.

Two decades of scholarship interrogating the role of anthropology in the colonial encounter also were ignored. Many Zaïreans perceive their status in European eyes to be that of the quintessential 'Other.' The subject has attracted post-colonial attention particularly with respect to ways in which anthropology has constructed African personhood. Study of cultural politics helps to situate Africans' 'underreaction' to AIDS in an international context.[9]

CULTURAL POLITICS, CULTURAL LOGICS

Research on representations of AIDS is a study of culture change, as well as of persistence. Meanings have developed on a complex international terrain of cultural logics, often unvoiced. The power to name and define the AIDS epidemic has not lain exclusively with the West. In Zaïre, meanings changed as popular knowledge and awareness of vulnerability increased. Knowledge spread most rapidly among elite urban young men. At first AIDS was rejected as 'an Imaginary Syndrome invented to Discourage Lovers.' Constructed from the acronym SIDA, this metaphor, which swept the country in 1986, encapsulates both historical knowledge of objectification and cultural defiance.

> Who was discouraging lovers? Europeans, of course.
> Which lovers were to be discouraged? Africans, of course.
> Why would Europeans seek to do this? Jealousy, of course.

The perceptions underlying the metaphor are not merely antique 'survivals' of colonialism. Kinshasa residents have witnessed European and Asian men who value African women as 'exotic' objects of desire. The metaphoric *Syndrome Imaginaire* combined defiance and denial; reduced to a humorous slogan, the disease was belittled; rendered mundane, it did not have to be dealt with. However, denial was a 'weapon of the weak.' It was counterproductive, since failure to confront the situation delayed prevention and so caused many new infections.

The next year, AIDS became more 'real.' Most of the more than 600 people interviewed in Kinshasa and Lubumbashi by mid-1987 had heard that AIDS is fatal and sexually transmitted. Awareness had increased with the beginning of a national information campaign. Detailed advice set to music by the late Franco (Luambo Makiadi) played throughout Kinshasa in June. Rumours circulating on the 'sidewalk radio' told of a growing number of people, including some well-known personalities, said to be dead or dying of AIDS. Deaths of high-status men were particularly visible. Many informants were touched personally by losing friends and family members. Some (mainly women) had to cope with problems of tending the sick and caring for orphaned children. The futures of surviving spouses were tainted by uncertainty, as families, friends, and acquaintances assumed that they were infected (Schoepf 1992d).

Laymen (but not women) tended to perceive AIDS chiefly as a threat to men. Although women predominated both among the ill

and among infected persons, the official, male-controlled information campaign focused on avoiding prostitutes. In the neighbourhoods, single women, especially sex workers, were pointed to as
AIDS transmitters. For women, especially, AIDS was shameful; its
symptoms, the stigmata of sin.

As awareness increased, Western speculation that the new virus
originated in Central Africa was rejected as one more evidence of
racism. A counter-hegemonic discourse arose in urban folklore. Had
the virus escaped from a US germ warfare laboratory? Many considered this plausible. Given the destructive role of US politics
throughout Zaïre's post-colonial history, it was easy to believe that
the virus had been deliberately planted. Others attributed it to environmental pollution, or to eating imported canned foods in place of
the more healthful traditional diet.

Scripts invented for the introduction of HIV to Zaïre and to Africa
varied. Some said it arrived by air with businessmen from Europe
who transmitted it to sex workers. Others said it came with sailors off
the merchant ships docked in the Atlantic seaports, where many sex
workers were dying. Still others said it came with US military men
engaged in supplying Savimbi's rebel army in Angola. Sex workers
were told that they were safe if they avoided European men; class
was implicated when women in Kisangani were warned against sex
with men arriving by air from Kinshasa, 1000 kilometres distant. Sex
with poorer riverboat travellers was said to be safe.

Just as Europeans had constructed Africa from erotic imaginings,
so Zaïreans elaborated fantasies about sex, money, and the special
proclivities of European men. Reputed to find Zaïrean women
desirable for their knowledge of sexual pleasures not available at
home, foreign men were said to pay fabulous sums of $50, $100, or
even $150 per night for these voluptuous delights. Another sexual
script linked AIDS to the desires of aging Europeans who paid
Zaïrean women to have sex with dogs and monkeys.[10]

In time, a socio-economic explanation was added. In 1988 the
initials SIDA were used by women to stand for: *Salaire Insuffisant
Depuis des Années* ('Insufficient Salary for Years'), or *Salaire Individuel
Difficilement Acquis* (Individual Salary Acquired with Difficulty'). In
anglophone countries, AIDS was the 'Acquired Income Deficiency
Syndrome' (SWAA 1989). This explanation has become widely accepted. At the same time, a social marketing project popularized
condoms among young men for sex with casual partners (Rukarangira and Schoepf 1989). Currently, popular discourse represents
AIDS as socially produced, a disease emblematic of Africa's deepen-

ing economic crisis and the situation of poor women forced to provide sexual services to multiple partners as a means of survival.
While this explanation has not supplanted others, it opens spaces for
a personal-and-political approach to prevention and to reducing stigma.

CULTURAL CREATIVITY AND EMPOWERMENT

Popular construction of AIDS as a disease of economic crisis and
sympathy for mothers unable to care for their children offer opportunities to build upon popular understanding. Anthropologists can
work with informants to deepen knowledge of situations and beliefs
that create obstacles to widespread adoption of safer sex practices.
Active, participatory learning methods in small groups enable
people to grasp the facts of HIV/AIDS in ways that are relevant to
their lives (Gordon and Klouda 1989; Aggleton et al. 1990; Lynch and
Gordon 1991). Role plays, especially, encourage groups to create
performances that shape common goals in support of prevention. In
Africa they resonate with the short dramas used by ritual specialists
to teach and enhance memory (Richards 1956), and with comic
sketches devised by popular theatre groups. Puppet performances
and pictures that provoke dialogue also can be used in this way
(Bone et al. 1991; Preston-Whyte, in this volume).

Sexual risk reduction requires that people talk about sex — not to
researchers, but to one another. Action-research enables anthropologists to combine theoretical concerns of the discipline with
humanist concern for the survival and empowerment of the individuals and communities studied. The cultural content of structured exercises generates emotions that help to overcome some of the
obstacles to cognitive mastery and value change. At the same time,
they produce new knowledge of culture and socio-cultural dynamics. The learning process used in 'training for transformation'
based on the work of Paolo Freire (1972, 1976), can generate critical
reflection and group action for social change (Hope, Timmel and
Hodzi 1984). Used in this manner, action-research is a form of what
Fabian (1990b) terms 'performative ethnography,' a means for oppressed people to reclaim their identity and power.[11]

Pictures that tell a story in readily understood metaphors are particularly appropriate for teaching complex information. The lengthy
period between HIV infection and sickness is a difficult but essential
concept; misunderstanding contributes to neglect of protection. Peo-

ple must grasp that healthy-looking individuals may be infected unknowingly and, if so, can transmit infection. Failing this, many have reinterpreted prevention messages in various ways (Schoepf 1988, 1991b, 1991c). For example, one hears men say: 'I'm not at risk; I only go with heavy women. Fat people can't have AIDS.' Pictures of a tree infested by termites and dying by degrees until it is completely dead help to convey the idea of delayed sickness.

A role play with emotional impact called *Mwana Mayi-Mayi* (literally, 'water child') helps to anchor this difficult cognitive material. A grandmother and her daughter take a sickly infant to the doctor, who takes a history and discovers that the baby's father has died of a wasting disease. The doctor draws blood and asks the mother to return for the test results. The next week she tells the women that the baby has AIDS, and that the mother, too, should be tested. Participants have played with a wealth of details in gestures and body postures, showing how they perceive health providers. This drama generally elicited gasps of astonished dismay, confirming that in 1987, maternal–foetal transmission was not widely understood.

Since healthy descendants are highly valued by both men and women, understanding the chain of transmission constitutes a powerful incentive to change. Constructed as a threat to family survival, male prerogatives such as multiple partners (spoken of as 'the Rights of Man') can be abandoned more readily than when they are attacked as a betrayal of the conjugal bond or Christian morality. The strategy was suggested by a woman television personality who lamented women's powerlessness to broach the issue of condoms with husbands (Schoepf 1988).

The links between HIV, sex, gender, and power emerge sharply from the experiential method. Culturally constructed meanings can be shared and critical consciousness of AIDS as a problem for families and communities developed. The next step is to place HIV risk reduction in a development context by asking: What keeps people from making changes? Why? This helps to remove the onus of guilt and stigma, emotions which, coupled with fear and anxiety, give rise to denial, avoidance and scapegoating.

One danger is that groups may give way to hopelessness in the face of the magnitude of the problems involved in surviving in a stagnant economy and political chaos. It is important, therefore, to discover limited changes that can be implemented immediately. For example, women in one group decided to check on sterilization of needles in local dispensaries; taking action was experienced as empowering. Sex workers who proposed condoms to clients found their status rising as people in the know. Female university students used discourse of traditions about pre-marital virginity to resist pressure to have sex. Some married women were able to address condom protection with husbands indirectly, through a discussion of family planning 'for the welfare of the children.' Husbands who agreed knew that their wives were attending an AIDS prevention workshop; they may have thought about AIDS but the talk was about family planning. These wives were careful not to bring up the subject of infidelity; instead, they talked about preventing pregnancy in view of the economic crisis and the hardships involved in educating the children they already had (Schoepf 1993a).[12]

Because many couples and their parents strongly desire children, it is unrealistic to expect them to use condoms on a continuing basis. Some protection is better than none. Thus, couples who believe that one partner might be infected can use condoms 'to space births' until they wish to conceive, and then use them again, following conception. However, many people believe that semen is needed not just once for fertilization, but to form the gestating infant, or 'to grow the pregnancy.' This problem, too, was solved when a nurse in a church Mothers' Club suggested a way to 'reinvent' culture by interpreting this belief metaphorically. What the ancestors really had intended, she said, was to prescribe frequent marital intercourse to provide a loving environment for the developing foetus.

I posed this problem with the President of the Zaïre Traditional Healers' Association. After considerable reflection, he agreed that this had indeed been the case and invited us to hold a workshop with his associates. They raised numerous objections. However, they convened a second workshop and eventually decided that they could advise clients that, actually, semen is a metaphor standing for frequent intercourse (Schoepf 1992a). The healers' collaboration in this reinvention of cosmology, which they could not but know to be a pure fabrication, suggests the possibility of other creative cultural adaptation to crisis.

CULTURE, ETHICS, AND METHODOLOGY

Some Africanists, sensitive to the history of racism that surrounds the subject of sex research in Africa, have intimated that researchers should 'just say NO' to studies of 'the sexual life of natives' (Packard and Epstein 1991). Sex research, however, can produce knowledge for disease prevention and sexual health. The issue is how to study sex in cultures that have been objectified and exploited, and how to use this knowledge.

For more than a quarter of a century, anthropologists debating professional ethics have argued that the sine qua non of ethical practice includes framing research questions within an adequate body of theory and methodology (Stavenhagen 1971; Schoepf 1973, 1991a). In bioethics this proposition is equally pertinent (Jones 1981; Curran 1992). Anthropologists extend their concern beyond individuals to consider the effects of research upon communities. The ethics of science are linked to the political realm. Not only are collection and interpretation of data historically contingent, but the power of knowledge calls forth questions about its use. Often science is 'politics by other means,' and epistemological questions about how we know are joined to the ethical questions of what we should know and what we should do with our knowledge.

To date the research and policy agenda has been determined by biomedicine. Anthropologists researching AIDS in Africa have worked chiefly in biomedical projects or been dependent on health units of development agencies for funding. Even when consulted on prevention, their advice may be ignored as contrary to medical 'wisdom.' Dominance and dependency relations narrow the scientific gaze. Although 'HIV prevention is first and foremost a problem of culture change ... too little attention was focused directly on the task of improving the design of educational efforts' (Bolton and Singer 1992:139–140). The major use made of anthropology in Africa continues to be collection of data on partner numbers, sexual networking, and frequency of intercourse, often by means of questionnaires. While research frequently is justified by the need to provide data for prevention campaigns, this claim seems dubious in seven proposals I reviewed in 1991–92: first, because a great deal already is known to anthropologists about how and why AIDS spreads; second, because in order to stop the epidemic, effective STD treatment, condom access, social support for risk reduction, and broad socio-economic change are needed; third, because informants need to talk about sex, not to researchers, but to one another.

None of these outcomes is likely to result from the reviewed studies, whether these use KAP surveys, sexual networking, diaries, or in-depth interviews. Nor are they likely to result from other research methods designed to capture data on 'who does what to whom, and how often.' Variations in frequency of partner change, styles and timing of intercourse, onset of sexual activity and so on are of particular interest to epidemiologists, demographers, and statisticians engaged in modelling the future course of the epidemic and its probable impacts. While they demonstrate to policy advisors the need for prevention to extend beyond conventional risk categories (Obbo 1993b), this should have been evident from ethnographic accounts and epidemiology. The proposed studies are of limited value for disease prevention. Moreover, if effective prevention takes place, the models will be outdated prior to publication.

The principal aims of large-scale biomedical projects are to study the natural history of HIV/AIDS and search for co-factors in transmission. They create cohorts of individuals of known serostatus useful for vaccine testing. Controlled trials are possible only in a large population cohort that can be followed over time and that is not significantly reducing its risk of infection. Otherwise, the research methodology would be as indefensible as that of the Tuskegee Syphilis Study, which purported to follow the disease in an untreated population of African-American men, despite the 'escape' of some individuals who sought care elsewhere (Jones 1981). As in Tuskegee, there would appear to be a fundamental conflict between research interests and disease prevention, between cohort development and effective support for behaviour change. In Tuskegee, racism served to obscure violations of ethical and methodological cannons. Could these reasons underlie the current 'obtuseness' with respect to effective HIV prevention?

An example from Eastern Uganda shows the tangle of interests involved. In this low-HIV-prevalence area a KAP study showed considerable risk behaviour. Informants highlighted circumcision ceremonies that attract relatives back to the villages, some from high prevalence areas, to honour the boys by dancing. Alcohol and sex are a valued part of the exchange between visitors and hosts. Suggestions were made by outsiders and local evangelical Christians to stop the ceremonies by decree. The district medical officer proposed instead to conduct condom distribution during the circumcision season and requested supplies. Following consultation with groups of local women, I suggested that this be done in conjunction with popular theatre and puppetry to open discussion of STDs and reproductive health issues. I also suggested that interventions at the market bordering a military base receive high priority as a means of protecting women and children. Interest developed in ethnographic action-research that would enable various groups to learn by doing.

An international health consultant visited for a day in the company of the agency director and staff. The expert's report stated that little is known about how to change sexual behaviour. He proposed a prospective sero-survey to determine risk factors for HIV in adolescent women. Although I and other women questioned the ethics of this research and pointed out that methods for change exist, the physician's authority and command of resources, including patronage networks, prevailed. The opportunity to demonstrate how to prevent the epidemic spread of HIV in a low-prevalence, high-risk district was lost.

Informants in Uganda expressed uneasiness over the rush to vaccine trials. The subject has interested me since 1988, when it became clear that Kinshasa was being used as a site for cohort development. Late in 1991, however, Zaïre's military rioted in Kinshasa and other cities; AIDS cohort data were destroyed and the social fabric unravelled. Uganda, with high prevalence and incidence, and with renewed political stability over much of its territory, is a much more favourable location for trials.

Scientific opinion is divided over the question of when to begin testing candidate vaccines, which ones show most promise, and whether it makes sense methodologically to test vaccines for particular strains in areas other than the ones in which they are found. Some researchers believe that testing is premature and that the fundamental biology of HIV should be more thoroughly understood before tests begin on humans. However, with high rewards certain for the first product on the market, methodology is the loser. 'There will be a temptation to design a trial for one year and to declare it a success.... when in fact the protection may disappear a year or two later,' an official of the World Health Organization's Global Program for AIDS (WHO/GPA) (Dr. José Esparza, quoted in Altman 1991:7). He added that since counselling is ineffective, the study methodology will not be endangered by behaviour change among the test subjects.

In 1988 I noted ways that 'culture' has been used in the past to blame African peoples for deficient health policies and lack of resources; that the same appeared to be occurring with respect to HIV prevention. This fear has been confirmed by observers at recent international AIDS conferences. Moreover, approval for vaccine testing is linked explicitly to lack of effective prevention. One reporter found that with rising HIV prevalence, many African and Asian 'health officials have become desperate. Countries that might have resented being guinea pigs in the past are eager to take part in an AIDS vaccine trial.... The trials may not work, [they say], but try anyway ... because there is no other way to stop the spread of AIDS' (Altman 1991:7). Leaders' anxiety is fuelled by unreleased data on seroprevalence in the armed forces of 30 to 70 per cent. The military probably will provide the first test volunteers.

The failure of AIDS education to effect widespread change has been ascribed by many biomedical researchers 'to the idiosyncrasies of African behaviour rather than to the possible inappropriateness of educational programmes and the research on which they are based' (Holmshaw 1991:448). The subtext leads back to culture: 'Those people can't change'; failure to provide funds for action-research has acted as a self-fulfilling prophecy. Whether AIDS policy-makers' obtuseness is intended or not, biomedical dominance and interests appear to have combined with the dependence of the anthropologists in their employ to retard prevention.[13]

CONCLUSION

Serving as a reminder that health and disease are social phenomena, the HIV/AIDS pandemic directs attention to relationships between things that frequently are depicted as mutually exclusive: rural and urban dynamics; macro- and micro-societal levels; formal and informal economic sectors; social structure and human agency; science and moral philosophy. It situates poverty, gender relations, and class at the centre of analysis.

thnographic research reveals numerous strong cultural constraints to prevention. It also provides examples of dynamic responses to crises and offers cultural materials useful to overcome obstacles to prevention. HIV/AIDS prevention requires dialogue on emotionally charged and culturally laden issues of sex and gender, and change in the wider societal contexts that shape these relations.

Once culture is viewed as offering possibilities for change, new vistas open. Popular knowledge and local social organization can be used to empower new value consensus in support of risk reduction. Useful in slowing the spread of AIDS, action-research also can serve to create critical understanding of persistent inequalities that hinder sustainable development. Anthropology has a double interest in participatory research. The first interest is ethical: to do no further harm to individuals and communities at risk; the second is instrumental: a quest for new knowledge.

Used together, performative ethnography and empowerment training constitute powerful tools for understanding and transforming the social relations and psychological dynamics that shape sexual behaviour. Researchers who facilitate performances and dialogue using participatory methods can collaborate in gathering data about sex as part of the intervention. This type of sex research is potentially more useful and less alienating than traditional methods, which, at this stage, are unlikely to contribute significant new knowledge essential to prevention.

Biomedical dominance of policy and resource allocation has deprived anthropology of an autonomous, creative role in AIDS research in many countries. Inadequate epistemology, concepts, and methods have resulted in ineffective prevention strategies, and have retarded progress in slowing the epidemic. Lack of behaviour change is invoked to justify the rush to vaccine trials. I argue that empowering forms of performative ethnography are an ethical way to conduct sex research in other cultures in 'the time of AIDS.'

ACKNOWLEDGEMENTS

Some issues were discussed with the Hon. Prof. Payanzo Ntsomo, Claude Schoepf, Dr. Rukarangira wa Nkera, Abbé Latchung Amen and Walu Engundu, of CONNAISSIDA/Zaïre; with Drs. Christine Obbo and Maryinez Lyons. While gratefully acknowledging these dialogues, I am solely responsible for this article.

NOTES

1. Based on fieldwork carried out in Zaïre with the CONNAISSIDA Project in 1985–1990, two-month visits to Tanzania (1991) and Uganda (1992), and upon responses of African and Africanist social scientists, health professionals, and laypeople to the work of CONNAISSIDA.

2. In 1985, organizers of CONNAISSIDA, a collaborative, trans-disciplinary medical anthropology project in Zaïre, set out to use culture and group dynamics to adapt community-based empowerment methods to HIV prevention and provide scenarios for mass media communications (Schoepf et al. 1986; Schoepf 1986). These documents were sent to numerous health and development agencies and research foundations. Experiential knowledge of social and sexual networking in various social milieux led us to propose the project when we learned of the presence of heterosexual transmission in Zaïre. Since Zaïre shares borders and cultures with nine other countries, we expected that many of the findings would be pertinent to societies throughout the region.

Moreover, while Central African cultures and belief systems are distinctive, they are hardly so exotic as to make the obstacles they pose to prevention unique to this area (Schoepf 1991a).

Constructed from the French word *connaissance*, or knowledge, and *SIDA*, the acronym for AIDS, the project's name has a double signification. CONNAISSIDA means knowledge of AIDS (a passive form), but it also means knowing, or getting to know about AIDS, an active learning/teaching process that engaged researchers and informants. The project developed a broad understanding of the spread of HIV infection and ways that AIDS was perceived and reacted to by the population. Action-research, devised in the 1940s by social psychologists, uses small group dynamics and active, participatory learning to stimulate individual and social change. We adapted the method to develop culturally appropriate ways to facilitate talking about sex and supporting prevention (Schoepf et al. 1991; Schoepf 1993b, forthcoming).

3. Falmouth, Massachusetts, where I live, is a case in point.

4. Critique and citations in Schoepf 1991a, 1991c.

5. A Ugandan woman said, 'The missionaries taught us that respectable women should not sing (utter sounds during sex), so now our husbands go to other women who do!' (Fieldnotes, March 1992).

6. This is the region in which Dr. Rukarangira grew up, and where he, Claude Schoepf and I did fieldwork.

7. Professor Buakasa Tula wrote in this vein in a 1985 brochure to which I have lost the reference. As in the US, both women and youth are the targets of control.

8. A similar situation obtains among many adolescents in the US.

9. A recent article on the subject by Caldwell et al. (1992) omits racism and male dominance as major contributing factors, and quotes selectively from my 1988 article to support the inevitability of 'tradition.'

10. A fable reported from the 1930s used the metaphor of sex between a European and his dog to comment on relations between colonizers and colonized (André Yav in Fabian 1990a:117–119).

11. CONNAISSIDA adapted the method to encourage risk assessment, decision-making, and risk reduction in a variety of community and workplace groups. First reported in 1988 (Schoepf and Rukarangira 1988; Schoepf 1993b), the experiments show how people can be empowered to understand the risks that AIDS poses to their lives, to their families and to cultural survival. Once they adopt the problem as their own, and examine possible solutions, people can decide how to respond.

12. When I drew this as a cartoon with explicit 'suspicion awareness' to illustrate the Draft Strategy for UNICEF in Tanzania, women secretaries in Dar-es-Salaam made photocopies to use to open dialogue with husbands.

13. Given persistent inequalities, it is a flagrant violation of human rights to bypass international and US ethical guidelines for individual informed consent by potential research 'subjects.' Family, community and national leaders are generally elder males; there is ample literature documenting how the interests of leaders frequently conflict with those of their dependents. Academic debates about the constitution of African personhood, about the strength of cultural persistence and change, or rural-urban linkages must not be allowed to obfuscate the basic issue as proponents of ethical relativity have attempted to do (recently, Christakis and Fox 1992). Moreover, consent can only be 'informed' if adequate methods are used to educate individuals, communities and national leaders about potential risks, probable (not merely possible) benefits, and alternatives to vaccine testing.

With this background, I have found myself saying 'No' to research proposals to study sex using only traditional methods. One review board requested another opinion, which came back with an even stronger critique than mine. Has this whistle-blowing resulted in change? Recent abstracts from one of the projects state that findings will contribute to the design of 'participatory community-based prevention.' Their staff has no experience in this, nor have they sought training. Another researcher proposes to use anthropology to design ethical vaccine trials. Without broad use of effective methods to reduce sexual risk, the phrase 'ethical trials' is an oxymoron, a contradiction in terms. Anthropological associations are better-placed to serve as effective 'watchdogs' than are individuals.

REFERENCES

Aggleton, P., C. Horsley, I. Warwick, and T. Wilton. 1990. AIDS: *Working with Young People*. Horsham, UK: AVERT.

Ahlberg, B.M. 1991. *Women, Sexuality and the Changing Social Order: The Impact of Government Policies on Reproductive Behaviour in Kenya*. Philadelphia: Gordon and Breach.

Altman, L.K. 1991. AIDS Vaccine to Be Tested on Humans. *New York Times*, 11 November.

Bassett, M.T., and M. Mhloyi. 1991. Women and AIDS in Zimbabwe: The Making of an Epidemic. *International Journal of Health Services* 21:143–156.

Bolton, R., and M. Singer. 1992. Introduction. Rethinking HIV Prevention: Critical Assessments of the Content and Delivery of AIDS Risk Reduction Messages. *Medical Anthropology* 14:139–143.

Bone, G., G. Gordon, P. Gordon, and E. Lynch. 1991. *Unmasking AIDS: A Different Approach to HIV Education*. London: International Planned Parenthood Federation.

Bruyn, M. de. 1992. Women and AIDS in Developing Countries. *Social Science and Medicine* 34(3):249–262.

Caldwell, J.C., I.O. Orubuloye, and P. Caldwell. 1992. Underreaction to AIDS in Sub-Saharan Africa. *Social Science and Medicine* 34(11):1169–1182.

Christakis, N.A., and R.C. Fox. 1992. Informed Consent in Africa. *New England Journal of Medicine* 327(15):1101–1102.

Corin, E. 1979. A Possession Psychotherapy in an Urban Setting: Zebola in Kinshasa. *Social Science and Medicine* 13B(4):327–338.

Curran, W. 1992. Scientific Ethics and Integrity. Paper presented at a Round Table on 'Professional Codes and Ethical Principles in the Sciences.' Marine Biological Laboratory, Woods Hole, MA, 1 July.

Douglas, M. 1966. *Purity and Danger: An Analysis of the Concepts of Pollution and Taboo.* London: Routledge and Kegan Paul.

Fabian, J. 1990a. *History from Below: The 'Vocabulary of Elizabethville' by André Yav.* Amsterdam: John Benjamins.

Fabian, J. 1990b. *Power and Performance: Ethnographic Explorations Through Proverbial Wisdom and Theatre in Shaba, Zaïre.* Madison: University of Wisconsin Press.

Freire, P. 1972. *Pedagogy of the Oppressed.* London: Sheed and Ward.

Freire, P. 1976. *Education, the Practice of Freedom.* London: Writers and Reading Cooperative.

Gordon, G., and T. Klouda. 1989. *Preventing a Crisis: AIDS and Family Planning Work.* London: International Planned Parenthood Federation.

Holmshaw, M. 1991. Editorial Comment on Papers of Outstanding Interest. *Current AIDS Literature* 4(12):488–489.

Hope, A., S. Timmel, and P. Hodzi. 1984. *Training for Transformation: A Handbook for Community Workers.* Gweru, Zimbabwe: Mambo Press.

Janzen, J.M. 1978. *The Quest for Therapy in Lower Zaïre.* Berkeley: University of California Press.

Jones, J.H. 1981. *Bad Blood: The Tuskegee Syphilis Experiment.* New York: Free Press.

Kisekka, Mere N. 1990. AIDS in Uganda as a Gender Issue. *Women and Therapy* 10(3):35–53.

Lindenbaum, S. 1991. Anthropology Rediscovers Sex. Introduction. *Social Science and Medicine* 33(8):865–866.

Lynch, E., and G. Gordon. 1991. *Activities to Explore: Using Drama in AIDS and Family Planning Work.* London: International Planned Parenthood Federation.

Newbury, C., and B.G. Schoepf. 1989. State, Peasantry and Agrarian Crisis in Zaïre: Does Gender Make a Difference? In: *Women and the State in Africa,* edited by J.L. Parpart and K.A. Staudt. Boulder, CO: Lynne Reinner.

Obbo, C. 1993a. HIV Transmission: Men Are the Solution. *Population and Environment* 14(3):211–243.

Obbo, C. 1993b. HIV Transmission Through Social and Geographical Networks in Uganda. *Social Science and Medicine* 36(7):949–955.

Packard, R.M., and P. Epstein. 1991. Epidemiologists, Social Scientists, and the Structure of Medical Research on AIDS in Africa. *Social Science and Medicine* 33(7):771–783, 793–794.

Pellow, D. 1990. Sexuality in Africa. *Trends in History* 4(4):71–96.

Quinn, T.C., J. Mann, J. Curran, and P. Piot. 1986. AIDS in Africa: An Epidemiologic Paradigm. *Science* 234(21 November):955–963.

Richards, A. 1956. *Chisungu: A Girls' Initiation Ceremony Among the Bemba of Northern Rhodesia.* London: Oxford University Press.

Rukarangira, wa Nkera, and B.G. Schoepf. 1989. Social Marketing of Condoms in Zaïre. *AIDS Health Promotion Exchange* (3):2–4.

Rukarangira, wa Nkera, and B.G. Schoepf. 1991. Unrecorded Trade in Shaba and Across Zaïre's Southern Borders. In: *The Real Economy of Zaïre*, edited by J. MacGaffey. London: James Currey; Philadelphia: University of Pennsylvania Press.

Schoepf, B.G. 1973. Ethics and the Politics of Anthropology. *Human Organization* 33(1):103–107.

Schoepf, B.G. 1978. Women in the Informal Economy of Lubumbashi: The Case of the *Ndumba*. Paper prepared for International Congress of Anthropological and Ethnological Sciences, Delhi, India, December. French version presented at IV International Congress of African Studies, Kinshasa, December.

Schoepf, B.G. 1980. Women and Development: Overcoming the Colonial Legacy in Africa. Background paper for the Women's Mid-Decade Conference NGO Forum, Copenhagen, July. Excerpt, 'Working for Change Through Projects.' In: *The Exchange Report: Women in the Third World*, edited by J. Kneering, and J. Shur. New York: The Exchange of Development Resources.

Schoepf, B.G. 1981. Women and Class Formation in Zaïre: The Informal Economy of Lubumbashi. Paper presented at the annual meeting of the US African Studies Association, Bloomington, IN, 25 October.

Schoepf, B.G. 1983. Health for Rural Women. *Community Action* (Zimbabwe) 1:26–27.

Schoepf, B.G. 1986. CONNAISSIDA: AIDS Control Research and Interventions in Zaïre. Proposal submitted to The Rockefeller Foundation. 12 November.

Schoepf, B.G. 1988. Women, AIDS and economic crisis in Zaïre. *Canadian Journal of African Studies* 22(3):625–644.

Schoepf, B.G. 1990a. AIDS in Eriaz. *Anthropology Today* 6 (3):13–14.

Schoepf, B.G. 1990b. Face au SIDA: Une situation nouvelle pour la jeunesse Africaine. Paper prepared for Colloque sur La Jeunesse en Afrique, Université Paris VII, 6–8 December.

Schoepf, B.G. 1991a. Ethical, Methodological and Political Issues of AIDS Research in Central Africa. *Social Science and Medicine* 33(7):749–763.

Schoepf, B.G. 1991b. Représentations du SIDA et pratiques populaires à Kinshasa. *Anthropologie et Sociétés* 15(2–3):149–166.

Schoepf, B.G. 1991c. Understanding AIDS in Africa: Political Economy and Culture in Zaïre. Cultural Studies Program (MIT). Working Paper 6.

Schoepf, B.G. 1992a. AIDS, sex and condoms: African healers and the reinvention of tradition in Zaïre. *Medical Anthropology* 14:225–242.

Schoepf, B.G. 1992b. Gender Relations and Development: Political Economy and Culture. In: *Twenty-First Century Africa: Towards a New Vision of Self-Sustainable Development*, edited by A. Seidman and F. Anang. Trenton, NJ: Africa World Press.

Schoepf, B.G. 1992c. Sex, Gender and Society in Zaïre. In: *Sexual Behaviour and Networking: Anthropological and Sociocultural Studies for the Transmission of HIV*, edited by T. Dyson. Liège: Editions Derouaux-Ordina.

Schoepf, B.G. 1992d. Women at Risk: Case Studies from Zaïre. In: *The Time of AIDS: Social Analysis, Theory and Method*, edited by G. Herdt and S. Lindenbaum. Newbury Park, CA: Sage Publications.

Schoepf, B.G. 1993a. AIDS action-research with women in Kinshasa. *Social Science and Medicine* 37(11):1401–1413.

Schoepf, B.G. 1993b. Gender, Development, and AIDS: A Political Economy and Culture Framework. In: *Women and International Development Annual* Vol. 3, edited by R. Gallin, A. Ferguson, and J. Harper. Boulder, CO: Westview Press.

Schoepf, B.G. 1993c. Political Economy, Sex and Cultural Logics: A View from Zaïre. *African Urban Quarterly* 5 (1–2), Special Issue on AIDS, STDs and Urbanization in Africa, 6 (1–2):94–106.

Schoepf, B.G. Talking AIDS and Sexual Health in Africa: An Exercise Manual. London: International Planned Parenthood Federation. Forthcoming.

Schoepf, B.G., Ntsomo Payanzo, wa Nkera Rukarangira, Engundu Walu, and C. Schoepf. 1988. AIDS, Women and Society in Central Africa. In: *AIDS, 1988: AAAS Symposium Papers*, edited by R. Kulstad. Washington, DC: American Association for the Advancement of Science.

Schoepf, B.G., and wa N. Rukarangira. 1988. Community-based risk reduction support in Zaïre. Paper presented at 1st SIECS, Ixtapa, Mexico, October.

Schoepf, B.G., wa Nkera Rukarangira and Mahoya Matumona. 1986. Etudes des réactions à une nouvelle maladie transmissible (SIDA) et d'un programme d'education populaire. Proposal submitted to Government of Zaïre, WHO, USAID, IDRC, others.

Schoepf, B.G., wa Nkera Rukarangira, C. Schoepf, Ntsomo Payanzo, and Engundu Walu. 1988b. AIDS and Society in Central Africa: A View from

Zaïre. In: *AIDS in Africa: Social and Policy Impact*, edited by N. Miller and R. Rockwell. Lewiston, NY: Mellen Press.

Schoepf, B.G., and Engundu Walu. 1991. Women's Trade and Contributions to Household Budgets in Kinshasa. In: *The Real Economy in Zaïre*, edited by J. MacGaffey. London: James Currey.

Schoepf, B.G., Engundu Walu, wa Nkera Rukarangira, Ntsomo Payanzo, and C. Schoepf. 1991. Gender, Power and Risk of AIDS in Central Africa. In: *Women and Health in Africa*. edited by M. Turshen. Trenton, NJ: Africa World Press.

Schoepf, B.G., Engundu Walu, D. Russell, and C. Schoepf. 1991. Women and Structural Adjustment in Zaïre. In: *Structural Adjustment and African Women Farmers*, edited by C. Gladwin. Gainesville: University of Florida Press.

Seidel, G. 1993. The Competing Discourses of HIV/AIDS in Sub-Saharan Africa: Discources of Rights and Empowerment vs. Discourses of Control and Exclusion. *Social Science and Medecine* 36(3):175–194.

Society for Women and AIDS in Africa (SWAA). 1989. Report of the 1st International Workshop on Women and AIDS in Africa, Harare, 10–12 May.

Stavenhagen, R. 1971. Decolonizing the Applied Social Sciences. *Human Organization* 30:333–357.

Taylor, C.C. 1992. *Milk, Honey and Money: Changing Concepts in Rwandan Healing*. Washington, DC: Smithsonian.

Vaughan, M. 1991. Syphilis, AIDS and the Representation of Sexuality: The Historical Legacy. In: *Action on AIDS in Southern Africa*, edited by Z. Stein and A. Zwi. New York: Committee for Health in South Africa (CHISA).

Walu, Engundu. 1991. Women's survival strategies in Kinshasa. MA thesis, Institute for Social Studies, The Hague.

Walu, Egundu. 1992. Women's response to AIDS in Kinshasa Zaïre. Paper presented at the conference 'Culture, Sexual Behavior and AIDS,' Amsterdam, 22–24 July 1992.

Yates, B. 1982. Colonialism, Education and Work: Sex Differentiation in Colonial Zaïre. In: *Women and Work in Africa*, edited by E.G. Bay. Boulder, CO: Westview Press.

Chapter THREE

Vulnerability to HIV Infection Among Three Hilltribes in Northern Thailand

Cornelia Ann Kammerer,
Otome Klein Hutheesing,
Ralana Maneeprasert, and
Patricia V. Symonds

Contributions to a recent issue of the journal *Anthropologie et sociétés* on AIDS clearly illustrate the variety of analytical angles adopted in social scientific discourse on the disease. With a slant towards African case studies, the emphasis centres on representations of AIDS (acquired immunodeficiency syndrome), stigmatizations, and values regarding sexuality. A central research question raised — and one which demands a nuanced analysis — is the transformation of the socio-economic and ethnic composition of those affected (Bibeau and Murbach 1991:5).

In Thailand, a country stereotyped as the 'epicentre' of Asia's exploding epidemic, investigative reports have largely emphasized two topics: the alarming statistics on HIV-seropositivity, and sexual behaviour related to prostitution. They have seldom touched on interethnic relations within the country or across its borders, nor have the sexual cultures of the people living at the nation's territorial fringes been adequately studied. Indeed, perhaps because of the enduring power of the myth of the isolated primitive, the vulnerability of tribal peoples — indigenous, small-scale, or Fourth World societies — to AIDS has been largely ignored around the globe. Yet given what Lindenbaum (1992:324) has labeled the 'undemocratic nature of the AIDS epidemic,' members of tribal minorities join members of other subdominant, marginalized, and stigmatized social groups worldwide in being particularly at risk. An enquiry into the ways the mountain tribes of the northern Thai periphery are being exposed to the threat of HIV would contribute to mapping the ethnic and class structuring of Thailand's epidemic and provide insight into strategies for effective prevention. Such a study would situate minority-majority relations within an exploitative political economy (Anan 1987). It might also provide a model for similar studies aimed at prevention of HIV transmission among indigenous peoples in other regions.[1]

While political and economic factors contribute to a better understanding of the causes underlying tribal vulnerability to the deadly virus, from the point of view of prevention, it is also important to consider the cultures of the tribal groups themselves (Kammerer and Symonds 1992). It is here that an anthropological eye can provide additional insights into such issues as sexual vocabularies, gendered power relations, 'talkability' and taboos concerning sexuality, and conceptions of disease and contagion.[2]

An introduction to Thailand's hilltribes and an overview of the nation's HIV/AIDS epidemic precede a discussion of the political economy of tribal vulnerability to HIV infection. The next section focuses on traditional sexuality and the changes wrought by recent politico-economic transformations. Finally, the conclusion contains prospective remarks about holistic anthropological work to facilitate culturally informed AIDS prevention.

HILLTRIBES IN THAILAND

The mountains of northern Thailand are home to numerous tribal minorities whose languages and cultures differ not only one from another but also from their lowland Thai neighbours. Totaling 562,139 persons, according to censuses conducted from 1986–89 by the government's Tribal Research Institute (1990), these minorities constitute some one per cent of the national population. The best known, as well as the focus of most governmental and non-governmental development programmes, are the so-called 'six tribes': Karen (279,183), Hmong or Meo (83,969), Lahu (61,128), Mien or Yao (35,652), Akha (32,758), and Lisu (25,251).[3]

While Karen may well have pre-dated Thai in the territory that is now the state of Thailand, the five other groups began to arrive in the area from the mid to late nineteenth century. Today, members of each group are also represented in nearby countries: Karen live in adjacent Burma (Myanmar), while Hmong, Lahu, Mien, Akha, and Lisu live in China as well as Burma, Laos, and Vietnam. Wherever they reside, these six tribes are minority groups, yet both within individual countries and overall their populations are substantial. For example, there are more than five million Hmong and perhaps 500,000 Akha in Southwest China and mainland Southeast Asia.

For centuries, tribal peoples in this region have depended on a combination of gathering, hunting, fishing, and agriculture. Although some mountain farmers plant irrigated fields, many rely on slash-and-burn (swidden) agriculture. They cultivate both subsistence crops, such as rice and maize, and cash crops, including the infamous opium poppy. Tribal oral traditions, which mention valley markets and trade in salt and iron, confirm that highland and lowland peoples have been in contact for centuries, even millennia (Alting von Geusau 1983). Yet contacts have increased and transformed drastically during this century with the creation of modern states with fixed borders.

HIV/AIDS IN THAILAND

Asia and Oceania could have the 'largest proportion of HIV infections by the year 2000' (Mann et al. 1992:4), despite the fact that full-blown AIDS hit the region later than the Americas, Europe, or Africa. Thailand's first recorded AIDS case, in 1984, was a Thai homosexual man who had lived abroad. Most of the ten known cases in 1988 were gay men, who were thought to have gotten the virus from foreigners; next an explosive growth in seropositivity was noted among intravenous drug users, with more than 40 per cent of clients at drug detoxification centres in Bangkok testing HIV-positive in 1988 (Muecke 1990). People remained complacent because they blamed others, in this case Westerners, and because they mistakenly believed that the epidemic was confined to the risk groups of homosexuals and intravenous drug users. Meanwhile, the epidemic spread via heterosexual intercourse, which now seems to be the major route of transmission nationwide.

Contributing to the speed of heterosexual transmission is Thailand's huge commercial sex industry. Although the industry expanded during the Vietnam War to service US servicemen, it pre-existed the war and continued after its end. Prostitution in Thailand dates back at least to the fifteenth century; nowadays many foreign tourists travel to Thailand on sex tours, but most clients are Thai. Indeed, having sex with prostitutes is a part of male Thai culture that crosscuts social class. By some estimates, four per cent of the women in Thailand — one million — are in the industry, in which they vastly outnumber male prostitutes. The commercial sex industry, while technically illegal, is an integral part of Thailand's economy, an economy which provides few employment alternatives to women.

The northern region, where most tribal people live, is particularly hard hit by HIV/AIDS (Weniger et al. 1991:S73–S77). According to the government's Sentinel Survey, which since 1989 has tracked seropositivity in selected groups, 1.9 per cent of patients at prenatal clinics in Chiang Mai Province tested HIV-positive in June 1990, while 4.9 per cent tested positive in June 1992. Similarly, 40 per cent of drug users tested in the province in June 1990 were positive, while 56 per cent were positive in June 1992. By that time, 37.3 per cent of direct prostitutes in the northern region tested HIV-positive, the highest percentage in the nation (Royal Thai Government 1992). No statistical data are available on the prevalence of HIV infection among tribal minorities. Yet, given that tribal people have never been isolated from their valley neighbours, there is no doubt that they are affected by Thailand's AIDS epidemic. In fact, a tribal infant infected perinatally was among the nation's first twenty-five reported AIDS deaths, and as of mid-1992 there were an estimated 100 cumulative AIDS cases among mountain minorities (Vichai Poshyachinda, personal communications).

UP AND DOWN THE POLITICAL AND ECONOMIC TRACKS OF AIDS

Hilltribe vulnerability to HIV is, in large measure, generated by state and capitalist penetration of the periphery by the centre. Transformations in the traditional agricultural and trading patterns of these minority people have led to a greater involvement with lowland lifeways and values. For hilltribe societies this confrontation between upland and lowland cultures has led to a breakdown in their material base and in their customary codes, including those regarding sexuality. The commercialization of cash crops and of sex has been caused, in part, by opium eradication policies emanating from the valley authorities.

The intricate intertwining of tribal economies with world and national markets necessitates a closer look at the migratory routes of goods and people, which at present contrast sharply with earlier movements across mountain trails. Roads cut through the hills since the 1950s carry military vehicles, logging trucks, vans for tourists, and pick-ups transporting people and produce from hill farms to valley towns. Underlying the spread of HIV among highlanders is the complex interrelationship between old and new cash crops, the eradication of poppy cultivation, poverty — both inadequate subsistence and a felt lack of desired consumer goods — and tourism, including sex tourism. This set of variables is caught up in an 'illicit economy' in which, among other things, the opium trade has been complicated by heroin trafficking (Klein Hutheesing 1992) and illegal migrants from Bangladesh who work the fields of Hmong farmers (Kunstadter and Kunstadter 1992:42).

The term 'illicit economy' helps to describe the economic activities of tribal societies enmeshed in the process of modern development. In the case of Thailand, it highlights the trading of heroin and of women and the practices of unlicensed injection doctors (Vichai Poshyachinda, personal communication). The concept could, however, be elaborated upon by placing it in an historical perspective which would demonstrate that border societies have always engaged in illegal enterprises like smuggling and cattle theft. It could be further elaborated to draw attention to the conflict between local legal systems of hilltribe societies and the legal codes of the states in which they now live. The illicit economy of modern states, on the other hand, involves the political manipulation of capital, labour, and nationality: officials might help entrepreneurs set up plantations on hill land that technically belongs to the Crown, benefit from illegal logging by lowland capitalists, or take bribes to issue national identity cards to tribal individuals.

During this century, ethnic minorities like Lisu, Akha, and Hmong in Thailand's northern provinces have been engaged in a cash crop economy besides being subsistence agriculturalists. Until recently, the livelihood of these fringe communities was obtained within a relatively closed economy in which goods, whether forest products, peppers, or opium, were traded in a localized setting by people who were often acquaintances and who knew the words in the other's language required for economic transactions. Contact with urban markets was limited, and transport was restricted to humans and pack animals traversing mountain tracks. Even the Lisu and Hmong farmers whose opium entered the international market traded in a vernacular context, where this commodity was either sold or exchanged for the labour of other tribal groups such as Akha and Karen.

Since the 1950s, integrationist policies from the centre, with their focus on security and development, and the introduction of mono-crop agriculture — often justified by the need to reform swidden farmers — and its attendant costly technological inputs have changed the structural relationship between hill-dwellers and valley-dwellers.[4] Government-supported programmes to replace opium poppies with other cash crops and the introduction of capitalist plantations have brought mono-crop agriculture to the hills. But it must be remembered that populations at the edge of Thai society have never been completely self-sufficient within a static environment; interdependence with other minorities and with lowland middlemen has long been maintained. Yet not only have degrees of dependency generally increased over time, but degrees of dependency in contemporary Thailand also vary across ethnic minorities as well as within a single group. For instance, a nearby tin mine links one Hmong village to the lowlands via itinerant Thai miners who come to smoke opium, while another village with its own pick-up truck has greater cultural independence from the town (Radley 1986:134, 211).

The basic change might be characterized as from a 'mini' to a 'macho' trading pattern (Klein Hutheesing 1990:166–168). Whereas both men and women engaged in the older form of localized 'mini-trading', trade outside the village is now largely becoming the monopoly of men. Thus as the mountain minorities have become increasingly hooked into the national and global economies, men have gained greater control. Farming systems geared towards production for larger markets have gone hand in hand with the opening of roads and inroads into highland cultures as their land, their men, and, to a larger extent, their women have been exploited. Tribal people have been drawn into a cash market in which sex for money has driven young women to seek employment in bustling urban areas as prostitutes and men to visit brothels in lowland towns and cities. The establishment of a coffee plantation in a Lisu village has led young women to sell sexual favours to the managers who have moved up from the valley. On a more subtle level, the tourist trekking enterprises have added the attraction of puffs of opium and the advertised eroticism of young, unspoiled tribal women (Kammerer and Symonds 1992:24).

Greater dependence on modern cash crops has increased indebtedness and poverty. The situation has been exacerbated by the decrease in acreage available to Thailand's tribal farmers, whether for subsistence production or cash cropping. Land previously used by mountain minorities has been annexed for roads, logging, government-sponsored reforestation, agricultural demonstration projects, plantations, and tourist bungalows. Meanwhile landless lowland peasants have moved up into the hills and immigrants have fled from war-torn Burma into Thailand's northern mountains (Chupinit 1988; Mirante 1988). Technically most hill land is property of the State (Sophon 1978:45–46), yet, in another example of the illicit economy, hill land is bought and sold, accelerating capitalist penetration as impoverished highlanders alienate their fields and house sites to entrepreneurs and speculators.

This breakdown in the material base of hill societies increases hilltribe vulnerability to HIV infection. Young people migrate to valley towns to work not only as prostitutes but as maids, waiters, and labourers on construction sites. There is a growing pattern of seasonal urban migration to earn wages to supplement inadequate highland incomes. For example, more than twenty young men and women from one Akha community went, often at their parents' behest, to find jobs in northern cities during the slack agricultural months of December and January of 1992–93. Again, we encounter the illicit economy, since many of these migrants lack identity papers, which by the government's own admission have been issued slowly to legal hilltribe residents of Thailand (McKinnon and Wanat 1983:xii). Moreover, the commercial sex industry, into which women are often sold or kidnapped, is illegal. Today, younger and younger women are sought by brokers in distant highland villages to meet the demand for 'AIDS-free' prostitutes (Kammerer and Symonds 1992:25; Mirante 1992:20).

In an ironic twist of events, the government's prohibition on planting poppies has resulted in grinding poverty for hilltribe families (Cooper 1984; Klein Hutheesing 1990). This poverty in turn contributes to vulnerability to HIV infection among tribal minorities. Whereas formerly among producers, such as Hmong and Lisu, the poppy harvest provided a secure livelihood without associated high levels of addiction, recent disturbances in both the traditional cash economy and social mores, including those that circumscribed opium use, have led to growing rates of addiction not only to opium but also to heroin. For instance, ten years ago in one Lisu village in Chiang Rai Province there were seven elderly opium addicts, but in 1992 there were twenty-one heroin smokers in addition to the elderly opium addicts. That same year in a nearby Akha village heroin addicts included not only smokers but also shooters. A similar situation is found in some Hmong villages, where children as young as ten use heroin (*Bangkok Post* 1991).

Increases in drug use due to economic and cultural disruption, first noted by researchers in the 1970s, have been characterized as a 'symptom of demoralization' (Hanks and Hanks 1978:21). Some tribal individuals have even pushed the drug habit on their own people (Klein Hutheesing 1992). Among Akha women, the wish to avoid marriage with an addict or future addict has been a catalyst for high levels of urban migration and with it increased risk of HIV infection (Kammerer forthcoming). Thus, it is clear that tribal vulnerability to HIV must be placed within the macro context — national, regional, and global — of changed commercial routes, the entry of urban-based governments and entrepreneurs into the hills, and the migration of the hill people into urban centres, as well as the political and economic chaos in neighbouring Burma which helps to foster the thriving illicit economy.

SEXUALITY IN HILLTRIBE CULTURES: SHAME, NAME, AND BLAME

In this section we explore hilltribe sexuality both in its traditional manifestations and in the transformations precipitated by recent state and capitalist intervention into Thailand's northern periphery. We do so by focusing on the 'outside' from three interrelated perspectives: (1) outside custom, sexual norms and practices that are contrary to or not recognized by tradition; (2) outside territory, which has both political and cosmological dimensions; and (3) outside ethnic groups, both lowlanders and other hilltribes. We interweave this focus on the outside with a focus on three complex and intersecting themes indicated by the terms 'shame', 'name', and 'blame'. Shame is a core value in many hilltribe cultures, Hmong, Akha, and Lisu included. It is central to the structuring of society, since it is implicated in relations among various types of kin, elder and younger, male and female.[5] In a synoptic fashion, the term 'name' communicates the whole issue of ethnic group, subgroup, and kinship identities. Together with the outside, particularly from our second and third perspectives, it points to the importance of intergroup relations, whether between communities or individuals, and of ethnic self-images, stereotypes, and prejudices in the construction of sexuality. This all, of course, intersects with blame, which, sadly, seems everywhere to enter into local conceptions of HIV/AIDS. In this, as we shall see, northern Thailand is no exception.

Sex in the traditional context of hill cultures was valued as leading to procreation, and women figured in this scene as precious resources. But just as economic dependency varies over time and both between and within ethnic groups, as we saw in the previous section, so the value of women varies along these same axes. To give an example of cross-cultural differences, among Akha and Hmong, whose kinship is strongly patrilineal, a heavier emphasis is placed on women as mothers of sons to perpetuate the male line than among Lisu, whose patrilineal bias is less intense. Among groups like Hmong, Akha, and Lisu, whose religions stress fertility in females and in fields, there exist strong cultural currents that will hinder the adoption of safer sex practices to prevent HIV's spread. Cultural resistance to condoms will no doubt be found among Akha, with their elaborate ancestral cult, since neither a man nor a woman without a son can become an ancestor (Kammerer 1988b). Similarly, condoms among Hmong will be seen as preventing the birth of the child that seals the marital union (Symonds 1991:135). Effective AIDS prevention among Thailand's hilltribes may well require the development of indigenous cultural arguments to motivate people to avoid HIV infection as a way to ensure continued reproduction and thereby generational continuity.[6]

In the days before the opening up of the mountainous areas to resident representatives of lowland government and businesses and to itinerant sex traders and tourists, premarital, marital, and extramarital sex were practised within a village context. This, of course, is not to say that there were no interethnic liaisons or unions in the past; these have, however, increased in recent decades. Among Lisu premarital sexual intercourse is labelled 'outside custom' and liable to anger the spirits. The forest, as the outside or wild space, is where illegal children or bush babies are conceived. Village gossip terms a loose girl lewd or bold. If she becomes pregnant, the 'outside child' is cared for and accepted by her natal family, even if no marriage takes place. At times a wedding ceremony is held at once, though the bridewealth might not be collected until after several children are born. What is shameful for Lisu is not that children are created outside marriage but that the bridewealth is not paid in due course. Akha have a similar category of 'outside child,' but, unlike among Lisu, a child conceived outside of wedlock — which for Akha means outside the father's house — cannot be born to an unmarried woman. If the child's progenitor will not marry her, before the child's birth she must marry another man, perhaps one whose senior wife is childless. In this way, an 'outside child' is born 'inside,' that is, within the father's house and beneath its protective ancestor altar. Hmong, Akha, and Lisu all have indigenous legal codes for handling cases of adulterers caught in their transgression. For example, among Lisu an adulterous man has to expiate his 'wrongdoing' by placing a large offering at the shrine of the senior village guardian spirit.

Public courting is part of the New Year celebrations of tribal minorities. Among Hmong, in the ball toss game between young men and women in lines opposite one another, the receiver intentionally drops the ball to indicate attraction to the thrower. And Lisu youth bedecked in festival finery dancing at New Year are admired by members of the opposite sex. Akha are renowned in popular publications for their courting ground — or 'embracing ground' in Thai — where young couples can be seen with their arms entwined, but, contrary to tour guides and tourist guidebooks, the 'level area,' as it is called in Akha, is not a place for wild and free sex. As Bolton (1992:11) observes, 'hypersexuality is often alleged for minorities and "others" of all kinds.' An additional factor in the Thai eroticization of the hilltribe 'other' may be a misreading of an embrace based on different cultural norms of public physical contact between members of the opposite sex. Whatever the reasons, tribal women, thought of by Thai as lusty lasses, are exploited for their supposed exotic and erotic qualities. It should be noted that majorities do not have a monopoly on seeing the 'other' as sexier or more highly sexed. White Hmong men, for instance, view Green Hmong women as good for a liaison, while they view women of their own subgroup as good for marriage, thereby dividing sex for enjoyment from sex for reproduction. And Lisu young men joke about the sexiness of neighbouring Lahu women and consider Thai women to be more pleasurable sexual partners than Lisu women (Niwat Tami, personal communication).

Among Thailand's tribal minorities the customary 'do's' and 'don'ts' of sexuality are intricately linked to concepts of shame. Complex codes exist concerning who can speak to whom about such matters. A general rule prohibits conversation about sex between or in the presence of father and daughter, mother and son, or brother and sister. This norm also applies to more distant cross-sex kin, including lineage or clan brothers and sisters. Here, of course, we encounter the issue of 'talkability' with its serious implications for AIDS education. Among Lisu, shame is involved when a girl is sexually licentious, when an unwanted child is aborted at a valley clinic, or when a man contracts gonorrhoea, while the shame complexes of other groups set their own standards.

Shame is also implicated in patterning sexual practices themselves. For example, traditionally only an Akha woman who 'had no embarrassment' would think of having sex in other than the cosmologically correct position: male atop female in vaginal intercourse. Normal sex for Lisu is when the male is above the female, since the men always have to 'work' harder during the sex act. In Thailand's hilltribe societies sex seems to include little foreplay or experimentation. Akha women, for example, remain clothed during lovemaking in the village context. Indeed, 'erotic scripts,' to borrow a phrase from Gagnon and Simon via Parker (1992:227), are limited in the hills. Among Lisu, oral sex, which they have become acquainted with from watching movies at Thai fairs, is looked upon with distaste. Some sexual practices are thus outside customs not in the sense of being forbidden but in the sense of not being culturally recognized at all. In the same way that 'lesbianism is not a culturally acknowledged possibility' in rural northern Mexico (Alonso and Koreck 1989:111), neither lesbianism nor male homosexuality are traditionally recognized — or named — among Akha, Hmong, and Lisu. Yet Thailand, with its transvestites, publicly presents the possibility of being homosexual (Jackson 1989). Foreign male tourists have tried to buy sex from young men in the hills, and some tribal youths are known to have engaged in male–male sex in urban areas.

Clearly a culture's scripting of the erotically proper does not encompass the universe of possible experience. There can, after all, be 'transgression,' which itself may be part of the 'ideology of the erotic' (Parker 1992:228). Moreover, in a context of interethnic contact, erotic scripts, transgression, and the universe of possibility can change. A young tribal woman who migrates to the city to sell handicrafts may learn new sexual practices, whether oral sex or full nudity, from a Thai lover. From this it is evident that it would be a mistake to focus exclusively on prostitution in an effort to understand transformations in hilltribe sexuality. Interethnic contacts in general are crucial to such an understanding. Thus what Alonso and Koreck (1989:113) call the 'regime of gender, power, and pleasure' must be situated not only in particular tribal groups themselves but in interethnic relations, both among hilltribe societies and with the dominant lowland society.

Gender and power are keys to understanding sexual behaviour. Despite the emphasis in tribal cultures on fertility and the cosmological value of femaleness, 'highland women ... are regarded as second class citizens in their own communities' (Ralana 1989:150; see also Tribal Research Institute 1985). Yet their positions vary from group to group, as one comparative example focused on women's place within kinship structures illustrates. Whereas among Lisu a divorcée is permitted to return to her parent's house and is given a field to cultivate, among Akha a divorcée can remain under her father's or brother's roof only for a few days and must therefore quickly find another husband. In fact, a number of Akha women who have migrated to lowland urban centres did so to escape an unwanted remarriage after divorce. Indeed, this aspect of traditional kinship may be a factor in Akha women's participation in Thailand's commercial sex industry.

For Hmong and Lisu, whose men 'buy' a wife by paying bridewealth — silver or money — there is a tendency to conceptualize a woman's value in materialistic terms based on future labour of the daughter-in-law or of her offspring. But among Hmong this seemingly economic transaction has a cosmological dimension in which a woman's male children 'will continue the lineage, feed dead ancestors and eventually propagate bodies into which the soul of dead lineage members will be reborn' (Symonds 1991:135; see also 1990). Lisu women may laughingly remark that their genitals are expensive, while in their songs they mention that 'brides are sold, the fee is paid, and the elders are satisfied.' As with Hmong, payment is not purely economic in nature: the cash paid by the groom's side to the bride's is compensation for the breast milk that nourished her as a child and for the use of her 'productive and reproductive power' and is intended to sustain Lisu honour (Klein Hutheesing 1990:128).

Akha, on the other hand, do not have brideprice. Interestingly, Akha women are more heavily involved in Thailand's commercial sex industry than either Hmong or Lisu. There are undoubtedly many reasons for this, one being the fact that Akha are the most populous tribe in the hills of eastern Burma adjoining the northern Thai frontier. Warfare between anti-government ethnic forces and Burma's national troops has devastated the region for decades. In this context of dislocation and dire poverty, Akha women have been lured, sold, or tricked into prostitution in Thailand. Another reason for the disproportionate number of Akha commercial sex workers may, in fact, be the lack of brideprice itself. Among Hmong and Lisu, a daughter is valued because the wealth received at her marriage enables what Lisu call the 'payment to acquire a wife' for the son. Without this essential cultural function of financially enabling her brother's marriage, an Akha woman is perhaps more easily parted from her family, which may indeed sell or indenture her into prostitution.

Despite the fact that hilltribe women are viewed as licentious by lowland men, prostitution is not indigenous in hilltribe cultures. Formerly, tribal languages had no terms for it; nowadays, Hmong, Lisu, and Akha phrases for it simply mean 'selling the body.' Yet the numbers of hilltribe clients and prostitutes are large and growing. Tribal men's visits to lowland brothels and the participation of tribal women, and to a much lesser extent, tribal men in the lowland commercial sex industry are contributing to reshaping the nature of sexuality in Thailand's mountain minorities. Hard data on the numbers of hilltribe clients or prostitutes are unavailable and would be virtually impossible to obtain. Men often do not talk openly in the village about their sexual flings in the valley. Lisu men can, however, be heard to jest that they are going looking for a wife or that they have accumulated the bridewealth needed to buy the services of a prostitute. For older men seeking sexual pleasures with a prostitute, the circumlocution is that they want a second wife. Such euphemisms should be seen as devices to understate the changed stance towards sexuality that engaging a prostitute entails. On the other hand, engaging in prostitution may be seen as a temporary move to earn quick cash or as part-time or occasional work. Young women working at brothels are said, perhaps euphemistically to conceal or avoid shame, to be washing dishes or selling chickens in the market.

The tribal groups differ in how participation in prostitution is treated. There are, after all, no traditional rules relating to it. Lisu mountain girls who sell their services to a brothel in the lowlands incur shame, but their loss of face does not result from getting paid for flesh; instead, it results from the fact that they no longer feed and fertilize Lisu culture. While men return from a visit to a valley brothel without evoking comment, ethnic groups, villages, and even families vary in their willingness to take back women who are thought to have been prostitutes. Some women have returned and married, and money earned by women in the commercial sex industry clearly returns to the hills. For example, an impressive Thai-style house of brick, concrete, and milled lumber in an Akha village is said to have been built from the money earned by a daughter sent into the trade.

Among Lisu a 'degeneration of repute' (Klein Hutheesing 1987) due to growing poverty may be patched up through concealing that shame with a materialistic display of a wooden house paid for by prostituting a daughter. Thus, the shame complex regarding sexual relations may be manipulated in novel ways.

The shame complex is implicated in male–female power relations, which are obviously critical to whether condom use can be discussed and, if so, effectively negotiated. From the point of view of AIDS prevention, it is essential to know who controls the sex act among couples of the tribal region. Shyness imposed by the shame complex may prevent women from being able to protect themselves. From impressionistic data, it seems that Lisu wives have succeeded in refusing to have sex with their husbands who had contracted gonorrhoea or syphilis. Two instances have been encountered where a wife ran back to her mother's home when she discovered her husband had something that 'ate his penis.' In the more patriarchal cultures of Hmong and Akha, such instances of female protest, let alone successful protest, are less likely.

Though non-HIV sexually transmitted diseases (STDs) such as gonorrhoea and syphilis have occurred among hilltribes as far back as the 1940s, cases are on the increase. Information about these can be obtained from district clinics where treatment is sought or from woman-to-woman talk during anthropological fieldwork. In a Lisu settlement of 54 households, it was found that eleven young men and four young women had gone for treatment for STDs during 1983–86; there may well have been additional infected individuals who did not seek treatment. Incidence of venereal diseases is relevant because biological and epidemiological research suggests that genital ulcers and perhaps also suppression of the immune system caused by untreated or frequent STDs contribute to vulnerability to HIV infection.

Tribal categories of ailments and theories of disease aetiology are complex and various. Akha, Hmong, and Lisu all consider some forms of illness to be contagious or infectious. Though the mountain people are viewed by the Thai majority as backward, dirty, and unhygienic, in reality they possess some practical knowledge of infection. Needles for ear piercing are first held to a flame, the wounds of a castrated pig are rubbed with ash, and dishes that were formerly scrubbed with ash are now scoured with soap. Yet these tribal groups also recognize myriad additional and not necessarily mutually exclusive causes of illness. Lisu, for example, see some ailments as related to the natural environment, whether the wind or the change of seasons, and others as inherited or inflicted by the supernatural.

Beliefs among Lisu, and perhaps among other hilltribes, about the relationship between blood and sickness (Durrenberger 1971:115–116) may be relevant to local conceptualizations of HIV, which can be transmitted by contact with contaminated blood.

Indigenous identification of the outside as the source of disease and disorder may also prove significant in local understandings of HIV/AIDS. Systematic data have not, however, yet been collected on how hilltribes are fitting the AIDS epidemic into their worldviews. Government broadcasts in both Thai and tribal languages about the dangers of AIDS are reaching mountain villages via radio and, less often, television. Coming as they do from beyond the hills, these may strengthen the notion that the disease is from the outside. Similarly, the phrasing of the broadcasts may encourage such thinking, since they admonish listeners not to visit brothels, which highlanders know are found in distant valley towns. AIDS is the latest in a series of intrusions into the hilltribes' damaged universe. Mountain minorities will gauge its danger within a world replete with threats perceived as coming from the outside: lowland authorities interdict their agricultural pursuits, unknown pests destroy their crops, pestilence wipes out their chickens and pigs, and chemical sprays affect their breathing.

Distrust of the outside is evident in the response among Hmong in Nan to the government's recent campaign advocating condom use. For years the government and non-governmental organizations have promoted family planning in the hills. Within the context of majority prejudice and discrimination against tribal minorities and of the disruption of traditional lifeways due to government and market intervention, Hmong interpret this new AIDS prevention campaign as a conspiracy aimed at curtailing population growth among hilltribes. There is evidence in the Thai press, with its many articles about HIV-positive prostitutes from Burma being sent back over the border, that the majority may also be blaming the outside in the form of illegal lowland and hilltribe immigrants. Whether this blame will be extended to Thailand's own tribal people remains to be seen.

PERSPECTIVES AND PERPLEXITIES

An understanding of vulnerability to HIV infection among hilltribes in northern Thailand requires a holistic and nuanced view which places this new viral threat in a fluid context in which linkages between upland and lowland societies are central. Some obvious linkages are development programmes and government-sponsored

elections for headmen in hilltribe villages; some less obvious
linkages are majority stereotypes of highland minorities and the
internalization of these stereotypes into tribal self-images. The fluid
context includes the globalized political economy in which Thailand
is situated. Furthermore, it encompasses a complex conceptualization of the village level wherein economic, political, and cultural
dimensions are seen as both rooted in local structures and embedded
in the larger structures of nation, region, and world. A qualitative
anthropology that is at once historical, materialist, and cultural can
contribute to effective AIDS education and prevention. After all, risk
behaviours are patterned by history, political economy and culture, a
sociological truth that has been elegantly documented for Zaïre by
Schoepf (e.g., 1992a, 1992b, and in this volume) and for Haiti by
Farmer (1992a, and in this volume).

For Hmong, Akha, and Lisu of Thailand, state and capitalist
penetration is implicated in their risk of contracting HIV. So also are
indigenous cultural values and practices such as the shame complex,
the religious celebration of fertility, and rules regarding residence
after divorce. Our previous research gives us some insights into
political, economic, and cultural factors that pattern hilltribe risk of
HIV; nonetheless, additional research is required. In particular, we
need to learn more about both traditional and transformed sexuality.
The collaborative project on which we are embarking will also investigate what information about HIV/AIDS is reaching Hmong, Akha,
and Lisu; how this information is being understood; what influences
are shaping this understanding; and which values and institutions
contribute to the spread of HIV and which might be harnessed to
help stop it. Our focus will be on tribal women because, like women
everywhere, they are more easily infected than men for physiological
reasons, and because they are less likely than tribal men to be
reached by ongoing educational efforts in the Thai language. In
addition, the 'regime of gender, power, and pleasure' places them at
a disadvantage to both highland and lowland men.

Our hope is that findings from this research can be used by highlanders themselves and by government and non-governmental organizations to facilitate more effective AIDS prevention among
Thailand's tribal minorities. Moreover, we hope that they may be
helpful to educational efforts for Hmong, Akha, and Lisu in China,
Burma, Laos, and Vietnam, where they also reside. The concept of
'talkability' suggests that adopting multiple educational strategies
may be superior to adhering to a single one. For instance, anthropological analysis of social organization may yield important data on

what Schoepf (1992a:89) calls 'naturally occurring interpersonal communication situations' or what Vichai Poshyachinda (personal communication) calls 'natural communication pathways' that could be used to channel information about HIV/AIDS. Information passed along these pathways, then, could complement more general, public discourse on AIDS prevention such as radio spots or village-wide lectures. In peripheral societies like Thailand's northern hilltribes, where there is distrust of outside powers and where many people, especially females, are mono-lingual in a minority language, these more local and informal channels may be essential to stopping the spread of HIV.

Members of marginalized groups, whether ethnic, racial, or tribal minorities in industrialized or industrializing societies, are particularly vulnerable to HIV. Deprivation — limited access to modern health care, technology, and education — impoverishment, and demoralization make them less able to protect themselves from infection even if they know how. Anthropological inquiry can uncover the sociological underpinnings of this increased risk, but by doing so it may contribute to precisely the type of 'risk group' mentality that has hindered effective prevention around the world and has fostered stigmatization, discrimination, and blame. Should social scientists, whose members have helped to deconstruct the notion of 'risk group' and to argue instead for the relevance of 'risk behaviours,' study the political, economic, and cultural factors contributing to such risk behaviours among members of particular groups if this may lead outsiders to see these groups as 'risk groups' defined in a misguided essentialist manner? If the view propounded by Schoepf and Farmer, among others, that political economy and culture pattern the local epidemics that form the AIDS pandemic is correct, as we believe it is, then social scientists *must* undertake such studies. We emphasize here that Thailand's hilltribes are *not* 'risk groups' whose vulnerability to HIV/AIDS rests on biology or genetics; instead, they are *social* groups *at* risk for reasons constructed in complex combination by history, political economy, and culture. Alonso and Koreck (1987:116–117), facing a similar ethical dilemma, published information about sexual practices among rural northern Mexicans that might invite further stigmatization because they concluded that breaking the community's silence would help hinder HIV transmission. We also hope that our work will do more good than harm.[7]

ACKNOWLEDGEMENTS

We take this opportunity to thank the many people who generously shared their time and knowledge as we formulated the project and wrote proposals for funding the research, which began in Thailand in January 1993. Our sincere gratitude to the following people who helped one or all of us: George Appell, Lauran Bethell, Barbara Boardman, Han ten Brummelhuis, Komatra Chuengsatiansup, Donna Chung, Ellen Cooper, Anan Ganjanapan, Jennifer Gray, Richard Herrell, Asue and John Hobday, Robert Hunt, David Jacobson, Don Joralemon, Peter and Sally Kunstadter, Elaine and Paul Lewis, John McDonald, Manus Maneeprasert, Barbara Millstein, Marjorie Muecke, Stephen O. Murray, Lucile Newman, Rick Parmentier, Usaneeya Pengporn, Vichai Poshyachinda, Howard Radley, Brooke Schoepf, Mike Sweat, Alan Symonds, Nikki Tannenbaum, Xoua Thao, Vicharn Vithayasai, and Michael and Susan Whyte.

For funding the previous research that informs this chapter, Kammerer thanks the Fulbright Hays Doctoral Dissertation Abroad Program and the Southeast Asia Program of the Social Science Research Council (New York); Klein Hutheesing thanks the Netherlands Foundation for the Study of South East Asian Mountain Peoples (Utrecht), and Symonds thanks the Watson Institute, Brown University (Providence, Rhode Island). Kammerer, Klein Hutheesing, and Symonds are grateful to the National Research Council of Thailand for permission to conduct past fieldwork. All four of us wish to convey our appreciation to the Tribal Research Institute (Chiang Mai) and its director Chantaboon Sutthi for their kind co-operation on our AIDS project. Gratitude to the American Foundation for AIDS Research (AmFAR) for funding this project (Award No. 001781-13-RG) and to Brandeis University for its institutional support for this grant is expressed by Kammerer, principal investigator, and the three other members of the research team. We are also grateful for the opportunity to participate in Amsterdam University's AIDS and Anthropology Group's conference on Culture, Sexual Behavior and AIDS (July 24–26, 1992), where Klein Hutheesing represented the team.

NOTES

1. The following remarks represent the preliminary reflections of four fieldworkers embarking on a collaborative research and applied

project on HIV/AIDS knowledge and education among three of Thailand's tribal minorities. They are based on general data collected during previous fieldwork among Akha (Kammerer), Lisu (Klein Hutheesing), and Hmong (Symonds and Maneeprasert). While our disciplinary specializations are various — cultural anthropology, sociology, medical anthropology, and public health — and our research foci have differed — ranging from missionization and political economy to cosmology and nutrition — we all have investigated gender, kinship, and marriage. Since the project is in its infancy, some of what we write here, particularly concerning hilltribe responses to HIV/AIDS, is speculative and suggestive.

2. During discussions in the work group on Sexual Subcultures and Cultural Minorities at the Amsterdam conference, 'talkability,' a term introduced by Paul van Gelder, proved to be a noteworthy concept. It encompasses, among other things, norms regarding conversations about sex and types of sexuality (homosexuality, paid sex, and the like). The concept further includes the family, community, or institutional contexts which set rules regarding how much can be said about sexuality, in which idiom, and with whom. Another facet of talkability conveys the meaning of communicability, which entails the possibility of transmitting knowledge about the AIDS epidemic and the type of media used, including body language. A Lisu announcer on the government's tribal radio station in Chiang Mai, for instance, had a frustrating time translating the Thai AIDS message into his own language because words related to sex would evoke feelings of embarrassment and consternation among his audience, while certain terms, like the Thai word for brothel, could not be adequately translated.

3. Ethnic labels are complex in the region. This paper adopts the auto-ethnonyms used by tribal people themselves in Thailand. Hmong are called 'Meo' by Thai, while in China they are members of the officially recognized national minority of Miao. Similarly, Akha are labeled 'Ikaw' by Thai, but in China they are members of the Hani minority.

4. Kammerer (1988a:9–11 and 1988c:275–278) discusses negative and damaging stereotypes of tribal minorities embedded in Thai government policies and in Thai popular culture. Hilltribes have been viewed as insurgents, drug producers and smugglers, destroyers of the environment through slash-and-burn agriculture, and illegal immigrants.

5. Symonds (1991) discusses the ways that changes in clothing dictated by the Hmong code of shyness indicate a female's sexual maturity and marital status. Klein Hutheesing's (1990) study of the emergence of sexual inequality among Lisu in Thailand demonstrates that the shame complex is essential to understanding the ordering and recent disordering of their society.

6. Schoepf (1992a:92) witnessed the development of an argument of this type among a group of clan elders in Zaïre seeking the 'protection of future generations.'

7. A further implication of the approach exemplified by the work of Schoepf and Farmer is that effective AIDS prevention requires change in those aspects of political economy and culture that contribute to risk. In the section on the political and economic tracks of AIDS, we illustrated ways in which intrusions from the dominant lowlands, such as crop replacement and other development programmes, contribute to hilltribe vulnerability to HIV infection. In the secton on sexuality, we illustrated ways in which traditional cultures, in particular the gender system, do the same.

Both Schoepf (e.g., 1992a, 1992b) and Vichai Poshyachinda (personal communication) stress development's impact as facilitating rather than inhibiting HIV's spread. Indeed, Schoepf (1992b:260) uses the phrase 'disease of development' to describe AIDS in Central Africa. Planners now see the AIDS pandemic as a crisis in development in that it disproportionately affects young adults, precisely the age group to whom development programmes have imparted knowledge and technology. At present, then, the crisis AIDS presents to development is narrowly defined; however, Schoepf's and Vichai's views suggest that a more fundamental crisis in development is required, one which questions and reworks the ideological foundations and analytical assumptions of the enterprise.

With reference to anthropological research on AIDS, Farmer (1992b:310) argues that '[i]n settings of significant social inequality, the success of the ethnographic project may depend on perceived opposition — which reflects, presumably, genuine opposition — to local authorities,' that is, representatives of law enforcement and government. Given inequalities of gender, it may also depend on opposition to the authority of local cultures, which, surely, places anthropologists in a perplexing position.

REFERENCES

Alonso, A.M., and M.T. Koreck. 1989. Silences: 'Hispanics,' AIDS, and Sexual Practices. *Differences* 1(1):101–124.

Alting von Geusau, L. 1983. Dialectics of Akhazan: The Interiorizations of a Perennial Minority Group. In: *Highlanders of Thailand*, edited by J. McKinnon and Wanat Bhruksasri. Kuala Lumpur: Oxford University Press.

Anan Ganjanapan. 1987. Conflicting Patterns of Land Tenure Among Ethnic Groups in the Highlands of Northern Thailand: The Impact of State and Market Intervention. In: *Proceedings of the International Conference on Thai Studies*. Vol. 3 (part 2). Canberra: Australian National University.

Bangkok Post. 1991. Hilltribe Heroin Crisis: A Post Enquiry. 15 December, pp. 8–9.

Bibeau, G., and R. Murbach. 1991. Présentation: Déconstruire l'univers du sida. *Anthropologie et sociétés* 15(2–3):5–11.

Bolton, R. 1992. AIDS and Promiscuity: Muddles in the Models of HIV Prevention. In: *Rethinking AIDS Prevention: Cultural Approaches*, edited by R. Bolton and M. Singer. Montreux: Gordon and Breach Science Publishers.

Chupinit Kesmanee. 1988. Hilltribe Relocation Policy in Thailand. *Cultural Survival Quarterly* 12(4):2–6.

Cooper, R. 1984. *Resource Scarcity and the Hmong Response: Patterns of Settlement and Economy in Transition.* Singapore: Singapore University Press.

Durrenberger, E.P. 1971. The Ethnography of Lisu Curing. Ph.D. diss. Urbana–Champaign: University of Illinois, Department of Anthropology.

Farmer, P. 1992a. *AIDS and Accusation: Haiti and the Geography of Blame.* Berkeley: University of California Press.

Farmer, P. 1992b. New Disorder, Old Dilemmas: AIDS and Anthropology in Haiti. In: *The Time of AIDS: Social Analysis, Theory, and Method*, edited by G. Herdt and S. Lindenbaum. Newbury Park, CA: Sage Publications.

Hanks, L., and J.R. Hanks. 1978. The Context of Opium Production in Chiangrai Province North of the Mae Kok Valley. Paper presented at the Conference on Opium Production, Trade, and Use in the Golden Triangle. Institute for the Study of Human Issues, Philadelphia, 3–7 April.

Jackson, P.A. 1989. *Male Homosexuality in Thailand: An Interpretation of Contemporary Thai Sources.* Elmhurst, NY: Global Academic Publishers.

Kammerer, C.A. 1988a. Of Labels and Laws: Thailand's Resettlement and Repatriation Policies. *Cultural Survival Quarterly* 12(4):7–12.

Kammerer, C.A. 1988b. Shifting Gender Asymmetries Among Akha Highlanders of Thailand. In: *Gender, Power, and the Construction of the Moral Order: Studies from the Thai Periphery*, edited by N. Eberhardt. Madison: University of Wisconsin–Madison, Center for Southeast Asian Studies.

Kammerer, C.A. 1988c. Territorial Imperatives: Akha Ethnic Identity and Thailand's National Integration. In: *Ethnicities and Nations: Processes of Interethnic Relations in Latin America, Southeast Asia, and the Pacific*, edited by R. Guidieri, F. Pellizzi, and S.J. Tambiah. Houston: Rothko Chapel.

Kammerer, C.A. Opium and Tribal People in the Golden Triangle. *Journal of Southeast Asian Studies.* Forthcoming.

Kammerer, C.A., and P.V. Symonds. 1992. AIDS in Asia: Hilltribes Endangered at Thailand's Periphery. *Cultural Survival Quarterly* 16(3):23–25.

Klein Hutheesing, O. 1987. The Degeneration of Lisu Repute. In: *Proceedings of the International Conference on Thai Studies.* Vol. 3 (part 2). Canberra: Australian National University.

Klein Hutheesing, O. 1990. *Emerging Sexual Inequality Among the Lisu of Northern Thailand: The Waning of Dog and Elephant Repute.* Leiden: E.J. Brill.

Klein Hutheesing, O. 1992. Distortions of Social Reality, Disorientations of Culture: The Lisu Case. Paper presented at the International Symposium on the Environment and the Regeneration of Culture, Penang, Malaysia.

Kunstadter, P., and S. Kunstadter. 1992. Population Movements and Environmental Changes in the Hills of Northern Thailand. In: *Patterns and Illusions: Thai History and Thought*, edited by G. Wijeyewardene and E.C. Chapman. Singapore: Institute for Southeast Asian Studies.

Lindenbaum, S. 1992. Knowledge and Action in the Shadow of AIDS. In: *The Time of AIDS: Social Analysis, Theory, and Method*, edited by G. Herdt and S. Lindenbaum. Newbury Park, CA: Sage Publications.

Mann, J., D.J.M. Tarantola, and T.W. Netter, eds. 1992. *AIDS in the World*. Cambridge: Harvard University Press.

McKinnon, J., and Wanat Bhruksasri. 1983. Preface. In: *Highlanders of Thailand*, edited by J. McKinnon and Wanat Bhruksasri. Kuala Lumpur: Oxford University Press.

Mirante, E.T. 1988. *The Victim Zone: Recent Accounts of Burmese Military Rights Abuse in Shan State*. Cranford, NJ: Project Majé.

Mirante, E.T. 1992. Silent Epidemic: Ethnic Minorities Are at Risk in Burma's Hidden AIDS Epidemic. *Cultural Survival Quarterly* 16(3):19–22.

Muecke, M.A. 1990. The AIDS Prevention Dilemma in Thailand. *Asian and Pacific Population Forum* 4(4):1–8, 21–27.

Parker, R.G. 1992. Sexual Diversity, Cultural Analysis, and AIDS Education in Brazil. In: *The Time of AIDS: Social Analysis, Theory, and Method*, edited by G. Herdt and S. Lindenbaum. Newbury Park, CA: Sage Publications.

Radley, H.M. 1986. Economic Marginalization and the Ethnic Consciousness of the Green Mong (*Moob Ntsuab*) of Northwestern Thailand. Ph.D. diss. Oxford: Institute of Social Anthropology.

Ralana Maneeprasert. 1989. 'Women and Children First'? A Review of Current Nutritional Status in the Highlands. In: *Hill Tribes Today: Problems in Change*, edited by J. McKinnon and B. Vienne. Bangkok: White Lotus-ORSTOM.

Royal Thai Government, Ministry of Public Health, Division of Epidemiology. 1992. Sentinel Surveillance, June 1989–June 1992.

Schoepf, B.G. 1992a. AIDS, Sex and Condoms: African Healers and the Reinvention of Tradition in Zaïre. In: *Rethinking AIDS Prevention: Cultural Approaches*, edited by R. Bolton and M. Singer. Montreux: Gordon and Breach Science Publishers.

Schoepf, B.G. 1992b. Women at Risk: Case Studies from Zaïre. In: *The Time of AIDS: Social Analysis, Theory, and Method*, edited by G. Herdt and S. Lindenbaum. Newbury Park, CA: Sage Publications.

Sophon Ratanakhon. 1978. Legal Aspects of Land Occupation and Development. In: *Farmers of the Forest:Economic Development and Marginal Agriculture in Northern Thailand*, edited by P. Kunstadter, E.C. Chapman, and

Sanga Sabhasri. Honolulu: The University Press of Hawaii, The East–West Center.

Symonds, P.V. 1990. Women and Birth in a Thai Highland Community. In: *Proceedings of the 4th International Conference on Thai Studies*. Vol. 1. Kunming, China: Institute of Southeast Asian Studies.

Symonds, P.V. 1991. Cosmology and the Cycle of Life: Hmong Views of Birth, Death and Gender in a Mountain Village in Northern Thailand. Ph.D. diss. Providence, RI: Brown University, Department of Anthropology.

Tribal Research Institute, Department of Public Welfare, and Faculty of Social Sciences. 1985. *A Socio-Cultural Study of the Impact of Social Development Programs on Tribal Women and Children*. Chiang Mai: Chiang Mai University.

Tribal Research Institute. 1990. *Tribal Population Summary in Thailand*. Chiang Mai.

Weniger, B.G., Khanchit Limpakarnjanarat, Kumnuan Ungchusak, Sombat Thanprasertsuk, Kachit Choopanya, Suphak Vanichseni, Thongchai Uneklabh, Prasert Thongcharoen, and Chantapong Wasi. 1991. The Epidemiology of HIV Infection and AIDS in Thailand. *AIDS 1991* 5(suppl. 2): S71–S85.

Part II

Contextualizing Sexual Risk

Chapter
FOUR

Gender, Age and Class: Discourses on HIV Transmission and Control in Uganda

Christine Obbo

Scientists working on AIDS in Africa have assumed that HIV transmission is a public health issue that may easily be solved by teaching people to change their behaviour, coupled with the promotion of condoms. The key to the transmission and control of HIV, however, is embedded in the traditional practices that need to be exposed. Researchers have re-read monographs in order to construct the traditional sexual practices of African groups. Some reports even predicted that certain groups would readily adopt or resist the adoption of condoms because of their sexual practices. Evidence has not supported these predictions (Obbo 1993a). Exotic practices, such as 'wet' and 'dry' sex, widow inheritance and funeral ritual intercourse were reported in newspaper headlines as being conducive to HIV transmission. Researchers continue to probe people to find out what they do during the sexual act and what they talk about.[1] This paper suggests that class, gender, religion, and age are not only important cultural definitions that have been overlooked by researchers, but also may be crucial to the transmission as well as prevention of HIV. Attention needs to be paid to the syncretic cultural practices resulting from the interaction between traditional Islamic and Christian ideologies. These, together with Western education (or lack of it), have created and exacerbated differences in perception that will be referred to here as voices of class, gender, and age. Thus, within societies or cultural groups or communities, the above divisions need to be taken into consideration when dealing with sexuality and HIV transmission.

In Uganda although a lot of progress has been made, complacency and indifference may prove detrimental to the efforts to control AIDS. The following sections of this chapter deal with the perspectives of men (politicians, professionals, and priests), women, and youth on the subject of HIV transmission and ways to prevent transmission. The discourse is presented in four voices: the dominant male and elite voices, purporting to articulate societal morals and cultural values, and determining the direction of research; the muted voices of women; the ignored, dissenting voices of young men; and the silent voices of girls in need of awakening. The sexual transmission of HIV makes it a disease of shame (Fee and Fox 1988), a taboo subject for conversation. New forms of discourse must be promoted to encourage 'talkability' in sexual education as well as sexual negotiation. The discussions on sex, HIV, and condoms must be seen as an exercise in using culture as a tool to negotiate societal survival while at the same time exposing the class, gender and self-serving indifference to societal survival.[2]

THE DOMINANT VOICES,
BOTH VOCAL AND SILENT

This section deals with the dominant elite (particularly male) voices. They determine the course of events because people react to them or are dominated by their silence in not promoting certain interventions or areas of research. Thus, while the acceptable sexual parameters are vocally alluded to in the discussion of condoms, the political economy of the foreign-dominated AIDS industry seems to render elites inarticulate. At the beginning of the AIDS pandemic it was thought that if people were told how dangerous the situation was, they would automatically observe interdictions, such as 'Zero grazing' (African Medical Research and Education Foundation

[AMREF]); 'Love carefully' and 'I am glad I said no to AIDS' (AIDS Control Programme [ACP]); 'Love faithfully' (church sermons); 'Those who play must pay' (priest); and 'Young girls must learn to say no to men' (men in general).

These messages were disseminated via posters, radio broadcasts, newspaper articles, church sermons, and general conversation. They assumed that, in order to change behaviour, people needed only their willpower in order to resist going astray. In fact, there was a suggestion in the messages that people either willingly expose themselves to AIDS or that they 'say no to AIDS' in different situations. While it is conceivable that truckers could go straight home to their wives and avoid the women along the way, it seems less likely that subordinates, such as secretaries or schoolgirls, can say no to the sexual advances of their supervisors or teachers. Thus, the interdicts ignored the social causes that surround many sexual encounters. The student who needs to receive good grades, a worker who needs to keep a job or to be promoted, or a poor woman with no alternative way to generate an income that constitutes a living wage are in no position to say no to AIDS. Thus, not only are some members of society coerced into having sex, but the majority of people discover their HIV status only when they have the disease AIDS.

The messages above must be seen in a condomless context. At first condoms were not available, but when their availability became a possibility the messages remained the same. Condoms were portrayed as foreign cultural villain: they would promote promiscuity, particularly among the young and women; men associated using condoms with eating sweets with the wrapping paper on; and as time went on condom use was associated with taking showers with a raincoat on. The latter association had diffused throughout all Eastern and Central African countries.

When it appeared that some people might be using condoms, concern was expressed about the promiscuity of the youth, as evidenced by the allegedly ubiquitous discarded condoms outside disco halls. There was concern over goats choking on used condoms and children playing with them as balloons. This would seem to be a straightforward case requiring instruction on how to dispose of condoms properly. However, stories and discussions surrounding condom use had a decidedly moral, disapproving tone: condoms promote promiscuity. Perhaps the hagiarchy and gerontocracy — i.e., the social power of religious men and older men — is best illustrated by a story that gained currency throughout Uganda between 1988 and 1990 and was used in sermons in both Anglican and Catholic churches by priests who sounded, with each telling, as if they knew the actors. The story concerned a headmaster of a school who one morning distributed condoms to the boys. Before school closed, some of the boys came to him and said, 'We have finished. We want more condoms.' This story was a setback for the school's AIDS programme. The attitude of the priests and some parents was that 'condom ignorance is bliss' which would protect the children from promiscuity.

It seemed that there was no acceptable way to educate school-children about AIDS. One of the most creative and sensitive attempts to reach children was devised in France by Libertés, a Danielle Mitterrand Foundation. Educational messages were put on the back of school exercise books donated to Ugandan schools and involved two mangos talking about the facts of AIDS prevention. Unfortunately, the notebooks were never allowed to leave the warehouse, and Ugandan schoolchildren missed an educational opportunity.

In 1991, women in the National Resistance Council organized a protest against the high incidence of sexual assaults, rapes, and seductions of young girls by older men in schools, communities, and families. The march in the capital city, Kampala, made stops at the Ministry of Education; the Ministry of Women, Youth and Sports; and regional and local government. The march was poorly attended and the women's organizations that bothered to respond sent a few underlings to carry placards. At several stops, men were heard to say that young girls seduce men by wearing provocative dresses. (One man in his twenties barely escaped from the women, who objected to this attitude and his effrontery in expressing it at the march.) Although a few 'progressive' National Resistance Council men marched with the women, they were anxious to change the issue on which they were marching; the sexual assaults on young girls by older men. At every opportunity, these men informed the press that too much attention was being paid to the 'sugar daddies,' when actually 'many boys' were also endangered by 'sugar mummies.' Soon after that march, stories about regional 'sugar mummies' and young men started to appear in the press. The question that was never addressed is: what is the percentage of Ugandan women, as compared to men, who have the economic clout to be 'sugar mummies'? The insignificant number of such women suggests that the 'progressive' men were railroading the women's protest. It is worthwhile noting that in our research schoolchildren in essays written in 1989 and in focus group discussions which took place in 1992 consistently mention 'sugar daddies' but not 'sugar mummies'

(Obbo 1993a). The rich women presumably attract men of 20 years and above and not children — as adult men do. However, invoking women as seducers of young boys is part and parcel of the general attitude of men from all walks of life, that women are the real vectors of HIV as compared to men. In fact there are three times as many girls as boys, in the age group 15–25, who are infected with HIV. The girls are being infected by older men, not women.

The use of condoms is fraught with many pitfalls. In 1988, newspaper reports suggested that Muslim men were snipping tips off condoms before using them, in symbolic association with their circumcised bodies. At the same time, fears were expressed that condoms would fall off and get lodged in a woman's vagina, with a harmful effect on the womb. This fear is understandable, and women were reassured when the researchers in focus group interviews stressed that a condom, if put on properly, should not fall off, and if it does it could be pulled out with a finger. In Kampala, the capital city, and Rakai, one of the most affected districts, focus group discussions were conducted with ten groups of 20 women to enable them to share their condom experiences. In all the ten groups there was no woman with first-hand experience of a lodged condom (because, in most cases, their men were not using them anyway), but 'a friend of a friend said that they knew a woman.' Several women traced the genesis of the womb and condom story to men. This is something that scared women because it threatened their reproductive health in an environment where barren women are pitied and mothers are respected. There is social pressure on women to prove their fertility. Women's *raison d'être* is to be mothers to men's children. All Ugandan societies practice patrilineal descent; i.e., children, whether legitimate or not, are affiliated with the man's group. This means that a woman gains access to social status and resources by getting married and bearing children for particular groups. But the control of men over women continues, even in the urban areas, where couples may be cohabiting in relationships that neither accord women access to land and status nor offer entitlements to their children. Patriarchal assumptions about women's sexuality as an extension of procreativity are forcing many HIV-positive mothers to opt for maternity, despite the dangers posed to them and their children. Some women are counselled by health officials or know of HIV-positive mothers whose conditions became complicated and who died of AIDS soon after the birth of their babies. In a focus group discussion, one young woman said, 'Look, I know I have no AIDS, I am pregnant.' Apparently her boyfriend had told her that HIV-positive mothers do not conceive. She died of generalized Kaposi's sarcoma three months after her baby was born.

Even when elites do not speak, their silence dominates. One international non-governmental organization (NGO) kept boxes of condoms in the toilet rooms to make them accessible to their youthful staff. However, condom use was minimal. In a group discussion with seven men and three women, the women revealed that they always carry condoms and the men concurred with the sentiments of one man: 'Why should we use condoms? Have you ever heard the President or any of the big men say that they use condoms? That is because they know that they are 99 per cent unreliable. The day I hear the President say he uses condoms, I will start using them too.' The suggestion here is that elites are regarded as role models by ordinary people. When elites contract HIV and die of AIDS, they generate a lot of anger because they are supposed to know better than to expose themselves to such dangers. In discussions with some women, it was suggested that women who came from prominent families and who were assertive usually warned their husbands about how their marriages would end (and some indeed did end) if illegitimate children showed up. Apparently, these men have always used condoms to avoid producing children not belonging to their legal wives. The issue is not about monogamy or protecting the other woman, but avoiding social scandal. However, many educated men are not condom users. In 1989, during a seminar, a prominent health educator, married to a medical doctor, screamed when she was shown a condom, 'What is that? My husband will kill me if I take it home.' At the same time, one hears a lot of statements about how the ordinary people will not know how to use and how to dispose of condoms. The uneducated and poor are the others in the elite AIDS discourse. And elites enjoy stressing how people might reuse the condom. (I have been investigating this widespread supposition since 1988 and no one has owned up to knowing anyone who has reused a condom.) Surely, the issue here is that of education. If one can put on trousers, then condoms should not be a problem. It is, admittedly, a new technology but, as an informant asserted, 'if the Karimajong can dismantle imported sophisticated guns, put them back together and use them without the benefit of Western education, then all of us in Uganda can learn to use condoms properly.'

Lastly, research as an aspect of the elite culture or 'dominant voice' deserves comment. About 600 AIDS-related studies are being carried out in Africa, and over half of them involve collaboration with outside researchers. Uganda is hosting many AIDS researchers. Here lies the danger: the research agenda on AIDS in Uganda is determined by outsiders. The Ugandan doctors involved in AIDS research have become rubber stamp collaborators who cannot set the agenda because they are paid by someone else. Several doctors have said:

'This is the only way I can make a living wage to support my family.'
'This is the only way I can keep in touch with international researchers.'
'This is the only way I can travel, I do not want to be an isolated scientist.'
'We are a poor country, our hands are tied.'

All this is understandable, but it does not explain why researchers are allowed to collect blood samples (the results of which come back to Uganda two years later) without counselling and educating people. One would hope that the purpose of undergoing a blood test is to enable people to take critical decisions about their behaviour. There seems to be a self-fulfilling prophecy which runs like this: people are not changing their sexual behaviour and, therefore, this is a good situation to study the natural history of AIDS. Many projects only pay lip service to intervention; people are not counselled by researchers who take their blood samples; people say they get their knowledge about AIDS from sources other than these projects. Examples from other parts of the world, for example, in California, show that changes have been drastic because gay communities have treated AIDS as a grassroots issue. Experts and outsiders can act as catalysts for change because they usually have resources and technical know-how.

In Uganda there seems to be an excessive dependence upon outside experts, and deference to foreign funding means that some projects that are ethically questionable are allowed to be conducted. For example, when it was announced in newspaper headlines that Uganda was one of the three countries selected for World Health Organization vaccine experiments, some were surprised that there was no discussion of the ethical issues, particularly as there were suggestions of anonymous control groups that would receive placebos. One researcher said, 'It does not matter one way or another; people have refused to change their sexual behaviour.'

Some foreign scientists and other researchers want to conduct research on human victims to benefit their careers rather than help AIDS sufferers. AIDS has become an 'industry' that is benefiting everyone, except the real victims. Sometimes rival organizations have been set up to help and share the AIDS wealth. The best illustration of this is the creation of the AIDS Commission in Uganda, whose functions are very similar to those already assigned to the AIDS Control Programme in the same country. Money is wasted on renting new, expensive premises, or paying directors inflated salaries and fringe benefits in dollars. AIDS control in Uganda is being sabotaged by complacency and indifference by those in a position to make a difference.[3]

MULTIPLE JEOPARDY: WOMEN AND THE CULTURE OF SILENCE

In the anthropological literature, women have been identified with the culture of silence, which can never be heard. Women's inarticulate voices may be real or symbolic (Ardener 1975). While some Ugandan cultures encourage women to have audible discussions with their husbands in public, in most cultures such discussions are branded as loud, rude, and unwomanlike. Women and children are best seen but not heard. Researchers who have tried to work with women know from experience that interviewing them in mixed-gender groups usually leads men to monopolize the answers, while women nod or shake their heads. Yet, when interviewed separately, the same women become articulate and informative.[4]

Women feel that it is important to break this culture of silence, which is compounded by poverty and renders them especially powerless and vulnerable in dealing with the AIDS pandemic. The accepted religious and social practices that allow men to enjoy multiple partners as wives or 'wives' (i.e., consensual relations), while strongly condemning women's expression of their sexuality, have been key factors in the spread of HIV. The dominant patriarchal cultural ideologies demand sexual monogamy in women, and women who wish to vary this prescription must contend with being branded 'bad women,' 'brazen faced,' promiscuous ('prostitutes') and 'bad mothers' (because they are not bearing children for their husbands only). Many women become enslaved by the social construction and demands put on 'good women' and always seem to see their sexual identity in relation to the opposite mirror image of the 'bad women.'

When Christianity was introduced in Africa the model woman was that of the good Christian wife who was a companion to her husband and acted to promote his social status. In Uganda it is no secret that nearly all the earliest converts to Christianity were chiefs who got rid of their older common-law wives and married young 'Christian' wives. Thus, from the beginning, chiefs who were the Christian role models for the masses had several families, distributed in different places. Ordinary men who were successful also married and distributed their wives to live on different lands. Those with no money to buy land started a system where co-wives lived in the same house and shared chores and child rearing. As more women became educated, the men who married them could not publicly justify 'polygyny'; after all, they were 'Christian and modern.'[5] Nonetheless, some men still had mistresses or casual girlfriends and thus continued to practice informal polygyny. The Christian 'ring' wives in the early 1960s campaigned for legislation to limit inheritance rights to legal wives only — i.e., in registered marriages — but the all-male Parliament (except for three women) laughed out the proposed legislation. At issue was the fact that some men dispossessed their legal wives and children in favour of mistresses. In addition, in some areas, upon the death of a man the relatives dispossessed the widow and her children. There was legal monogamy, but it was not well connected with other social expectations and, therefore, made women vulnerable to poverty and sexually transmitted disease (STD). During my research in the early 1970s, women often complained of STDs they had contracted from their husbands. In the villages, women associated miscarriages with STDs. Now scientists are saying that STD is a co-factor in the susceptibility to HIV transmission.

Ugandan women have become cynical even of recent 1990 laws that require a life sentence for rape conviction and a death penalty for having sex with a girl younger than 13 years. The women insist that those who will be caught are poor men who touch the sisters and daughters of rich or powerful men. As one elite woman in her 70s observed,

> There has not been a drastic change in the reported rape patterns since the 1990 sex law. In every community a few people have always been accused of rape, usually marginal, unmarried men with no family; since the beginning of this century male teachers have been known to be a hindrance to girls' education because of their lecherous activities. A few mothers have complained that while some men have been prosecuted the majority of women are still not protected.

Women are not protected in their families, in the work place or in any other place. Women revealed anger, fear and vulnerability during focus group discussions: 'We live in daily fear for our daughters and ourselves.' 'We fear what our husbands may bring home.' 'Women are going to perish through no fault of their own.' 'Women are innocent of sexual transgression, they are dying for nothing.' 'I will not allow my daughter to be married without she and her boyfriend being tested first.' 'I wish they would invent a drug that women could use for their own protection.' 'Men, now more than ever, think marriage to young women (and sometimes girls) is the solution to AIDS.'

Women's concern here is with the need to have a means to protect themselves from unnecessary infections and death. This is a recognition that women are totally dependent upon men's co-operation and willingness to use condoms. It also underscores the fact that women are 'coerced' into having sex with men by the social expectations that accord men the power to 'choose' sex partners and for women to be subserviently 'available.' Women's availability is dictated by the expectations surrounding spousal and maternal roles; the need to prove that they are normal women, attractive to men, and able to procreate. These are all vestiges of the dominant patriarchal ideologies that both men and women support. On top of this, most women now need to survive in a commodified money economy, but often they have no marketable skills. There are many examples to illustrate the perils faced by young girls who are seduced by older men, by married women (or women not yet married) attached to unfaithful men, and by poor women doing sex work for survival. Below are brief illustrations of the interconnections of how sexual availability and vulnerability are experienced by women. Two newspaper stories were the subject of women's focus group discussions during our research.

In a village not far away from the capital city, Kampala, a husband was enraged when he found his wife sleeping with a diviner who was treating her for infertility. He complained to the all-male Resistance Committee, which dismissed the case because the diviner said this is how he treats infertility. The women traditional healers who were interviewed and studied in a 1992 Save the Children Fund Kampala Primary Health Project always examined women's stomachs above the pubic hairline. They said this was sufficient to diagnose the infertility problem. Apparently male traditional healers deliberately examined women below the pubic hairline, thus 'leading themselves into temptation,' a male AIDS researcher and sympathizer suggested (Obbo 1992). This is the region of high HIV seroprevalence, but no one seemed concerned about the dangers faced by women in such situations.

Another incident was reported to have taken place in the North. A war widow had won custody of her children as well as those of her dead brother. A living brother felt that this eroded his authority because he should have been in charge of the children. He sought every opportunity to discredit her as a good guardian simply because she was a woman. One day he went to her home, quarrelled, beat her, and took her to an army prison. She was locked up and during the night she was raped by soldiers. In reaction to public admonitions that his actions had virtually sentenced her to an AIDS death, the brother said that he had only wanted to have her locked up for one night to 'teach her a lesson! but not to be raped.' Epidemiologists and local people suspect that soldiers are primarily responsible for transmitting AIDS to the North.

Women in focus group discussions felt that these two reported cases were not isolated incidents and that these are things that can happen to any woman at any time because social power is in the service and the hands of men. In one instance the woman was endangered while on a quest for reproductive health so she could bear children for her husband and thus validate her social worth; in the other, the woman was endangered by the male need to control women and to resort to force when traditional practices seem to be changing — in this case allowing a woman to be guardian to children in a patrilineal society.

THE IGNORED VOICE OF THE YOUNG

Men assume the responsibility of stating what societal norms are and what the women and the young are expected to do. Older women often support this dominant voice. So the young rarely get heard. In this research we sought to learn at first hand the students' views and perceived solutions to the AIDS pandemic.

In 1989, 98 high school students between 15 and 18, when asked to complete three projective essays, raised similar issues. Of the boys 74.40 per cent, and of the girls 42.10 per cent, mentioned the issue of rich men enticing young girls with money and gifts; 92 per cent of the boys and 52.60 per cent of the girls said that boys pressure girls to have sex with them. Also, to distinguish themselves from the dominant elite culture, which they presumably aspired to, 97.45 per cent of the boys and 52.60 per cent of the girls asserted that elites should know better than to contract HIV and die of AIDS. Most interestingly, the young wished to be tested, but our anthropological research project lacked blood testing or counselling resources, so the students were never tested.

The predominant view among adults is that parents cannot talk to young people about sex and condoms because they fall in the category of proscribed, taboo subjects, which cannot be broached without appearing to be promoting promiscuity among the young. The young people interviewed said that they know that older people disapprove of their knowing about sex, but they had in fact learned from their peers. This is true even in cases where parents are not taboo bound. One girl in a rural school said, 'By the time my mother talked to me about menstruation, sex, and pregnancy, I already knew about them from friends, but I did not tell her.' Another girl said, 'Once, when my mother was away for a long time because of an illness, my father told me to be careful and avoid sleeping with boys because I would get pregnant.' Still another girl gave credit to a Catholic priest for having taught her and her peers, 'that since sex seemed to be unavoidable, that it was important to learn ways of protecting ourselves.' These are important testimonials because they suggest that while in the dominant ideologies the sex education responsibilities are assigned to fathers' sisters or grandmothers, some parents in fact do talk to their children about sex and its consequences. Furthermore, some priests do not engage in moralistic escapism and are willing to deal with the reality that young people engage in sex and offer them alternatives to the inevitable pregnancies and ruined educational opportunities.

This was an encouraging finding. The point here is that young people learn from their peers, and the sex taboo words are learned as early as 10 years of age. In Rakai, a Luganda-speaking district, schoolchildren, women, and men in segregated focus groups said that they had learned the rude body and sex words at an early age. For example, *kutoomba* (to fuck) and *kuziina* (to dance a woman) were often cited. But we found that people found it acceptable in mixed gender and age groups to use *kwegatta* (to unite, to come together) in reference to heterosexual acts. This represents a triumph for Victorian prudery. The bible translation used this sanitized word, and it is acceptable. The point is not to shock people with the rudest words, but to encourage parents, children, men, and women to talk about sex in ways that are not uncomfortable for them. It is important for researchers to discover how parents impart to their children correct information about sex and sexuality so as to discourage most of the peer misinformation imparted *sub rosa* during attempts to master rude words tabooed by adults.

The young regard the older men as hypocritical because they are aware of their peccadillos with other women and young girls. One of the influential priests who is most vocal in condemning condoms and promiscuity is regarded, even by some parents, as a hypocrite. He wants the young to control their sexual urges, but people point out that he was promiscuous even in his 30s when he was already a 'saved Christian' (Mulokole). His moral crusade irritates his colleagues, who are privately contemptuous of his zealotry.

In 1992, in order to gauge the way young people conceptualized sex, sexuality and HIV transmission, a catholic school near Kampala was selected. This choice was influenced by the fact that the headmaster was concerned with the issues of AIDS and the young, he had a good relationship with both the lay teachers and the nuns, and he enjoyed the respect of the community.

There were focus group discussions with students in the cohort age groups of 9 to 13 and 14 to 18. The 9 to 13 age cohort was selected because it was presumed that they were on the threshold of sexual involvement (although, in fact, some had already experienced sex). The 14–18-year-old cohort was assumed to be sexually active and, therefore, most vulnerable to HIV infection. A total of ninety students were involved in focus groups of 15 each. In all groups the general question for discussion was: 'What should we do about the problem of AIDS that is threatening all of us, particularly the young people?' Below are the answers provided by thirty 9 to 13 year olds. There were only four girls in this age category, and they did not talk.

'We hear AIDS is spread through sex; let's give up sex.'
'Our priest says sex is bad for our salvation.'
'I hear sex is good and I do not think we should miss out on it.'
'I think it is only adults who get AIDS.'
'I will avoid anything that might expose me to AIDS.'
'We are still young, nothing can happen to us.'
'I think we are all going to perish.'

There were 60 students in the 14–18-year-old category and thirteen of these were girls.

'Sex is fun and we would not have been born without it.'
'We are told AIDS is spread through sex so we must protect ourselves.'
'We will not marry.'
'If you say you don't want sex, then your friends will abandon you.'
'We cannot forego sex when everyone among our friends is enjoying it.'
'All young people should be forced to use condoms.'

'But condoms are only 98 per cent protective so they are not a
solution.'
'One should have sex with people one knows well.'
'It is difficult to know everyone well.'
'It is sad when we are told that sex is dangerous and there are so many
beautiful girls around.'
'It is difficult for us girls because boys are always pressing us to sleep
with them.'
'We boys must stop pressuring girls to sleep with us.'
'We spend all the time tricking, begging and making girls have sex.'
'I think it is the adult men who spoil girls. Teachers, businessmen
and politicians are stealing girls from us.'
'Rich mean are a menace. They give girls money and AIDS and
then we get it.'

After the first focus meetings with each group of the 14 to 18 year
olds, 100 condoms were left in the room and some students took
some. In the second meeting, some male students raised issues about
the proper way to put on condoms and whether, instead of one, one
should use two or three for maximum protection. By the fourth
meeting, 100 condoms did not seem enough for the male students in
each group. The girls were curious but they never took the condoms.
In subsequent meetings, students were showing up with their non-
school male friends — houseboys, gardeners, hawkers, etc.[6]

It would seem that all the students had knowledge about sex and
that it was the primary mode of HIV transmission; and they were
willing to protect themselves. The students had heard of condoms
through the public debates, but few had actually seen them. They
were curious and open-minded. They discovered that until a cure for
the HIV virus is found, condoms offered the best solution. Consequently they voluntarily sought advice on how to use condoms.
Perhaps the results would have been different if we had merely
lectured about the dangers of sex and the need for protection against
HIV. They also believed that it is adults only who die of AIDS. The
students had heard from their peer groups and some even from
experience that sex is enjoyable. They felt that it was worth doing
something about something one enjoyed. If the students were indeed
using the condoms they were taking, we were pleasantly surprised
that they had not learned and internalized the view about sex being
less pleasurable with condoms (as adult men who feel that it is a
man's right to have pleasurable sex no matter what may occur). All
this suggests that, despite the anti-condom stance of the religious
leaders and indifference by politicians, young people are willing to

take a chance with condoms because they say it is a matter of 'our survival.' Interestingly, the girls were shy of taking condoms even after the boys in the discussion groups said that they would put on condoms if asked by their girlfriends. The girls said that men do not want women who use condoms because they are not good women. These girls, probably like all other girls, had internalized the assumptions of the dominant ideology. The boys insisted that they were willing to work on saving the youth but that the greatest danger was the older men who are both unwilling to wear condoms and to leave the younger girls alone.

What is needed is transformation education, whereby the youth learn about the mechanism of wearing and properly disposing of condoms; social analysis of the social practices that can result in HIV transmission, and the effective way of practising safe sex. Above all, the young, particularly the girls, must learn the social skills of negotiating safe sex. AIDS education programmes must promote the engagement of both girls and boys in identifying the issues and solutions. The true adaptation of condoms depends upon both boys and girls (future men and women) feeling comfortable about introducing them in a sexual encounter.

CONCLUDING REMARKS

This chapter has mapped out the different cultural ideologies manifested as voices that must be understood in order to devise strategies for curbing HIV transmission. The dominant ideology stresses morality, chastity, and monogamy as more effective solutions to HIV transmission than condoms, which are deemed to promote promiscuity. In the final analysis, those who break the sexual moral code must pay with death. On the other hand, there are the silent voices of women and the private voices of the young. These seem to be unarticulated cultural voices, based in the realm of action. Women feel powerless and vulnerable because they are dependent upon the willingness and co-operation of men to wear condoms in order to be protected against HIV transmission. Because men have the power to 'choose' women and women are socialized to be 'available,' men have access to young girls, their wives, as well as other women. Women feel that these practices overexpose them to HIV transmission. Because of the dominant ideology that divides women into 'good' and 'bad,' most women are unable to insist that men wear condoms without risking being thought of as promiscuous. The silence of women starts when they are young girls. Education for transformation must break this silence. When women can discuss their sexuality with men, and the threat of HIV to their health, then they will not solely be vehicles for men's sexual desires and procreativity. This is a great opportunity to deconstruct the cultural constructions of male and female sexuality. In this way, self-respect, honesty, and social responsibility to one's sexual partners and community become an aspect of the ongoing process of cultural change. After all, culture is a dynamic instrument for survival.

NOTES

1. Researchers, in an attempt to use accurate words for sexual intercourse so that condom programmes would not carry ambiguous messages, have often ended up with words that are offensive and taboo. Little attention has been paid to the impact of Christianity and Western education in shaping people's sensibilities. In our research we found that sanitized words, which were the product of Victorian prudery at the turn of the century, were acceptable as unambiguous by different groups and also suitable for mixed intergenerational group discussions.

2. This chapter is based upon three field trips between 1989 and 1992, totalling 20 months. Research has been done in two rural areas in the central and eastern provinces; in two factories in the industrial town of Jinja and the capital city Kampala. In Kampala work has been done among elites and adolescents.

3. A social scientist working for a Foreign Medical Council project illustrated the detachment of researchers at the 1990 AIDS in Africa Conference in Kinshasa, Zaïre: 'We are only doing research to know what is going on. If people ask us, we all give them condoms or tell them the HIV test result.'

4. In recent years the Uganda government has encouraged the participation of women in politics; yet in village meetings, women sit behind the men and usually say nothing unless prompted. In the urban areas in elite neighbourhoods, women sit alone and are expected to be knowledgeable, even when they occupy such positions as local treasurer.

5. In the capital city, Kampala, two elite men who live openly as polygamists are the butt of ongoing amusement among elites, especially the women. The men both claim to be practising Catholics, they are active in many civic organizations, they are well travelled and do not drink alcohol. One is a civil servant; he has two wives who rotate between his rural homestead, and his city home. The other is a busi-

ness tycoon with four wives, including a French one; one wife is in charge of the rural homestead which is as grand as the city one.

6. The next stage of the research project is to involve the parents and other community leaders, particularly the priests and the resistance committee members in deciding the solutions.

REFERENCES

Ardener, E. 1975. Belief and the Problem of Women. In: *Perceiving Women,* edited by S. Ardener. London: Dent.

Fee, E., and D.M. Fox, eds. 1988. *AIDS: The Burden of History.* Los Angeles: University of California Press.

Obbo, C. 1992. *Needs, Demands and Resources in Relation to Primary Health Care in Kampala.* Kampala: Save the Children Fund.

Obbo, C. 1993a. HIV Transmission: Men Are the Solution. *Population and Environment* 14(3):211–243.

Obbo, C. 1993b. HIV Transmission Through Social and Geographic Networks in Uganda. *Social Science and Medicine* 36(7):949–955.

Chapter
FIVE

Sexuality, AIDS and Gender Norms Among Brazilian Teenagers

Vera Paiva

The low efficacy of attempts to reduce sexual transmission of HIV is basically due to mistakes which have already been globally identified in many countries of the Third World. Decisions regarding public prevention policies have not taken account of the relevant sexual culture, particularly the social and cultural context of sexual decision making. Public prevention measures have not gone beyond providing general information on HIV transmission and have not stimulated the development of skills to ensure protection. The emphasis has been on individual decision making and motivation, based on notions of autonomy and the individual's sense of responsibility — notions which are not appropriate in many countries (Elias 1991).

In Latin American countries like Brazil, we have apparently forgotten our tradition of popular education for freedom — the experience of grassroots movements in dealing with health and counselling. Where, for example, were the representatives of the Brazilian feminist tradition, who have done so well for at least a decade in dealing with sexuality, the erotic and the reproductive body? I believe that we were paralysed by the way this disease has been socially constructed; a construction based on fear and promiscuity, perceiving the disease as life-threatening while simultaneously seeing it as a problem faced only by the 'different others,' by 'groups at risk.' People in my country who have received a long training in popular education or community development have followed a path which can be typified in the words of a leader in a community of poor women:

> I used to think AIDS had to do only with rich people and TV stars. I had to worry about food, violence, unemployment, street children, homeless people ... lots of things! Poverty, that's it. But one day I realized that people around me were getting ill and were dying. Goodness gracious! It's such an ugly death! So I spent a lot of time thinking without wanting to think.... And now this!!!

Developing the tools required to face this challenge has been a hard task. For the feminists who fought to claim a woman's right to pleasure, questioning the narrow limits imposed on feminine sexuality, it was difficult to maintain a defence of sexual and reproductive freedom in this new, restrictive context.

> How can one suit one's speech to the new, perturbing reality of statistics that show a progressive spread among women? How can one provide information to 7 million sterilized women who must now use condoms? How does one convince sexual partners to use a method they have systematically refused? For many years, feminism has aimed to dissociate condom use from disease and prostitution, so how do we relate its use to the prevention of AIDS and other STD's without going back to where we started? How do we deal with the information that sexual and menstrual fluids also transmit the virus when we fought so hard to deconstruct the image of the feminine genitals as something dirty and related to disease? (Barbosa 1992)

Some changes in this scenario, especially in São Paulo, have to do with the frightening growth and the profile of this new epidemic: impoverishment; the increasing number of young people, women, and children becoming infected and the rapid spread of HIV due to (hetero)sexual intercourse, which is a proportionally rising trend. In São Paulo in the period from 1980 to 1994, there were 5,894 AIDS cases among women (out of a total of 34,215). In 1985 38 men were infected for every woman. In 1994 the ratio was 4:1. Among women, 50.1 per cent of newly notified AIDS cases in 1994 were sexually transmitted, while drug use accounted for 28 per cent, and infected blood for around 1.7 per cent. In 12 per cent of the cases the means of transmission has not been determined. Notifications of the disease have revealed that 47.1 per cent of infected women are between 15 and 30 years old, compared to 35.8 per cent of men in the same age range. The fastest spread of AIDS within the female population is found among married women and women whose partners use intravenous drugs (Centro de Vigilancia Epidemiológica 1994).[1]

Which social and cultural context forms a background to all this? How is it possible to induce the psychosocial changes which may help people understand the risks of HIV infection and identify acceptable options for themselves and their partners among the safe sexual practices which prevent AIDS? How can we offer support to people who have decided to change their sexual practices? These are, in my opinion, the challenges faced by researchers in the psychosocial field.

THE CONTEXT OF SEXUAL DECISION MAKING IN BRAZIL

To even begin to address these problems in Brazil, we must understand the hegemonic sexual subculture, made up of multiple ideological subsystems (see Parker 1991). We can point to at least five distinct subsystems: (1) a patriarchal gender ideology with its feminine/passive and masculine/active polarities; (2) the Jewish/Christian discourse based on the Iberian tradition, the important values of which are marriage, monogamy, and procreative sex; (3) the discourse on social hygiene dating from the 19th century, which defines sexuality as either healthy or sick; (4) the discourse on 'the modern science of sex,' which emphasizes scientific information about sex, individual choice, and personal truth; and (5) the erotic ideology which defines the Brazilian people as sensual and seductive, with a 'breach-the-norm-to-have-pleasure' principle. This latter subsystem became more powerful with the rise of the great urban centres in the 20th century, but has always worked as a counter-system together with the other subsystems.

The first four subsystems are well-known, since they were introduced by the white colonizers' culture. The erotic ideology has to do with carnival, body exhibition, and sex and seduction, and has been shown for the last decade without restriction and at peak viewing times by the nationwide TV networks. It is this attitude that allows the popular culture to assert, 'There is no sin under the Equator' or

'Within four walls, everything is permitted.' Private life is considered to be sacred (see Parker 1991). The ideology of the erotic body and *sacanagem* (a sometimes playfully used Brazilian slang expression for amoral acts especially of a sexual nature) is interwoven with a sense of individual responsibility and citizenship. It cries out against corruption and the double moral standards of, for instance, politicians, but ignores the individual's own small acts of corruption in the everyday life of the Brazilian social world (O Estado de São Paulo, 20 June 1992). The individual never asks himself, 'What can I do for my country?' but always demands what the country, meaning the state, 'can do for me.'

When the public sphere is penetrated by the private sphere, a well-known script is repeated: the appropriation of what is impersonal by what is personal. The abstract is captured by the concrete, the subjective conquers the objective, the collective is surrendered to the private (see Holanda 1986). The reader may imagine how little legitimacy public authorities acquire in the sacred domestic ambience, where sexuality and love games reside.

Data collected during our research seem to show that seduction is a prerequisite to convincing oneself or one's partner to use a condom. No silence; talking is a must. It is not natural to stop the stream of passions, to rationalize feelings in the context of sexual life. The condom causes feelings of strangeness; it symbolizes an accusation. When proposing the use of a condom, one has to ask, kindly and charmingly. It is impossible to demand because then one becomes disagreeable and unreliable. 'I don't use condoms because I know him.' In Brazil, an acquaintance rapidly becomes an intimate. Based on the same confidence that allows one to see small infidelities as 'natural things,' risk is won over and denied — by affection in the women's case or by blind impulsiveness, which is more common among men. A dual morality is accepted naturally in the world of men, the public world. A woman must be more responsible for the coherence between the public and private worlds. She is a prey to coherence. She belongs either to the mundane world with its double standard, or to the household world. In a large city like São Paulo, unwanted pregnancy is quite easily solved by (illegal) abortion. AIDS remains someone else's problem.

The majority of studies that attempt to clarify the social and cultural context within which decisions about sexuality and/or reproduction are made have many points in common. They indicate that the changes which are publicly recommended to protect people against HIV infection directly threaten the notions of virility and femininity shared by almost all the subgroups within the Brazilian population, especially those belonging to the lower classes.

Condom use confronts the basic notion of virility which asserts that *being a man* is to possess less control over one's sexual and aggressive impulses — to feel them more strongly than a woman. To wear a condom, to rationalize or rule one's sexual drive, or to take the female partner into consideration is to betray one's masculine nature. *Being a woman* is to be more fragile, less aggressive and to be able to control one's sexual drive — to be ignorant about sex until one gets married, and then to conform to one's husband's desires.

> A man learns about sex on the street, his domain, and a woman learns about it at home with her man. A man learns about sex with the street woman, a slut or a whore. The single young woman must *always* say *no* and the married woman must *never* say *no*. For a woman, talking about sex or offering a condom is to show that she is wiser than the man and means that she will be taken for a street woman. It is to abandon the traditional feminine discourse focused on dating and getting engaged followed by sexual activity. (Brasil 1992)

A woman has to be ready for sex but should also be naïve and never take the initiative (Coureau 1992). Despite several — partly TV-induced — changes in notions about sexuality and gender among the more liberal urban middle classes, the woman's negotiating capacity is still limited by a lack of power within the relationship. Men still determine the modality and the rhythm of sexual intercourse. 'Dealing with a risk associated with the exercise of sexuality is something that belongs so closely to feminine identity and everyday life that if the social, economic, and cultural costs are too high a woman will naturally decide to take the risk' (Barbosa 1989).

Safe sex is sex without conception. The decision regarding the use of condoms or other contraceptive methods is taken in a cultural context in which motherhood is still essential to the construction of the feminine identity (Barbosa 1989; Paiva 1990). We know that condom use is more consistent when the desire to avoid pregnancy is added to the purpose of preventing AIDS. But in Brazil use of condoms is frequently restricted to short periods when the existence of a pathological process in a man or a woman requires the interruption of other contraceptive methods (Barbosa et al. 1991; Guimarães et al. 1991). Condoms are associated with the prevention of pregnancy — for which they are not considered to be particularly effective — and with promiscuity, clandestine sex, and AIDS — in which case they are considered efficient.

The AIDS epidemic also influences decision making about sex. Everyone knows about AIDS and knows that sexual intercourse can cause infection. Virtually all studies point out that talking about AIDS involves talking about the fear that AIDS brings to mind. It is like a frightening shadow — the materialization of the old spiritual or psychological contamination that comes from 'impure' and 'dangerous' people. Within the context of a love affair or of sexual passion an attitude of denial, restricting consciousness in order not to feel guilt in the face of the sensual body, is still common. Furthermore, most official authorities on prevention guidelines, in particular the majority of medical doctors, have constructed an idea of AIDS based on a morbid and accusatory attitude towards the 'promiscuous practices' of those infected. They are representatives of the collective ignorance, prejudice, and taboo surrounding sexuality. Criminally, this causes many people to remain at risk while believing that they are not (see Paiva 1992).

THE SEXUAL CULTURE OF POOR ADOLESCENTS IN SÃO PAULO

The remainder of this chapter is based on research and intervention work aimed at AIDS prevention among 14–20 year olds in a poor region of São Paulo City.[2] Our aim is to develop a proposal that will have an impact on teenagers' everyday life. Therefore we need to talk about pleasure as much as about responsibility. We need to deal with AIDS prevention in a way that will not drive away their curiosity about sexual experience but which does convince them of the risks involved in not protecting themselves against HIV — a way that offers creative spaces where individual choices can be made. We need to provide information, counselling and discussion on relationships between the sexes — a key obstacle to changing unsafe practices.

In August 1991 we began a two-year study, interviewing 30 boys and girls for about two hours, with a schedule of questions encompassing six major topics. Each interview began with free conversation, without direct questions from the interviewer, whose initial request was, 'Tell me about your life.' The interview then developed according to a semi-structured script covering gender ideology, dating, sexuality, drug use and AIDS. In 1992, using information based on analysis of these interviews, we set up 'face-to-face' groups with nearly 5,000 teenagers from this community and from other poor districts of São Paulo.[3]

The first association made by these young people in relation to AIDS is with 'death,' 'disgrace,' and 'fear.' The city districts where they live have a high incidence of AIDS. Almost all of them know someone who has died of AIDS. They think that everyone is at risk, but paradoxically the majority also believe that *they* themselves are not at risk because of their way of life. They choose their partners carefully ('not a whore, a drug addict, or a homosexual'), and they have reduced the frequency of intercourse as a protection against HIV. They do not use condoms, however. Reasons given by the boys include confidence in the female partner, dislike of condom use, or even simply because they forgot to buy them (they are expensive!). Among the girls the main reasons for not using condoms were confidence in the male partner or his reluctance in using them (see Bedoian et al. 1992).

Girls

We can observe some similarities in the subjects discussed by the girls in the interviews and groups, despite individual differences. Families still bring up their girls basically in the old-fashioned way. They stay at home where they belong, and their going out is controlled, as well as their virginity. These are families of rural origin that depend on the income of all their working members, so girls are allowed to work and study but they may not stay out too long. One of the girls interviewed reported that her mother took her to the doctor in order to get a certificate of virginity because she stayed on the street too much and everybody gossiped about her.

When we asked, 'What does being a woman mean to you?' the answers varied: being dedicated to love and home life, keeping away from certain places, moderating their language, being fragile and crying easily, controlling their impulses, keeping themselves for the right man. Men, according to the girls, are all alike: they are naturally more aggressive, with no control, they do what they want to do, they think only about sex, they want to take advantage of women, they are more suited to heavy work and to street life. When choosing a boyfriend, criteria such as being steady, honest, serious, and having a family are important to the girls, as is being a loving and understanding person. Many girls think about what a man has to offer in 'exchange' for their fidelity, virginity, or dedication. They are attracted to the idea of 'equal rights' for men and women, and so they think that being a woman also means that they 'have to be strong' in order to face this new reality.

In relation to their own bodies, girls know very little about the way reproductive or contraceptive processes work — and even less about the erotic body. The changes occurring in the boys' bodies are also a mystery to them. They get no information at home and they are ashamed to talk about it with friends. Most of them have already had sexual intercourse (65 per cent) but they either do not know what an orgasm is or have never experienced it. They do not masturbate, do not like anal or oral sex, and believe that when sex is involved the man must take the initiative. Sex for them means penetration (Antunes et al. 1992).

The majority think that virginity is worthwhile. They clearly distinguish street life from home life. A woman who loses her virginity is at risk of becoming a 'street' woman or a 'slut.' To be a 'slut' is to be prohibited from choosing a man to save her from the family's poverty, to climb to a higher status. The street woman, the slut, is also a threat to other women; she's the one who never says no, who 'steals my man and passes on diseases,' including AIDS, from the street to home. The girls think faithfulness is important, but they accept a certain degree of male infidelity.

The first thing that these girls associate with sex is 'love' or 'prohibition.' The majority grow up listening to other women who say that sex is bad, that it hurts the first time, and that it is dangerous because of the risk of pregnancy, but that they have to do it well since, 'if a woman doesn't know how to do it, a man will search for another woman.' The girls themselves consider sex to be something good, but nevertheless feel themselves to be under pressure to comply with male demands. One 'has to pretend to be willing to avoid being deserted.' 'A man thinks only about having fun, and a woman only about getting married.' If they do not allow a man to 'caress' them, they are accused of being 'cold.' If they object to the fact that the man has to take the initiative, they are nonetheless ashamed to make the first move. They endorse the rule which asserts that a woman always has to say no and a man always has to conquer, to besiege, since a man who doesn't behave this way is a 'queer' — he doesn't like women.

There is a great deal of ambivalence among the girls who have lost their virginity outside the context of dating or engagement. Almost all of them assert that they were deceived or forced, but usually describe situations that they helped to create. They seem not to feel responsible for their own desires. In stating this, it is not our intention to deny the extensive violence existing in this community. Pressure to exchange sex for money or gifts is always present. Many girls, when asked, 'What is normal sex?' replied, 'Sex without violence.' The majority also found heterosexual sex to be normal.

Some complain quite a lot about the boring life of a housewife. They want to be independent of their parents, although they are devoted to them, with much respect and obedience. Others want to play, to enjoy life, hiding it from the family. Sometimes beauty and sex appear to be a way to seduce and to achieve a higher status — to be a model or to marry a rich man. They want to have children. Some say, 'A woman stays alone at home,' 'A child is a companion,' or 'Dating and a child are things to pass the time.'

Boys

The boys' discourse is perfectly meshed with that of the girls. Being a man is 'being born this way': having a penis, liking women. They distinguish themselves as men in front of other men: 'I'm a man because I don't like queers and I like women' — not because they are different from women. Being a man is behaving and speaking like a man, being strong, thinking a lot about sex, having fun: 'playing ball, catching a woman.' But also, in the future, being a man means being respectful, restrained, tender, and patient with women simply in order to get married. Then he must improve professionally, keep his word, be honest, and work hard. Being marginal or a drug addict, which is common within this community, is a danger which everyone knows well. It means the end of illusions about a future, which already seems something fragile and of little hope to them.

Most boys have already taken part in fights or have been involved in other violent or illegal activities as accomplices. Many are acquainted with cases involving confrontation between the marginal outsider and the honest man. They know about police abuse and violence among bandits. Almost all of them know someone — whether a family member or a neighbour — associated with murder or other forms of illegal activity. Many talk of having 'a confused past' including the use of drugs, which they fortunately rejected. Clearly they also need to control their impulses — which are aggressive and consumption-oriented: 'We want to have things.' They rebel against the lack of leisure and work opportunities.

With regard to their gender identity, boys have a precise idea of what it is to be men in a male world, where their values fit in well. What they think and do is what every man in the world does. There is little margin for doubt — it works like this and that's it. Girls are more likely to question their world, its values, its truths.

The boys think that sex is something good. All of them masturbate and like all kinds of sex (oral, anal, vaginal). They feel a great deal of anxiety until they do it for the first time, and afterwards they feel more experienced, more in control. They learn about it on the streets, talking to friends and to the 'street women.' Sex is something 'everyone does.' They distinguish between sex with love and sex for 'relief.' There is a strong belief that not having sex for a long time is harmful: 'It goes up to your head.' That is why women must be available. Masturbation is viewed as something natural. Sperm is almighty, it is pure fecundity: 'If you come into the girl, she gets pregnant.' Their greatest concerns are to 'come outside' and to choose their partners well in order to avoid an STD or AIDS.

For the boys, there are two kinds of women. The first kind includes the women they can date or marry. She must be honest and steady in character, show herself only to him, be marriageable, have a beautiful face and body, and be well known. The other kind are the 'bitches' who stay on the street. They are easy to 'get,' promiscuous and pass on diseases. They are a good target for unleashing one's aggressive impulses. The boys do not want to marry young. They want experience and to have many women. They complain about women's jealousy since they intend to be faithful only after getting married, to find a good job, and to be able to 'give my children a better life.' A woman has to be tough but not necessarily a virgin. A virgin is preferable, but the boys do not believe that there are many left.

The boys believe they must have their wits about them, know about everything and not be fools. They are afraid of peer pressure; that became very clear during the group discussions. They do not easily admit ignorance of topics related to sex — they prefer either silence or fabrication. Only after much perseverance from us did they start to reveal their doubts, and then only in the absence of the girls. It is important to them not to be a virgin, to be a lady-killer, and not to be gay. They know very little about a woman's body (most boys think the fertile period is during menstruation, and that a woman ejaculates every time she has sex, just as boys do). Pregnancy is, in general, a woman's problem. Neither girls nor boys admitted to having an STD. But 25 per cent of the boys and girls have either caused pregnancy or become pregnant. Half of the pregnancies ended in spontaneous or induced abortion, the other half were brought to term either within or outside marital union.

'SAFER SEX, REPRODUCTION AND
AIDS' WORKSHOPS

What sort of intervention is most suitable on the basis of analysis of this data? We chose face-to-face intervention, with separate groups for boys and girls, but ensuring at least one final session where they could work together. It was clear that we had to go beyond a discussion of AIDS and deal with the erotic and reproductive body and with contraception.

We carried out four 3-hour sessions with boys and girls in separate groups. This makes it easier to explore gender roles, which can be especially rigid during adolescence. Only in the fifth session did the boys and girls work together. This final session, suggested by the young people themselves, was an exceptionally creative learning process.

After a pilot study, we began to develop our workshop model — a face-to-face group for 15 participants, chosen from 100 students from the district. During the first session, after introducing and discussing the rule of respecting each other's differences and the need for confidentiality, each participant answers a questionnaire (which has been evaluated as being a powerful instrument for promoting thought on sexuality and risk taking). We ask them questions about gender roles, dating, sexual partners, frequency of unsafe practices and condom use, knowledge and use of contraceptive methods, alcohol and drug use, attitudes towards AIDS and preventive guidelines, their own efficacy in communicating and negotiating about sex, and HIV testing. On completing the questionnaire participants are often visibly moved, especially concerning their doubts and feelings.

After this self-awareness exercise we develop the sessions further, using various techniques to identify vocabulary, knowledge, prejudices, group norms etc. These techniques are based on Paulo Freire's (1982) method, the work of Pichon Riviere (1988), and psychodrama techniques, and are inspired by other Brazilian community-based education and intervention procedures. We take advantage of techniques employed by the women's health and reproductive rights movement when dealing with the discovery of the erotic body, and providing information about AIDS, reproduction, and contraception (see Núcleo de Investigaçao da Saúde da Mulher/Casa da Mulher do Grajau 1992). We encourage free debate between the participants, making up stories, using a clipboard to introduce AIDS-related topics, videos, activities with flour and salt paste to shape the reproductive body and the genitals, role-playing, and games with contraceptive methods. We talk about safer sex practices and fantasize about pleasant ways to have safe sex between men and women, men and men, and women and women. We play with condoms, attempting to make the condom a commonplace. We stimulate the use of words and slang which they normally use to refer to things, as well as providing them with the 'scientific' names.

The goal of the workshop, previously discussed with the group, is to get to know more about AIDS prevention, working through feelings and acquiring tools to live a normal life (whatever 'normal life' means to each participant) in a world where AIDS exists. The discussion leader has a script in his head and some tested techniques, but works according to the themes as they emerge in each group. He organizes information, stimulates exchange, and ensures that emotions, prejudices, and difficulties are made clear and understandable. The group itself carries on the discussion, confronting and elaborating and creating individual or collective answers. At the final meeting reactions are usually enthusiastic. Some students cry because it is over, while others encourage us to carry on with this work. They also help us with work in their community. A statement made by one of the teenagers was adopted by everyone as a synthesis of this process: 'I feel more mature, lighter, and broader.'

The differences between the girls' and the boys' groups are remarkable. The girls, virgin or married, conservative or liberal, are more spontaneous and tend to remain in the group until the end. The virgin boys always pretend to be smart or experienced and are more tempted to leave the group. If we did not work through the theme of homosexuality, the boys with bisexual experiences would be practically expelled from the group. A typical speech (made at the opening of a session involving a pact of secrecy and respect for differences) was, 'Don't take me wrong, but if there's a queer in here he'd better leave 'cause I hate queers.' This was followed by silence in the group.

In the girls' groups, on the other hand, the tendency is more towards acceptance. For example, after a debate with lots of complaints about men, their indifference and infidelity, their lack of responsibility towards sex, one of the girls declared she liked women and actually lived with another woman. It seemed strange at first and aroused much curiosity but no repression. In the next session when the group came back to this subject, another girl told the group she was a lesbian. We worked as always: suggesting that they personify the characters who are their imaginary companions and speak through them to the group. We sometimes use pillows or any other thing we can put in the middle of the room. Anyone can change and be the character represented by the pillow (the lesbian in this case). Everybody does it. They can have discussions with their own internal characters, feel themselves in the place of the other, understand their own fantasies, etc. In this way, the participants do not need to fight with each other directly. They can also speak out while preserving their own privacy by speaking through an 'imaginary' character. The group in our example ended by abandoning the expression *sapatao* (a derogative word for lesbian) and replacing it with *entendida* (the native word used in both the male and female homosexual world).

The girls usually become friends and accomplices, with many secrets that they could not share with men. They love to learn how the body works, in particular the parts that can provide pleasure. Many of them go home and look at their genitals for the first time. They are happy to get more information about contraceptive methods and the condom. Thinking about men's infidelity is painful, as it makes them realize that they are at risk. Role-playing activities which show the difficulties of negotiating condom use or contraceptive devices are less confrontational than those performed by the boys, showing very clearly that the girls have little power to face male accusations of being street women if they seem knowledgeable or can communicate freely about sex. Girls do not want to be seen in this way, even if they are already classified as street girls by the boys. The typical scene where they have to demand the use of a condom by the husband or regular partner is generally resolved by asking him to wear a condom in his extramarital relationships.

In the boys' group the pressure is much greater: they have to like women very much, they have to be quick-witted. It is hard for them to ask for information or to admit to ignorance. They take less advantage of the opportunities to clarify points. They are well aware of the reasons for wearing a condom but are often heard to say such things as, 'Ah, it's just like having a candy without unwrapping it.' On the other hand, they are fascinated with games and proposals for making the condom erotic, with the use of lubricants to lessen contact with the latex, and with debates on the feminine orgasm, the clitoris, and the vagina's elasticity (they think it gets loose when used often). They can grasp the discussion on cultural differences regarding gender, and they love role-playing activities involving safe sex negotiation. Talking about desire, convincing and seducing a woman is what they mostly want to learn. The greatest difficulties arise when negotiating deals with giving up penetrative sex, blind impulses, and replying to female accusations of being gay.

Among both boys and girls there is an especially strong conviction that if one knows and likes somebody there is no danger of contamination — the virus simply vanishes. Love makes it difficult to keep a critical distance.

Some scenes are emblematic during the process, marking the weight of gender differences. After a session in which we introduced the idea of making condom use erotic, the boys gathered at the school gate and talked excitedly. Suddenly they besieged our car playfully and asked, 'Are the girls talking about the same things? Do they use the same words? Condom, having a good fuck and everything? Look, we're gonna turn over this car.' In the following session they denied any feelings of aggression, agreeing that a woman must also be informed. They were very enthusiastic about the day the two groups were to come together. They denied feeling threatened by the girls' knowledge, or being influenced by the attitudes of their parents.

When the boys and girls did get together, the girls remained accomplices in their secrecy, apparently protecting themselves against the eternal classifying attitude of the boys: 'That girl is like this (a good marriage prospect, beautiful), the other is like that (a slut, ugly), etc.' The girls accused the boys several times of being irresponsible about love, the girls' desires, or pregnancy. When asked by the boys why they preferred older men, they said that more mature men did not make a habit of telling everybody about the relationship or about what they did with the girls. The girls exchanged meaningful looks, expressing their revenge.

Another remarkable scene occurred when I told the boys that we thought it would be better to have the next groups conducted by the male members of my team. They insisted that the feminine presence (myself and my student, who played the auxiliary ego in the role-playing) would be very much missed. In such situations, a woman's presence seems to suppress the atmosphere of competition and exhibitionism among men — they drive men to take things more seriously. In contrast to this, the girls do not want men in their group. It seems that the girls, isolated in the domestic world and separated by the classifying gaze of men, find pleasure in participating in something larger than their everyday experience. They can learn and share their doubts and feelings, whereas the boys seem to use this sharing within a male group in order to increase their perception of themselves as individuals.

Both boys and girls find enormous pleasure in revealing what they have learned, being able to talk freely about sex, being less ashamed, etc. They would come to us after a session to tell us about their experiences. They love the atmosphere of *sacanagem* (sexual mischief), foolish talk, eroticization, and excitement which arises in the group. Girls tend to experience these feelings more easily. Both boys and girls feel that they can remain faithful to their own values and ideas, whether liberal or conservative, during the process. We also received the support of both parents and teachers, with whom we have continuously discussed our ideas and methods.

When we decided to attempt this model of intervention we were aware of the danger of affecting an excessively conservative or patriarchal tone, but we nevertheless hoped that there would be openness on both sides, given the influence of the media and the erotic ethos that continually influences more traditional ideas. Although the weight of migrant, rural, and patriarchal culture is still enormous in this community, there is a permanent feeling of personal inadequacy. This is especially true among women, who find an opportunity to expand their boundaries in our groups, to escape from the seclusion of their home, to be in touch with new ideas, and to review attitudes.

It must be noted that the social and political context helps us understand the joy of participating in this work. The boys and girls who took part in these workshops see the neighbourhood as 'the ugliest place in Brazil.' It is violent, with lots of drugs, outsiders, weird things: 'tranvestites, whores, all kinds of marginal people.' They relate the legend that, 'down there' in the place called Baixada do Glicerio (the lowest part of the district) there is a cemetery 'because there are so many suicides and violent murders.' When they talk about their lives they refer to their youth as something which has already gone — too fast. They cannot play anymore, or have fun, for fear of becoming a marginal person who will suffer the everyday violence more intensely. Risks are permanent: lack of jobs, a bad health care system, unstable living conditions. AIDS is just another risk. The pleasures of sex, which are easy and free of charge, are seen as compensation by the men. Dating and having children give women a meaning in life.

In addition, in Brazilian culture, unlike that of North America, a person is considered to be worthiest because of his hours of fun and pleasure, and not because of his hours of work. We offer them the opportunity not only to have fun but also to regain some sense of citizenship, of 'belonging' to something and not feeling 'left out.' Typical reactions to the interview and the questionnaire were, 'I've learned a lot' (about myself) ... or 'I got things off my chest, I feel lighter.' Talking sets people free. They feel their worth as citizens.

The message presented by the slogans of the Health Ministry over the last decade, namely, 'If you're not careful enough, AIDS will catch you' or 'You cannot see HIV just by looking at a face,' are pointless. They provide no helpful instruments, and that is what people need, particularly in a society where fatalism abounds. 'After all, if I'm going to catch it, I'll catch it anyway, there's nothing I can really do about it,' stated one of the boys. This is consistent with the attitude that there is nothing to be done individually about hunger, poverty, and violence.

A face-to-face group seems to provide a creative space if one can guarantee respect for individual differences. Providing information and preventive guidelines, developing skills, and working through emotions can help us break down the socially constructed prejudices and fears that in the case of AIDS can literally be fatal. Outside this context, calls for individual responsibility are a waste of time.

In Brazil, we have no translation for the word 'empowerment.' The most effective tradition of popular education and grassroots organization speaks of 'oppression against liberation,' of 'rescuing (collective) dignity.' It speaks in terms of solidarity in the search for a better standard of living for everyone. It is nevertheless empowerment that this tradition of popular education actually proposes. And it is sexual empowerment, at least according to our experience in São Paulo, that offers the only effective response to the risks posed by HIV and AIDS.

ACKNOWLEDGEMENTS

I would like to thank Richard Parker, an inspiring mentor on this project, especially for his comments on this chapter. I would also like to thank the MacArthur Foundation for their support of this work.

NOTES

1. Approximately 71 per cent of Brazilian women with a partner between 15 and 54 years old do use some kind of contraceptive method. Out of this total, 44.4 per cent have been sterilized, and 41 per cent make use of hormonal contraceptives (pills) while only 1.8 per cent use condoms. Some studies indicate that the dream of many women today is sterilization, although this is illegal and often badly carried out in poor regions throughout Brazil. Brazil's fertility rate has dropped from 5.7

children per woman in 1970 to 3.3 in 1985, while population growth has dropped from 2.9 per cent in 1980 to 1.8 per cent in 1990 (Berquó 1989). We also know that 52 per cent of Brazilian women become pregnant before they are 22 years old and that, even though abortion is illegal, the number of women admitted to public hospitals in the City of São Paulo due to problems caused by induced abortion is higher than the number of women who give birth to a child in the same hospitals (Araújo 1991).

2. The first stage of the project involves students at an evening elementary school. Their mean age is 18.9 years for the girls and 17.6 years for the boys. Together, 90 per cent work during the day. The majority (55 per cent) come from families with an average income of up to 5 times the minimum wage (US$ 280 per month). Another 30 per cent come from families with an income ranging from 5 to 10 times the minimum wage (US$ 280 to 560 per month).

Half of these teenagers are migrants or children of migrants from the Northeast of Brazil. Most of their parents never went to school or did not complete their elementary education. The majority are non-practising Catholics, and 20 per cent have no religion. Other significant religions are Protestant/Evangelical, Buddhist, Afro-Brazilian religions, and spiritualism.

Among the girls, 33 per cent define themselves as negro, mulatto or dark-skinned, 53 per cent as white, 6.5 per cent as indigenous and 6.6 per cent as Asian. Among the boys, 45 per cent consider themselves to be negro, mulatto or dark-skinned, 47 per cent white and 5 per cent Asian. The remainder is unknown.

These young people come from a neighbourhood known for its large numbers of immigrants. It is considered to be a slum district with a high concentration of prostitutes, drug users, and dealers. Transvestites and homosexuals live here more openly than in most other districts.

3. This project is financed by the MacArthur Foundation and developed together with my students at Universidade de São Paulo: Camila Peres, Fernando Cipriano, Fernando Silveira, Graziela Bedoian, Maria Cristina Antunes, Odonel Serrano e Vladimir Stempliuk.

REFERENCES

Antunes, M.C., V. Stempliuk, F. Silveira, and G. Brajão. 1992. Sexualidade, Normas de Gênero e Crenças sobre AIDS entre adolescentes. Paper presented at XXII Reuniao Anual de Psicologia.

Araújo, M.J. 1991. A escolha de metodos anticoncepcionais para programas de planejamento familiar: a perspectiva das mulheres. Paper presented at the meeting of the Special Program for Human Reproduction by the World Health Organization, Geneva, February 1991.

Barbosa, R. 1989. Mulher e contracepção: entre o técnico e o politico. Ph.D. diss. Instituto de Medicina Social. Rio de Janeiro.

Barbosa, R. 1992. Feminismo e AIDS. Paper presented in the Women and AIDS Seminar, Instituto de Medicina Social, UERJ, June 1992.

Barbosa, R., A. Kalckman, T. Lago, and W. Villela. 1991. Aceitabilidade e efetividade de uso de diafragma entre mulheres de baixa renda em São Paulo: Resultados Parciais. São Paulo: Instituto de Saude.

Bedoian, G., F. Cipriano, and O. Silveira. 1992. A fala expontânea de adolescentes do centro de São Paulo. Paper presented at XXII Reuniao Anual de Psicologia da Sociedade Brasileira de Psicologia.

Berquó, E. 1989. A Esterilização feminina no Brasil hoje (Sterilization in Brazil today). Paper presented in the International Meeting on 'Women's Health: A Right to Be Conquered,' Brasilia, June 1989.

Brasil, V.V. 1992. Percepção de risco e possibilidades de prevenção da AIDS em mulheres. Paper presented at the Seminar Women and AIDS, Instituto de Medicina Social, UERJ, June 1992.

Centro de Vigilancia Epidemiologica. 1994. Boletim Epidemiologico (dezembro). São Paulo: Health Secretariat in the State of São Paulo.

Coureau, S. 1992. Mulheres, a epidemia do HIV e direitos humanos. Paper presented at the Seminar on Women and AIDS, Instituto de Medicina Social, UERJ, June 1992.

Elias, C. 1991. Sexually Transmitted Diseases and Reproductive Health of Women in Developing Countries, Working Papers No. 5. The Population Council.

Freire, P. 1982. *Pedagogia do Oprimido*. Rio de Janeiro: Editora Paz e Terra. (Published in English as *Pedagogy of the Oppressed*. London: Sheed and Ward, 1972.)

Guimarães, C.D., and V.V. Brasil. 1991. Criacao do Programa de Apoio Visando o Incentivo do Condom. Relatorio Fase I. Rio de Janeiro: BENFAM/ AIDSCOM (mimeo).

Holanda, S. Buarque de. 1986. *Raizes do Brasil*. Rio de Janeiro: Jose Olympio, 18th edition.

Nucleo de Investigaçao da Saúde da Mulher–ISSP e Casa da Mulher do Graja. 1992. Seguro Morreu de Velho. Video e manual de Treinamento. Projeto Mulher e AIDS: Sexo e prazer sem medo.

Paiva, V. 1990. *Evas, Marias e Litiths ... As voltas do feminino*. São Paulo: Brasiliense.

Paiva, V. 1992. *Em tempos de AIDS*. São Paolo: Summus Editorial.

Parker, R. 1991. *Bodies, Pleasures, and Passions. Sexual Culture in Contemporary Brazil*. Boston: Beacon Press.

Riviere, P. 1988. *O processo grupal*. São Paulo: Martins Fontes.

Chapter SIX

The Dynamics of Condom Use in Thai Sex Work with *Farang* Clients

Carla van Kerkwijk

Wholesale sex tourism, occurring since the 1970s from the industrialized West to Third World countries such as Thailand and the Philippines, has only in recent years become an important vehicle for the spread of AIDS. In Thailand the idea that AIDS was a *farang* or Westerners' disease to which Asians were genetically immune prevailed until the late 1980s (*The Nation*, 11 November 1987). Statistics seemed to support this belief. Infection was indeed noted in Thailand, but on a small scale and mainly among long-term foreign residents, in the homosexual circuit, and among hard drug users (see also Kammer et al., in this volume).[1]

Since then both the myth of immunity and the ideas concerning propagation have undergone drastic change. The breakthrough coincided with an anthropological field study which I carried out in 1989 and 1990 in Bangkok. This period was characterized by a relatively rapid change in disclosures concerning AIDS. At first, reports concerning HIV infection were reassuring for the average sex tourist, but towards the end of this period the first figures on widespread HIV infection among sex workers were made public. In February 1990 the first reports of high percentages of seropositive sex workers in Chiang Mai appeared in the *Bangkok Post*. An important distinction was made between the degree of infection in the brothel circuit, catering mainly to Thai clients (44 per cent), and the 'free' circuit for *farang* (5 per cent).[2] Although these unsettling statistics related mainly to the circuit for Thai men, they brought the risk of infection in the *farang* circuit much closer to home. At that time large-scale government information campaigns were already taking place, as well as education on the spot by EMPOWER.[3] In most Western countries mass media campaigns had been going on for some years.

At least towards the end of this period the necessary information concerning care to be taken when involved in unprotected sex was available in the sex tourist scene. The fact that care was not taken in many cases has to do with a number of diverse factors which will be analysed in this chapter. The specific character of this sex scene can be discovered only if one approaches the field with a minimum of prejudice, and attempts to operate as closely as possible to the people and places concerned. The complex of factors influencing actual condom use cannot be sufficiently charted by means of macro-research and surveys.[4] Microlevel data, for example longitudinal case studies on the daily practices of sex workers, provides indispensable supplementary information. Condom use can be effectively influenced only if one has a good picture of the specific characteristics of this particular sex work in this particular environment.

The most important aim of my study was to obtain the best possible overall view of the real daily lives of a small number of sex workers. For this purpose, it was necessary to be in long-term close contact with the scene, to hear the stories, and wherever possible to keep up intensive contacts with the actors in question. Diverse locations and working conditions are to be found within the tourist sex scene, depending on the nationality of the client. My focus groups were bar girls, free-lancers, and their Western customers. The style of the sex circuit for Arabs and Japanese is completely different from that of the *farang* circuit. The establishments catering mainly for Thai men are much more modest, although this circuit is much more extensive than that for the *farang*. It is mainly made up of brothels and massage parlours. The contacts are often short-lived and the sex workers service a large number of different clients. Prices are much lower than for *farang* clients and coercion is often used, both for entering and remaining in sex work and for not refusing clients. Unhygienic working conditions prevail.

Because working conditions were considerably better, condoms were used more in the *farang* circuit than in sex work with Thai men. Compared to heterosexual sex work in the West during the same period, safe sex was practised much less. This fact poses a number of questions relevant to AIDS prevention. The next sections outline the Thai sex scene for *farang*. In this context, the question of how analysis of the specific dynamics of this scene can provide indications leading to direct prevention will be answered.

THE TOURIST SEX SCENE

The Thai sex market for *farang* is a large field of commercial enterprise that is very important for the local economy. Its commercial nature can be seen in the numerous different settings where tourists can meet sex workers: in bars, discos, hotels, coffeeshops, barber shops, massage parlours, on the beach, or on the street; for 'high-class' encounters there are escort bureaus and international brothels. This particular market caters to human differentiation in sexual preferences: heterosexual men and women, homosexual men and lesbians, paedofiles and transsexuals — there seems to be something for everyone.

The sex market is large, easily accessible, flamboyant, and very cheap by Western standards. In Bangkok alone the sex circuit is very differentiated. The Patpong area represents the most extravagant scene for tourists. Sex on stage is a normal occurrence. Swindling customers is also routine. Areas like Nana's Plaza and Soi Cowboy are more moderate and in the bars customers are cheated less. Nevertheless, these stand in marked contrast with the composition of brothels for Thai men. The visibility of sex is greater in Western than in Thai culture. The circuit for *farang* makes specific use of this behaviour. All references to sexual excitement are much more explicit in this circuit: bare breasts, naked dancing, vibrator shows, and other 'on stage' sexual practices are not to be found in the circuit for Thai men. Thai behavioural norms prohibit the public show of sexuality. The appearance of the sex scene for *farang* is moreover based on a rather vulgar stereotype of Western taste, as can be seen in the 'banana' bars, 'ping-pong' shows, and the use of explicit language ('I love you, I fuck you'). On stage almost anything is possible.

The clothing worn by many sex workers is not distinguishable from that of the average Thai woman. One does not come across 'whorish' clothing, except in places where 'sex working clothes' are worn, e.g., in 'gogo' bars. Bras are still worn. The girls do their best not to look like prostitutes but are often dressed glamourously. Sexy lingerie is almost unknown; if nudity is unnecessary, girls do not undress. Thai norms play a strong role.

The relative openness of the sex business poses the question of how much sex work is institutionalized in the Thai society and to what degree sex workers are stigmatized. Officially, sex work is forbidden in Thailand, and sex workers can in principle end up in jail. The extent and visibility of the sex work circuit, however, makes it clear that the government operates a double standard. Even before the rise of sex tourism there was widespread and culturally tacitly accepted sex work for the inland market. As far as stigmatizing of sex workers is concerned, one needs to distinguish between their formal and their actual status: their formal status is at the bottom of the social ladder; their actual status is in practice partially defined by the fact that economic contributions to both the family and the state are recognized, a fact which ensures more 'behind the scenes' tolerance than would otherwise be expected. Of course the abundance of women on the employment market and the fact that 'ordinary' occupations are very poorly paid makes sex work attractive to many. Nevertheless sex workers often lead a double life. Relatives, parents and daughters have an unspoken rule that sex work activities are not to be mentioned. The women themselves say that they work in a restaurant or hotel, which is often partly true. Acquiring city ways and making acquaintance with foreigners, other countries, and other languages also compensate for the fact that they are sex workers (see also Meyer 1988:371).

Most Thai girls who work as prostitutes with *farang* are of rural origin. Some begin at the age of fourteen. The beginners are often naïve and modest and have little education. The circuit, however, has a clear formative influence. Girls who have worked longer on the scene are often assertive and have an eye for money and pleasure. This can also be associated with social class and level of development. Sex workers above thirty are seldom found. As a rule, one must 'make it' before reaching that age. My impression is that many girls come from broken families, are divorced themselves, and/or have children (see also Meyer 1988:321).

Country girls are presented with an example of a life of luxury by family or friends. Some go to visit a friend and 'acclimatize' themselves without beginning directly with sex work. Others begin with work in the tourist circuit or go on trips to 'guesthouses' for tourists. There they discover that sex can earn them a great deal of money. Some students have a 'sugar daddy.' How often this happens is difficult to document. The financing of a pretty dress is often repaid with sex. The step from here to real sex work is therefore not a large one. On the islands in particular, one finds many girls who associate with *farang* and are content if he pays for their food and lodging. These islands are also a holiday spot for girls who deal in sex tourism. Many girls 'acclimatize' themselves to the sex circuit here.

Women in the *farang* circuit are employed by a bar at a basic wage (often not enough to live on: between 700 and 2500 baht) as 'playgirls.'[5] The only addition to their wage is a percentage of the 'lady drinks' bought by their clients. If a client wishes to take a bar girl with him he has to pay a 'bar fine' (250 to 350 baht). The bar girl receives none of this money. The sexual transaction takes place exclusively between customer and bar girl. The average price for a night is between 500 and 1000 baht. In principle, sex takes place in his hotel room, except on Patpong, where rooms can sometimes be hired by the hour from the bar itself. Most bars have a manager who supervises the girls and helps them with problems. Free-lancers are not welcome in bars employing sex workers. They are tolerated only when brought by a customer or if they have worked in a certain bar and in that way are acquainted with the other girls. Otherwise, free-lancers frequent after-hours bars and coffeeshops that do not employ sex workers. If girls do not know each other, they don't talk to each other, even if they find themselves in the same workplace.

Particularly in the off-season, the relationship between supply and demand is such that the many who do not excel in beauty or assertiveness do not earn a great deal of money. The need to keep one's head above water leads to strong competition between the girls, which in turn influences the style of action: go for the customer and try to win him over as quickly as possible. There is also a great deal of rivalry as far as the customers themselves are concerned. The sex worker often does not see herself as a real 'prostitute' and considers her customer to be a boyfriend. She pressures him not to be a 'butterfly.' Nevertheless, the rule about keeping away from one another's customers is often broken. Where competition is strong the tendency is to advertise oneself by waiving the use of condoms if the customer so wishes.

The sex worker who services *farang* clients, in contrast to her colleague who services the Thai, is relatively free in her actions. She can, in principle, refuse a customer. Her relative freedom does, however, have its drawbacks. Protection from the bar is not available if she goes to a customer's hotel.

Characteristic of the role image of the Thai sex worker is that she provides a much broader service than her Western counterpart: varying from brief encounters exclusively for sex (she is often prepared to do more than her Western colleague) to comprehensive, providing a wide range of other nonsexual services. The Thai sex worker is very much a companion who provides a variety of services: from washing his socks to acting as travel guide and interpreter. This veils Western eyes to a certain extent to the commercial character of the sexual transaction. This form of service is a regular occurrence, but by no means all the girls are prepared to go this far.[6] On the level of sexual practice, kissing takes place which is considered to be unprofessional by Western sex workers and also not usual in Thai culture. A sex worker who does kiss is therefore easily regarded as not being engaged in work by her client. The Western sex worker keeps her contact limited and stylized. Within such strictly defined margins, wider emotional interactions are given less chance to develop.

A continuous stream of new girls at certain sex spots is also characteristic. The girls have quite a large degree of mobility in their sex work, both in terms of changing workplace as well as their extensive travels with foreign clients. Mobility is stimulated by the dominance of short-term goals (fun, food, etc.), changing clientele, development of relationships with clients, and the need to escape from time to time.

Such an extensive and richly variegated sex industry with such an important position in the employment market attracts girls with a great variety of personal characteristics. Nevertheless, Thai sex workers in general follow the rules of the 'modal' Thai personality model: easy-going, without too much emotional investment except in matters of pleasure, and not too articulate. Thai appear very friendly to Westerners. The function of this attitude is to remain aloof, but it gives the Westerner a very different impression. 'Paradoxically, emotional distance turns out to be perceived as affective closeness in the context of brief holiday encounters' (Meyer 1988:263). Emotional distance ensures a minimum of conflict during contacts. In this way, contacts between Thai sex workers and *farang* clients are supple and directed towards pleasurable activities. In this, Thai body language also plays a leading role. For the Thai this language provides an emotional screen, whereas the Westerner sees it as an expression of emotion. Most Westerners are neither prepared to look nor capable of looking behind this façade (ibid.).

Farang sex tourists come from a wide variety of backgrounds. Yet some patterns are visible. Composition of the client population differs to quite a large extent from the group that visits sex workers in their home countries. It is interesting that there seems to be little overlap between those who visit sex workers in the West and those who do so in Thailand. Sex tourists are often recidivists: many have made more than one sex trip to Thailand, 75 per cent also visit other exotic lands, and 50 per cent of these visit sex workers there (Kleiber et al. 1991:17–19).

Expansion of the tourist industry into the low-income countries has benefited from the growing interest of European blue-collar workers who have shifted the setting for their holiday pleasures from Spain to Thailand. The average educational level is lower than that of customers in the West (Kleiber et al 1991:14–15). The specific composition of the sex tourist group is important. For example, Western research has shown that socio-economic status and level of education and income are important factors influencing both knowledge and use of condoms in clients (Vanwesenbeeck et al. 1992).

It is striking that more unmarried and divorced men are involved as customers than in the West. This undoubtedly has to do with the nature of the services offered. Kleiber, in a study of German sex tourism found that customers describe themselves as 'losers', 'daddies', 'playboys', and 'lonesome riders' (Kleiber et al. 1991:20–21).[7]

AIDS: INFORMATION, MOTIVATION AND PREVENTION

In the sex scene for *farang*, information available on AIDS has been put into practice only to a limited degree by sex workers and their clients. I found little evidence of consistent condom use. Less than 20 per cent of the sex workers observed used them regularly, and then often only with short-term contacts. Even experienced girls used condoms not as protection against AIDS but against pregnancy, and even inconsistently. On more than one occasion a sex worker claimed to have used them while her client denied it. A majority used condoms occasionally for the first contact, but after a few days with the client they disappeared from the scene. Many sex workers became pregnant, despite the resulting considerable loss of income. Women who used the pill were inconsistent now and then, mainly due to the irregular lifestyle inherent in the *farang* sex scene: all-night binges with drink and drugs. One typical girl, despite years of sex work experience and two pregnancies, was anything but consequent in her use of contraceptives, certainly when it had to do with her own safety. Remarkably, she sometimes used condoms to avoid AIDS. She usually used one the first time with a client, but there were exceptions if she or her client had too much to drink or if she had none with her. If she slept more than once with a client she stopped using them except if her client insisted. Her own personal safety was not an important criterion. It was striking that sex workers were well-informed about 'visible' venereal diseases and probably took some measures to avoid them. That was logical, not just because these diseases have been present longer on the scene but also because, through its visibility, infection caused immediate loss of income.

Condom use on the part of the client was mainly dependent on nationality, social class, type of tourist, and general acquaintance with Thailand. The better educated clients in particular used condoms much more consistently. But numerous clients in the circuit used condoms inconsistently or not at all. From my observations relating to condom use in the period 1989–90 it appears that a significant risk of infection existed among Thai sex workers in the *farang* circuit. One can not rule out the possibility that also quite a few tourists went home with HIV. During this period, Thailand was not internationally recognized as a country with a high incidence of AIDS/HIV infection.

Why was condom use apparently so rare despite the information about AIDS that was available from press reports and actively spread by campaigns at that time? Certain factors impede safe practices. Sex workers have a great degree of mobility and operate in a relatively free sex market. The continuous necessity to compete with a large number of others influences condom use because many clients prefer not to use them. There is also a constant supply of beginners. Aside from this, a number of personal, professional and contextual (in particular, cultural) factors are indicated.

At the beginning of the period there was some public knowledge concerning AIDS, but this was loaded with prejudice and misconceptions. Sex workers were apparently aware of the existence of AIDS as a 'disease' but it is obvious from their behaviour that they were not fully aware of the danger of infection or the exact means of transmission. They certainly did not know the difference between safe and unsafe sex. Many, both in the countryside and in the city thought that AIDS could be avoided by paying attention to the appearance, especially the personal hygiene, of their clients. This opinion was not drastically changed by the alarming statistics on HIV infections in Chiang Mai. If faulty assessments are made about the means of transmission (like kissing, skin contact, saliva etc.), there is no reason to believe in the efficacy of condoms in preventing disease.

Clients provide incentives not to use condoms, offering girls more money. Poverty is perhaps the most important reason for taking risks. The necessity of supporting her family lays a heavy responsibility on the shoulders of a daughter. This is one reason why some girls keep on working even when infected. Economic pressure also brings about a tendency towards short-term thinking. This attitide is amplified when one leaves the family and begins a whole new life.

The working conditions of the sex worker were at least partially conducive to unsafe sex. In Bangkok there were a reasonable number of VD clinics where AIDS tests were also carried out. The bar girls were obliged to undergo tests for venereal disease and to keep a VD book, where these tests were noted. An AIDS test, however, was not compulsory in this period. Very few bars worked with a compulsory AIDS test because this involved a substantial financial investment. Many relieved themselves of responsibility by hanging a sign behind the bar stating that all their employees were AIDS-free. A sign could hang there for months and did not mean a thing. In terms of Thai living standards a condom is rather expensive. In Bangkok a condom costs on average 10 baht — as much as a simple meal.[8] Besides this, the quality of the condoms available was generally bad and variety was limited. For example, no condoms were available for anal use. Historically, in contrast to Japan, for example, the condom was never popular in Thailand as a contraceptive (Sairudee and Cash 1992).

Working conditions can in the long run cause apathy and indifference in some sex workers. Constantly compromising their moral standards, prey to perpetual social insecurity, and at the mercy of the vicissitudes of their clients, these women often turn to drink and/or drugs. Amphetamines are particularly popular to keep up the energy levels. Some girls develop an indifference to danger. The constant obsession with having to hunt for clients can exacerbate this apathetic attitude.

The attitude of many sex workers toward safe sex can also be partly explained in terms of Thai cultural beliefs. Self-protection was not of primary importance to most Thai sex workers, but money and the promise of a profitable relationship were. AIDS is 'far away,' not immediately visible, and clients leave the country anyway. The concept of 'karma' also plays a role. According to Allyn and Collins,

AIDS is often connected with this idea of Buddhist retribution in the Thai homosexual world. 'If I'm fated to have AIDS, then I'll get it anyway' (1988:93). I heard this statement several times in my contacts with sex workers, though I do not know how representative it is of the attitude of sex workers in general. The attitude of many girls I met was certainly a little fatalistic. Many sex workers presented an indifferent façade concerning their personal welfare. They made it known to me that they were not afraid of the AIDS virus and that they were not worried about inconsistent condom use. This indifferent attitude (*choey*) is associated with strength. Defying bad karma and ignoring risks is regarded as a strong attitude.

The differences in HIV infection rates found between domestic and *farang* facilities offered both clients and sex workers in the *farang* circuit the possibility of convincing themselves that the danger of infection was not so great. There is a general tendency in the Thai culture to ignore unwanted information, particularly if it could lead to loss of face. Another factor hampering the development of adequate general knowledge is the taboo on explicit communication concerning sexuality. Typically, sex workers hardly ever talked about it among themselves. When they did it was in a giggly manner. Even EMPOWER's 'Honey Bee Show' (AIDS education) was affected by this unease, making full use of humour (playfulness, pleasure). Because explicit communication concerning sexual matters does not even take place amongst the girls themselves, adequate transfer of information concerning safe sexual practices is difficult to bring about.[9] The girls also often find themselves in a communication vacuum with regard to their clients. Negotiations about safe sex are subtle business, and the possibilities are severely limited by the absence of a common language. When play begins in the hotel room and the client makes it obvious that he does not wish to use a condom, her line of defence is often limited to 'I no do. No good.' Every verbal nuance is absent, and nonverbal communication causes many misunderstandings.

Unsafe sex resulted not only from the mistaken beliefs and attitudes of sex workers themselves; clients were equally responsible. Sometimes it seemed that clients approached this sex scene specifically with the idea that 'Thailand is AIDS-free so I can have sex here without a condom.' Sometimes feelings of superiority also played a role. Clients considered themselves to be much smarter than the girls. If they indicated that they wished to use condoms it was often assumed that this was not for reasons of general safety. It was even interpreted as an indication that the girl in question was suffering from some form of sickness herself. Many clients, sometimes through this feeling of superiority, were under the false impression that the AIDS virus could not affect them. I met other clients with an overtly indifferent attitude. Some Australians, for instance, made remarks like: 'I will probably die of skin cancer anyway.' In the following paragraph I shall discuss another complex of factors, namely those concerning the relative unrecognizability of Thai sex work as such and the experience of a holiday as a 'cultural time-out.'

Sex workers are influenced considerably by their clients' reasons for not using condoms, primarily because Thai sex workers are inclined to trust the client's judgment. Sex workers who see the *farang* as a sort of patron with worldly knowledge are likely to accept his attitude towards condom use. This can have as much a positive as a negative influence on sex workers' general attitude towards their own protection. The more the client can be persuaded to accept the use of condoms, the more willing the sex worker will be to consider condom use as a general practice. If the client finds condoms unnecessary and the girl herself has no definite viewpoint, then she is more easily persuaded to leave her condoms in her bag. Sometimes clients have considerable power, exerting extreme pressure — including physical violence — not to use a condom. Pressure is especially brought to bear by drunken clients. In the Thai culture drunken men are seen as dangerous: it is better to submit and avoid problems (Mulder 1990:54). This notion also plays a role in contacts with *farang*.

CULTURAL TIME-OUT

In a number of respects the sex market functioned as a 'cultural time-out' for both sex workers and their clients. A specific analysis of this time-out is important in that the needs catered to by this phenomenon increase the tendency towards unsafe sex. The nature of this time-out is different for the sex worker and the *farang* because it involves either a reversal or an accentuation of their own particular cultural norms and behaviour. Despite, or even because of, a lack of insight into one another's motives, this can lead to the development of a shared time-out in the form of an emotional relationship.

It was not until the 1980s that Thailand revealed itself as a sex paradise in the ideology of the Western male. The Thai sex worker as presented in the Western media was an exotic beauty, an Aphrodite in comparison to the Western sex worker, who is presented as a 'whore' (Meyer 1988:252–254). She is a person close to nature. It is a fact that *farang* see Thai sex workers as different from those in their homeland.

There are currently a number of different hypotheses concerning the motives behind this new Western interest in 'exotic' sex, each influenced by its own scientific or ideological orientation. The feminist explanation is fairly well-known: the male urge towards exploitation of women is becoming more and more difficult to satisfy in Western countries but can be satisfied cheaply in the Third World. Other writers see the motivating factors in terms of cultural developments in the West. Motivation research on mass tourism is particularly interesting in this respect. According to Yiannakis and Gibson, Western tourists need to create 'pseudo events' (1992:290). An adventure with a Thai sex worker can satisfy this need. Gottlieb emphasizes the attraction of role reversal and accentuation (1982:165). It is indeed clear from conversations with clients in Bangkok that they consider themselves to be generally better treated as consumers, despite the considerable amount of theft and swindling with which they are confronted. A man can feel like a king, even if he is a construction worker at home. He is massaged, taken to expensive restaurants and he has a permanent sex partner at his beck and call. Another side of his personality appears. Psychoanalytically formulated: the dominance of the superego is displaced by that of the id. With impunity, he casts off the financial and sexual reins that he wears at home. Calculation makes way for impulse, also when it comes to taking precautions against infection. Another very different type of client is the intellectual, whose social status at home prevents him from being associated with 'exploitation.' He is more inclined to take more care of his own safety.

In Western culture individualistic values are predominant: be assertive, look after your own interests, respect the individuality of others, etc. Men who don't do well with women are given new chances in a climate where different values are prevelant. Indeed, a relatively poor capacity for verbal contact or a lack of subtlety or assertivity can contribute to the experience of a cultural time-out. It is striking how many clients are content to associate for long periods of time with a very simple girl. Attention, warmth, humour, company, and pleasure in bed seem to be enough. Lack of depth is compensated by the fact that she acts as a connection with Thai culture, at least in as far as the client wishes to become acquainted with it. In the long term, however, one sees a great deal of boredom. The basis for understanding is often so tenuous that possibilities for communication, apart from the physical, are soon exhausted. Barter of a body for money remains the main binding factor: a girl exclusively for oneself is apparently more acceptable to some than a deeper relationship at home with an emancipated woman. The fact that the Thai sex worker forms part of a foreign culture is considered important by Meyer amongst others. In the post-modern age more and more values which were taken for granted in the past are being questioned, and the resulting doubt leads to a search for the values and practices of other cultures.

The variety and the disguises of the Thai sex scene cause the sex tourist to develop a blurred view on the phenomenon of paid sex. He may come across sex workers and not recognize them as such. He may consider the possibility that his foreign status and relative wealth make the ground for a real intercultural love affair. His scope is limited by his Western ideas about how to recognize a 'whore' (for instance: calculating, time-bound, emotionally distant). Even if the tourist is aware that there are many sex workers in Thailand, he can nevertheless come to the wrong conclusion about 'his' girl. Part of the explanation of the success of the Thai sex business is possibly that, to Western eyes, there is no clear boundary between paid sex and free love. Even on the first evening of a bar encounter the client hear the words, 'I love you,' time and time again. There are clients who wish to believe it. Often no clear negotiation concerning the price of the transaction takes place beforehand. If she is a bar girl, then he needs to buy her out. Even then it is not always clear that the girl receives none of this money, and that the tourist must carry out a transaction not only with the bar, but also with the woman. A client may even be convinced that he has done a good deed by buying out a go-go dancer without taking her with him for sex. She earns nothing for this, however.

At first, many sex tourists allow themselves to be cheated and duped. There is a great deal of theft on the circuit. Some more experienced clients continue to allow themselves to be swindled, while others become strict and suspicious. Others attempt to learn from their bad experiences or seek new sex spots where they are just as likely to be cheated, but then in a different way. The client is under immediate pressure. He is plied with hard-luck stories and caresses or undergoes a collective attack by numerous sex workers. On the other hand one also comes across clients who have seen it all. These men are hardened, and they make this obvious in their behaviour towards sex workers. Respect is hard to find.

In terms of this cultural time-out, it is possible for a Thai sex worker to be treated with respect by her *farang* client. The Thai sex worker has more freedom and demands more respect in her dealings with *farang* than she could normally do with Thai men. According to Sukanya, Thai women who break the existing sexual rules are condemned and held in contempt (1983:116). They are brought up with the idea that if they overstep the boundaries they risk negative attention and violence. 'So a girl learns to narrow her gaze, mask her face and close her body' (Thitsa 1980:16). Women are expected to be obliging, docile, and submissive. Their sexuality is also characterized by passivity. Within marriage women are allowed a limited sexual freedom, but for the unmarried there is very little freedom indeed. Open sexuality is reserved for the Thai man, not for the 'ordinary' Thai woman.

Sex workers who work with *farang*, on the contrary, form a group who earn relatively well for not working very hard. Their work is much less taxing than that of their colleagues in the brothels that serve Thai men. Sukanya confirms the autonomy of the sex worker: 'It is interesting to watch an innocent and obedient young girl turn into a sophisticated and rebellious woman in such a male dominated society.' She can escape from all that hard work for little pay without the necessity of schooling. Many *farang* clients pay for her hotel, her food, her social life, and her travels, and she accepts this as perfectly natural. This is understandable if seen in the context of a patron/ client relationship. The *farang* is seen as a patron because he has money, and in return for his money she gives him what he needs: sex, illusions, affection, company, and sometimes love. Such a relationship is based on reciprocity; you give some, you take some. Seen from the poverty aspect, it is a pragmatic approach: catching a rich man who is willing to share some of his riches.

Women in the scene for *farang* often say that a Western man shows more respect and offers a better chance for personal fulfilment than a Thai client. In this way the *farang* is often more attractive than the Thai man. He is strange and represents adventure. Because it deals with tourists, the *farang* scene offers the sex worker an active social life and the possibility of a much freer life-style than in the traditional woman's role. This is true in terms of both emotional expression and sexuality. Moreover, the *farang* sometimes offers her the chance of marriage, long-term freedom from poverty, and even the chance of schooling and social development. This provides her with the security that she needs to continue to support her family.

Sex workers create their own work and make their own decisions, which gives them a great deal of freedom and thus a degree of independence. In general, this means that they are in a stronger negotiating position than their brothel colleagues when it comes to condom use. Through their work, these sex workers often become tourists themselves. They can also be affected by role reversal or accentuation. Going out (*pay thiaw*) is a favourite pastime in Thailand. As sex workers, simple country girls can visit expensive hotels and restaurants. They have the chance to travel throughout Thailand — to places where people do not know them personally, allowing them more room to be themselves and to take on more assertive roles. In this way they can come to imitate Western behaviour and to break with local customs.

The most important effect of this commonly experienced time-out is that in many cases experiments are made with forms of relationships that combine paid sex with love. Cohen speaks of 'open ended prostitution' (1987:225–226). Thai girls are considered to be compliant and are led by the Thai norms concerning feminine docility. This is also an important factor in the frequent choice of Thai wives by *farang*. Expressing jealousy when she discovers him with another sex worker, though often a case of professional rivalry, is one way for her to give the impression that she cares for him. A good example of how ambiguity can lead to the development of an emotional relationship involved a sex worker with whom I had long-term contact. She met an Australian client on holiday, travelling with friends through Thailand, joined their group, and began to develop emotional ties with him. After a few weeks they parted temporarily, arranging to meet in a week's time in Bangkok. In the meantime they would not have sex with others. She returned to work directly on arrival in Bangkok, and had a number of clients in that week, even though she claimed to miss her Australian. He went to the islands and was involved with a number of women. He did not appear at the agreed time in Bangkok. A few days later she met him by chance in the company of another sex worker, made a scene, and won him back. This was the start of a deeper relationship, eventually leading to her departure for Australia.

In this way the start of a relationship is characterized by a lack of insight into one another's motives, or on an ambiguous attitude. Ambiguity exists particularly in relation to the question, 'Does this have to do with me (personally) or with the exchange of sex for money?' In the West, love and financial motives are considered incompatible. This is much less so in Thai culture. For the Thai sex worker it remains the question whether her Western friend is interested in only her for the sex or whether he is in love with her and wishes more from their relationship. Her previous experiences also

play an important role. Many women in the circuit have had relationships with, or have been married to, a *farang*. Sex workers themselves
have also had to deal with cheating or broken promises. In the first
flush of excitement many clients say things like, 'Come with me to
Germany. There we can build a perfect life together.' But the client
often then leaves and is often never heard of again. After a number of
these experiences she becomes increasingly disillusioned. As long as
she hopes for a profitable relationship, part of her routine will be to
make the client feel that he is special and that she would do anything
for him. Not using a condom then functions as a sign of the transition
from commercial sex to love.

CONCLUSION

In the introduction, I posed the question of how analysis of the
specific dynamics of the Thai sex scene for *farang* can provide indications leading to prevention. In attempting to answer this question
one must bear in mind that since my research period, both the AIDS
problem and preventive practices have undergone swift development. In a relatively short time the percentage of infected individuals
in diverse social groups has increased markedly. This has led to both
large- and small-scale prevention projects, a number of which are
directly related to the *farang* sex scene. The dangers of unsafe sex are
better known today and as a result the rate of condom use has
increased.

An important problem which arose in the above analysis was the
lack of a feeling of responsibility for oneself and the other that was
characteristic of both sex worker and client. It is possible that this has
improved in the meantime, but it nevertheless remains a bottleneck,
because the underlying causes (for the sex workers, economic pressure, lack of education, gender roles, karma; for the client, racism,
sexism, rancour towards women, indifference) are still in force. It is
necessary to address these underlying factors if prevention is to be
effective.

The Thai sex market is extremely customer-oriented. The customer
is treated like a king, the girls are easily influenced by their patron
and often develop a dependent relationship with him. The client is in
a relatively powerful position and decides what happens to a large
degree. For this reason, a great deal of preventive activity should be
aimed at the client. There are still quite a number of men who are
willing to pay more for unsafe sex (Mann et al. 1992:374). Being
extremely mobile and generally only present on the scene for a short

time, clients are difficult to reach. The efficacy of educative campaigns is increased when the cultural origins of clients are taken into consideration and when they are specifically aimed at the sub-scenes that cater to their needs. The degree to which sex is visible varies quite strongly between the locations studied. The scene for *farang* is the most explicit in public displays of sexuality. In Patpong, the most 'un-Thai' of the various sub-scenes, a more explicit form of prevention would therefore be possible than in other places, incorporating it, for example, in the sex shows.

Given the characteristics and motives of clients, effective prevention is problematic but is in any case strongly dependent on an approach that is specific to the target group. One problem is posed by the effects of a cultural time-out, where role reversal occurs to such an extent that the tendency to irresponsible behaviour is increased. Many clients also take part in sex tourism in other exotic lands and in this way can provide an important vehicle for transmission. For this reason, explicit information on Thai sex work should ideally be supplied in the land of origin. Access routes to Thailand (planes, taxis from the airport) could also be utilized as sources of information. Relatively large numbers of men are divorced or unmarried, and therefore possibly in search of a relationship. Educational material could provide factual information on the grey area between paid sex and relationships, as well as on inter-cultural relationships. The general level of education is relatively low, so material should be simply worded and available in a number of *farang* languages. The presence of subgroups with diverse motivations (e.g., 'daddies' and 'losers') should influence the psychological approach: 'You wouldn't want to give your daughter AIDS.' or 'Don't be a double loser.' One could also make use of the 'feeling like a king' effect or of feelings of superiority.

Although educative material should provide information on the nature and differentiation of Thai sex work, care should also be taken when addressing the potential client as a client. There are a large number of clients who initially had no intention of becoming involved in the scene but were drawn in through the relatively unrecognizable nature of the work. Contactual status between sex workers and *farang* clients is often ambiguous and unclear. The novel form of the sexual contact allows the client not to define it as prostitution. Furthermore, development of an emotional relationship is not uncommon.

As often as not, even the sex worker does not wish to consider herself a prostitute, and the variety of services that she provides makes it easier to continue in her denial. It is clear that sex workers in this circuit are in a stronger position than those in bonded prostitution with Thai men. Nevertheless, their position needs to be strengthened further in order to guarantee that they put their own safety first and to enable them to be consistent in their transactions with clients on the subject of safe sex. In general, inconsistent behaviour on this point is associated with a lack of resilience and a poor self-image. Drug and alcohol addiction can exarcebate this effect. For these reasons wide-ranging empowerment is necessary. It is important to transcend the cultural ideologies that impede the development of resilience, such as the link between power and indifference, the tendency to ignore unwanted information, and the taboo on explicit communication around sexuality. In principle, empowerment can be brought about in a number of different ways, such as through peer education and training of new sex workers. A sex worker will participate in a training scheme only if it is worth her while — if it enables her to improve her market position, for example. This is why such programmes should not be directed exclusively towards prevention but also towards schooling: developing assertivity, improving dealings with money and officialdom, learning better bargaining skills around payment and condom use, gaining insight into the cultural background and motives of the client, becoming better informed about the advantages and risks involved in inter-cultural relationships. English language education is vital because development of deeper communication enabling effective discussion on the theme 'safe sex' is dependent on this.

It is important to organize this schooling as much as possible on the spot. In this, mobility of sex workers and a continuous stream of new girls poses a problem. On-the-spot schooling cannot reach everyone in time. It should be augmented with educational projects in the rural areas where sex workers originate and in the 'acclimatization zones' which act as a transitional step on the road to sex work.

An important problem when organizing education programmes, including peer education, is that in the setting investigated the girls had only superficial contacts with each other and that there was very little open discussion concerning the work involved. In this situation it is necessary to find means of improving communication between sex workers themselves and to strengthen collective representation. Such a development could also have a positive effect on the unregulated competition between sex workers, which stimulates unsafe sexual practices.

NOTES

1. In this chapter I will avoid the use of 'prostitute' (and 'prostitution') and use the more neutral 'sex worker' for a person who earns an income from providing sexual services. Sex tourism can be circumscribed as a form of tourism which, at the tourist's side, is primarily motivated by the prospect of engaging in temporary (commercial) sexual liaisons.

2. Sex workers who cater to *farang* clients are at less risk than sex workers who serve Thai clientele, if only due to the fact that sex work for farang is in general not 'production line' work. Thai men are also said to be less likely to use condoms than *farang*.

3. EMPOWER is a woman's organization working with female sex workers through direct contact and (street) theatre.

4. For reasons of brevity I give no further consideration to the methodological shortcomings of surveys, particularly in transcultural application. Especially in the socio-cultural climate of Southeast Asia there is a relatively heavy preoccupation with 'proper' public behaviour. This may give inaccurate information on actual condom use. For 'proper' behaviour see Mulder (1990:48).

5. One baht is approximately $0.05.

6. The general gender relations in Thai society are an important factor in the role obligations of a Thai sex worker.

7. In the literature on Thai prostitution clients are presented as pathetic, ugly men with psychological shortcomings (e.g., Latza 1987). They are supposedly the 'leftovers' who cannot find a woman, who have an unattractive personality. A marginal power to attract women in one's own society can undoubtedly provide a motive to look elsewhere, but in my experience clients were so diverse that this sort of description is only relevant to a minority.

8. In Western countries the price is about the same, but average wages are much higher.

9. Furthermore, reciprocal information transfer is a process whereby essential elements are easily lost or distorted in a network situation.

REFERENCES

Allyn, E., and J.P. Collins. 1988. *The Men of Thailand. Noom Thai*. Bangkok: Bua Lang Publications.

Cohen, E. 1987. Sensuality and Venality in Bangkok. The Dynamics of Cross Cultural Mapping of Prostitution. *Deviant Behavior* 8:223–234.

Gottlieb, A. 1982. Americans' Vacations. *Annals of Tourism Research* 9:165–187.

Kleiber, D., M. Wilke, and E. Kreilkamp. 1991. *AIDS and (Sex) Tourism.* Berlin: Sozialpädagogisches Institut.

Latza, B. 1987. *Sextourismus in Südostasien.* Frankfurt am Main: Fischer Verlag.

Mann, J., J.D.M. Tarantola and T.W. Netter, eds. 1992. *AIDS in the World. A Global Report.* Cambridge: Harvard University Press.

Meyer, W. 1988. *Beyond the Mask. Toward a Transdisciplinary Approach of Selected Social Problems Related to the Evolution and Context of International Tourism in Thailand.* Saarbrücken: Breitenbach.

Mulder, N. 1990. *Inside Thai Society. An Interpretation of Everyday Life.* Bangkok: Editions Duang Kamol.

Sairudee Vorakitphokatorn, and R. Cash. 1992. Factors that Determine Condom Use of Traditionally High Users: Japanese Men and Commercial Sexworkers in Bangkok, Thailand. Paper presented at the VIII International Conference on AIDS, Amsterdam, 19–24 July.

Sukanya Hantrakul. 1983. Prostitution in Thailand. In: *Development and Displacement: Women in Southeast Asia,* edited by G. Chandler, N. Sullivan, and J. Branson. Monash Papers on South East Asia 18, Clayton: Monash University.

Thitsa, Khin. 1980. *Providence and Prostitution. Image and Reality for Women in Buddhist Thailand.* London: Change International Reports.

Vanwesenbeeck, I., et al. 1992. Beschermingspraktijken van prostituanten. Intenties, gedrag en overwegingen in verband met AIDS. *Gedrag en Gezondheid* 20(2):82–93.

Yiannakis, A., and H. Gibson. 1992. Roles Tourists Play. *Annals of Tourism Research* 19:285–301.

Chapter SEVEN

Risky Business? Men Who Buy Heterosexual Sex in Spain

Angie Hart

You can always tell when a puta's (whore's) got something. The face is the mirror of the soul.

Manuel, 43, divorced waiter

El sida (AIDS) is women's [i.e., prostitutes'] fault in many ways, because they should tell their clients if they had it and then they wouldn't go to them.

Alfonso, 63, married, retired carpenter

Arturo had kept up the deception for over 35 years. 'Still,' he told me, 'I think my wife probably guesses. Saves her having to do it with me anyway. She's always ill and never wants sex. What's a man supposed to do?'

Early in February 1991, Arturo and I were standing outside a religious waxworks museum in the *barrio* (neighbourhood) in which

I was doing ethnographic research on street prostitution. Whilst we talked, a couple of prostitutes interrupted us to say goodbye to me — most of them were going home for the night. Of the 40 or so prostitutes who worked in the *barrio*, only a handful stayed to work past 8 p.m. 'Watch old Arturo,' laughed Matilda, 'he looks sweet as shit, but he's dangerous.' Arturo voiced his disagreement. I played along, assuring her that I would be careful.–Arturo and I were discussing how he fitted into the barrio's prostitution scene. His story was a familiar one, versions of which I had heard many times during my research. Nevertheless, in some respects he was quite different from other prostitutes' clients whom I had interviewed. The way in which he talked about HIV was quite typical of the way he voiced opinions on other things. Arturo created the impression that he got what he could out of life: he lived for the moment.

When clients talked to me about HIV, although most of them never had protected sex and were extremely adept at demonstrating that they were not at risk, they did at least pretent that they were concerned about the dangers. Arturo was different. He told me that life was full of risks, even if you weren't always aware of them, so why bother about HIV?

Arturo's truism — that we live in a 'risk society' — is one that has been intellectualized by social scientists concerned with the 'consequences of modernity.' Many of them have written about this at a general, theoretical level (for example, Giddens 1990; Krimsky and Golding 1992); others have examined this notion in more concrete ways, for example, by considering major risk incidences such as Chernobyl (Beck 1987). Despite the wealth of social-scientific writing on modernity and risk, very few writers have linked these concepts to HIV (but see Douglas and Calvez 1990).

One of the most prolific writers on modernity and risk is Ulrich Beck. Amongst others (for example, Giddens 1990), he argues that in order to survive, we must learn to mistrust our senses. He suggests that there is no longer a simple and direct relationship between perception of risk and actual risk occurrence.

> In matters of risk, we have been disenfranchised.... Our notions of individuality, of 'self-determination,' of 'one's own life,' are founded upon personal access to reality. To the extent that we are cut off from this access, we are driven — in the full flower of individualism — into a *collective existence* at the height of modernity. Of this fact we can deceive ourselves only by refusing to recognize the danger, insisting on the continued functioning of our senses. None are so blind as those who will not see. This adage is true in a revised form: none are so

blind to the danger, as those who continue to trust their own eyes. (Beck 1987:156, his italics)

Beck also calls for those who create the risks to be held responsible: 'Autonomy of risk avoidance should be subsumed by the autonomy of sub-politics.... [We must insist that] those who create the risks take responsibility' (Beck 1987:164).

The material presented below on HIV and men who buy sex could be construed as a story about risk resistance: it is largely a story of men who, come what may, continue to 'trust their own eyes' and who do not represent themselves by way of a collective existence. However, these particular men who buy sex do not simply trust their own eyes; they often trust other people's, with potential effects that are as detrimental as trusting their own.

The story I am telling, might also be seen, à la Beck, to be about locating those who create the risks and making them take responsibility. In this case, the very men who take risks might also be responsible for creating them. However, few of them ever see it like this. Take Arturo; he saw HIV as just another risk in the great scheme of things. Typically, he did not ever stop to think that he might be placing others at risk. Perhaps Matilda was right, perhaps he was dangerous. If we were to follow Beck in seeking those responsible for the (potential) creation of HIV risk in this context, who, if anybody, would we blame? Would we blame clients, prostitutes, governments, and/or the amorphous collective 'society'? At different historical locations, in varying contexts, they have all had the finger pointed at them. Even if we accept that clients should take responsibility for their actions, it is difficult to see how this might be implemented without causing more futile stigmatization of those who choose to sell and to buy sex.

In HIV research, the issue of responsibility and blame has become a thorny one, intertwined with the politics of health promotion or education and the 'groups vs. behaviours' debate. This chapter discusses how men who buy sex construct themselves in relation to HIV risk, linking their stories to the 'groups vs. behaviours' debate. It shows how prostitutes' clients accommodate health education messages to fit in with the ways in which they choose to construct risk. Whilst agreeing that there are considerable difficulties with discussing risk and HIV in terms of 'risk groups,' I suggest that there are also problems with discussing 'risk behaviours.' Simply changing the semantic framework of the debate does not necessarily mean that people will respond. Before I consider my own data in some detail, I briefly outline the parameters of the 'groups vs. behaviours' debate.

PROBLEMATIZING RISK 'GROUPS' AND 'BEHAVIOURS'

In order to tackle the complex 'groups vs. behaviours' controversy, I think it is important to be clear about the particular context in which one is considering it. Clearly, 'groups' or 'behaviours' have different meanings depending on whether one is talking about them primarily in relation to, for example, health-education messages, pressure-group lobbying, lay beliefs and behaviours, or the design of anthropological research projects.

For some time now, health educators and many researchers have been arguing that talk of 'risk groups' does nothing to encourage people to change their behaviour. They suggest that individuals will merely construct themselves as not belonging to a 'risk group.' In addition, they argue, the use of such a concept merely reinforces people's prejudices against certain 'groups,' most notably 'black people,' '(male) homosexuals' and 'drug addicts.' Thus health promoters argue that, rather than defining people as belonging to 'risk groups,' educational messages should aim to define 'risk behaviours' (basically, any that result in exchange of body fluids) and target individuals who practise them.

However, there is growing evidence of moves towards this practice being reversed in certain contexts. In Britain, for example, a powerful pressure group, Gay Men Fighting Aids (GMFA), is lobbying for the reinstatement of gay men as a 'risk group.' This reflects the burgeoning contradictions in HIV/AIDS discourses. Whilst at the lay level it may well be the case that HIV/AIDS is negatively associated with gay men, GMFA have elected to trade off the increased financial benefits of defining gay men as a 'risk group' with the possible negative effects of increased stigmatization. This is a clear indication of the power of GMFA to steer health provision and services to some extent, despite the negative representations of gay men in many different contexts.

What is happening in relation to the groups controversy is a kind of pushing and pulling, a battle over group representations. 'The group' is constructed in opposition to 'the rest,' by both those who claim to represent 'the rest' and those who claim to represent 'the group.' This practice is often played out as a struggle over positive and negative group representation. Individuals claiming to represent one side blame 'the group,' and 'representatives' of the other side hit back, representing the group in a positive light. This has happened in many spheres of HIV research, including gay men's issues and those of prostitute women. However, such attacking and defensive push-and-pull contestations of representation do little to tease out the complexities of risk contexts.

More than many other social scientists, anthropologists have conventionally been most comfortable studying small 'groups' of people, definable as having something — culture? — in common. Choices about which 'group' to ethnographize, in which context, and how to do it, are necessarily political. However, given the issues of 'group' stigmatization, it might seem that political significance in relation to HIV research is particularly problematic.[1]

The dangers are obvious. By concentrating research on 'risk groups,' it is likely that they will be further marginalized and stigmatized. Anthropologists and other social scienists called in to explain the 'culture' of these 'risk groups' have repeatedly called into question their very construction (for example, Glick-Schiller et al. 1991).[2]

For anthropologists there is then the enormous problem of identifying a body of people (dare I say group?) that is appropriate for study. Given that, at least in applied work, HIV prevention is our aim, and given that we are generally constrained (both economically and politically) by funding, it is often the case that this 'body of people' is seen (by both funding bodies and by anthropologists?) to be at relatively more risk than some others.[3]

PROSTITUTION AND HIV RESEARCH

Prostitution research is an area that is subject to these kinds of ethical and methodological complications. Although prostitution involves a number of different roles (clients, prostitutes, procurers, madams, etc.), 'prostitutes' have historically been the most consistently well represented of these in HIV research and health promotion literature. Much of this literature has concentrated on whether or not prostitute women insist that clients use condoms.

This has provoked a number of responses. Many texts have pointed to the connections between the historical scapegoating of prostitute women for venereal diseases and current preoccupations with HIV (see, for example, English Collective of Prostitutes 1988). Others (e.g., Alexander 1989, *El Pais* 1 December 1990) have attempted to make a positive example of 'the group,' pointing to low rates of HIV transmission amongst prostitute women, especially non-intravenous drug use (non-IDU) prostitute.

Some researchers, such as Sophie Day (1993), have deconstructed the notion of prostitutes-as-a-group in relation to HIV, both in terms of its negative (push) and positive (pull) representations. Such researchers have pointed to the great variation in prostitution, concluding that statements about whether prostitutes do or do not use condoms should be understood on a context-specific basis.

Whilst the roles of prostitute women in relation to HIV have been researched and discussed at great length, those of clients have received rather less attention. Male clients are often part of the (at least apparently) heterosexual white majority and have not been constructed as a 'risk group.' It is certainly no accident that they have been consistently under-represented in research on prostitution.

Historically, men who buy sex have enjoyed a relatively privileged status both in the eyes of the law and in sociological, theological, medical, and psychological texts. Whilst women who sell sex have been the objects of consistent regulation, there is no evidence to suggest that customers (in Spain, at least) have ever been sanctioned. In many texts on prostitution, lay and academic, the work, psychologies, and lives of prostitute women have been scrutinized and sensationalized. Clients have been either ignored or stereotyped, precluding an analysis of precisely who these men are and where their responsibilities lie. Hence prostitution has been seen to be the realm of prostitute women. Customers have been given (and have taken) a back seat.

This applies equally to studies of the links between prostitution, HIV, and drug use. IDU prostitute women have been consistently represented in this type of research — perhaps justifiably, because it may be that there is a higher incidence of injecting drug use amongst prostitute women than amongst male clients. However, this is simply taken for granted; to my knowledge no research has been conducted to investigate it.

As far as I am aware, there has been no epidemiological or other research published on incidences of HIV amongst customers of prostitutes in Spain. This lack of information is due to a number of factors. Customers have a much lower profile at sexually transmitted disease (STD) clinics than do prostitutes, who are carefully monitored. This low profile is perhaps connected to the fact that, whilst clients may consider themselves as 'at risk,' they do not see themselves to be potentially infected. Thus they would not voluntarily have an HIV test. In addition, many customers do not go to STD clinics because they treat themselves for STDs with drugs purchased directly from pharmacists. There are also complicated socio-cultural taboos with regard to researching prostitutes' customers. This would mean that even those who do frequent STD clinics would not generally form part of a research project, at least not in Spain. This was certainly the case with regard to the HIV/AIDS prevention centre to which I was attached in Spain.

Male Clients: A 'Risk Group'?

Thinking about prostitutes' clients in relation to risk groups drives home the fact that these groups are ideologically constructed, even by those who purport to be members of them. Whilst gay men and prostitute women have been targeted from the outside, it is also to a degree true that they have been involved in targeting themselves for HIV prevention. This does not appear to be true of prostitutes' clients. It would seem that they do not want to be liberated as a political lobbying force.

Are male clients a sexual subculture 'group'? Is it enough simply to talk of the 'behaviour' — buying unprotected sex? If they can be seen to be a 'group,' is it right to talk about them as such at a research level? Should the semantics change when health education is being implemented? Once again I think that, in this regard, issues of power are most salient. In some respects it might be challenging to expose clients as a 'group.' They have not, historically, been stigmatized. Hence their exposure by certain sectors (feminists? prostitutes?) potentially becomes a political act of resistance.

Some feminists have begun the task of exposing clients; in some cases they have even suggested that clients be criminalized (see, for example, Higard and Finstad 1992). However, I do not see this as a positive step. What these kinds of studies seem to be doing is further-ing the stigmatization of prostitution as a whole. The value of target-ing 'groups' for HIV prevention research might work in some con-texts, but perhaps it is better to leave clients as a kind of compliant 'muted group' (Ardener 1975). Their involvement in HIV risk could then be discussed in relation to risk contexts, rather than risk groups.

But how do clients themselves construct their HIV-significant be-haviour? Do they see themselves as a client group? Would they be persuaded by health education policies that targeted them as such? Or are they, like Beck's blind fools, content to rely on their own perceptions, persistently individualistic. And if they do construct risk on an individualistic level, would they be persuaded by health education messages that targeted their behaviour? Below, in my account of men who buy sex in Spain, I examine these questions. Before I consider these in detail, I first present the local context within which I am discussing HIV.

PROSTITUTION IN THE BARRIO

The local context of buying and selling sex in the *barrio* was typical of street-prostitution areas in Spain: poor health and sanitation, low attendance at the STD clinic (by prostitutes, and even more so by clients), general unsafe sex, and low condom usage. The *barrio* was a site of poverty, drug dealing (primarily cannabis and heroin), drug taking, violence, and crime.[4]

There was also a substantial number of men who rarely bought sex from the prostitutes. They simply stood around watching the women in the streets and appeared to gain sexual satisfaction from this activity. Some of these men tried to take advantage of a prostitute new to the patch by attempting to obtain cheap sex. The prostitutes were mostly between the ages of 35 and 65 and had little formal education. Each had an average of two customers per day, receiving anything from 1,000 to 3,000 pesetas per transaction. Approximately 10 to 15 per cent of the prostitutes were intravenous drug users (IDUs), and a minority were alcoholics.[5]

HIV/AIDS IN CONTEXT

Whilst I was in Spain, HIV/AIDS was a much-debated issue in the media. Spain has the third highest number of AIDS cases in Europe, the majority connected with the sharing of needles during intravenous drug use. Increasingly, the infection is spreading through those people having sexual relations with infected drug users (*Anuario El Pais* 1992).

It was not until 1990 that the government, alarmed at the rate of infection amongst the 'general public,' addressed the issue at a national level by implementing a general advertising campaign aimed at heterosexuals. This encouraged condom use as a measure against all STDs. The Catholic Church condemned the campaign, and the Catholic organization 'Accion Familiar' even attempted to bring out an injunction to stop it (*El Pais*, 18 December 1990).

Prostitutes (and not clients) have been highlighted as a 'risk group' by numerous Spanish epidemiologists, including those I worked within Spain. However, the construction of this 'risk group' belies the complex patterns of infection. It has been said that the consequences of sharing needles to inject drugs, rather than the direct consequences of prostitution, lie behind HIV transmission in Spain (as in other European countries). In a study carried out between 1985 and 1989, 9.3 per cent amongst 2172 prostitute women were found to be infected. However, a more detailed study revealed that most of this infection was amongst prostitutes who were IDUs (*El Pais*, 1 December 1990). This is unlikely to remain static. The concentration of prostitutes, clients, and others in socio-geographical networks will no doubt change the pattern of spread, leading to wider infection.

HIV/AIDS has proven to be a considerable problem in Spain, and much of this has thus far been connected to intravenous drug use. The results of the local health authority quantitative HIV study are not yet available; however, from a qualitative angle, one can certainly see some devastating effects.[6]

In my fieldsite, HIV and AIDS were apparent, both at the level of discourse and as biological realities. Both sellers and buyers of unprotected penetrative sex knew that *el sida* (AIDS) was not simply an issue debated at a distant national level. Most customers were to some extent aware that a number of people in the *barrio* (so far, to my knowledge, IDUs and their partners) had died of HIV-related diseases (although they always talked about *el sida*, never *VIH* (HIV). The recent decline in prostitution trade was often attributed in part to fears about *el sida*. In fact I knew of a few men who, although they continued to use the *barrio* as a social venue, no longer had sex with any of the prostitutes because they were scared of 'catching *el sida*.'

The subject of customers' attitudes toward *el sida* frequently arose in the course of my research. Their attitudes left me with a number of puzzles, the possible solutions to which might help in looking at how people construct their own senses of risk. Why was it that most customers in the *barrio*, who appeared to have significant knowledge of HIV/AIDS and some experience of its local effects, did not use condoms for penetrative sex, despite the fact that they were widely available for purchase? In addition, why, in this area of extreme distrust, did customers not only trust their own eyes but also often purport to trust prostitutes with regard to HIV/AIDS? Answers to these questions are of direct relevance to the 'groups vs. behaviours' debate introduced earlier in this chapter.

STRICTLY NOT PART OF THE GROUP?

Most of the men who bought sex in the *barrio* lived outside of the immediate vicinity. When they went to the area, they generally went alone, although they sometimes had conversations with other clients once there. Those who did linger to chat also talked to prostitutes or to Pedro, one of the local barmen. In *El Atlantico*, the main bar in which prostitutes and clients met, a small group of men played cards together three afternoons a week. However, they were not all clients; some had been in the past, and another was the partner of a prostitute who worked in the *barrio*. Another member of this group had never had sex with any of the prostitutes in the *barrio*. He told me that he went with prostitutes in a different part of town. A couple of men who worked locally took their morning and afternoon breaks together in *El Atlantico*. However, they did not always go there to have sex with a prostitute. For many clients, the *barrio* was a place in which they socialized; they did not have sex on every occasion they went there. Thus there seemed to be no feeling amongst men of a specific 'client group' identity in relation to their *barrio* visits.

However, this had not always been the case. Venturo, a client well into his 80s, described to me how different it had been 'in the past.' He used to go to the *barrio* specifically to have sex with prostitutes, but he used to go with his male friends. I had observed this activity in many other prostitution locations in Spain. Nevertheless, clients in the *barrio* were different, they did not physically manifest themselves in groups.

It was also the case that most clients in the *barrio* did not see themselves as belonging to a client group. Indeed, many of them had trouble with accepting the label of 'client,' and would often refer to themselves as a 'friend' of a particular prostitute.

Client Groups, Behaviour and HIV

As many men who bought sex in the *barrio* were unwilling to describe themselves as clients, it is hardly surprising that few of them saw themselves as belonging to a 'risk group' defined as 'prostitutes' clients.' In fact many clients latched onto other, more prominent, ideologically constructed 'risk groups' to show that they were not at risk. On numerous occasions individual clients told me a similar story: I'm not a 'homosexual,' 'drug addict,' 'black' or 'prostitute,' so I've got nothing to worry about.

Whilst they did not necessarily construct themselves as part of a risk group, some clients saw themselves as at risk precisely because of the high prevalence of perceived 'risk groups' in the *barrio*. For example, a 51-year-old married factory worker said that he was 'terrified of AIDS because black people and Arabs come round here.' Despite his fears, he did not use condoms because he had difficulty getting an erection.

Clients and HIV Prevention

Most clients I spoke to about HIV prevention seemed to juxtapose ideas about HIV prevention behaviour and HIV risk groups. On the one hand, some did in part see HIV (or rather AIDS) prevention in terms of the avoidance of 'high-risk behaviour.' Thus they perceived there to be a connection between prevention of '*el sida*' and 'safer sex.' For customers, 'safer sex' generally meant using a condom for sex that involved penile penetration of the vagina. Penile penetration of the female anus was not something that customers appeared to request with great frequency, although it was offered, often unprotected, by a small number of prostitutes.

On the other hand, unprotected sex with any sexual partner was not generally viewed by customers as 'high-risk behaviour.' Many customers classified potential sexual partners according to the degree of risk that they appeared to represent, in categories that often corresponded to epidemiological ones. Thus for most of them high-risk behaviour meant sex (even protected sex) with '(*barrio*) prostitutes,' perceived as a 'high-risk group' by many of these customers. However, customers were also liable to divide this 'high-risk group' into subgroups, placing the particular woman or women with whom they had or wanted to have unprotected penetrative sex into a 'safe(r)' subgroup.

Much of this group-division practice was tied up with the idea of status, in relation to both the client's perception of the prostitute and to his self-perception. Clients who perceived themselves to be regarded as having high status in the *barrio* often did not like to be seen to be having sex with 'lower-class prostitutes.'

Joaquin, a divorced self-employed plumber in his 40s, was one such individual. He owned two flats, had been educated to the age of 18, and employed two other plumbers. Consequently he was considered to be, and considered himself to be, of relatively high status in the *barrio*.

In response to my vague question about 'prostitution in the *barrio*,' he told me: 'These women have got too many problems: diseases, they're drug addicts, thieves. Nobody wants them except men who can't get any other women. But for somebody who wants status and a family, it's no good.' Although he told me that he saw the prostitutes in the *barrio* as a 'diseased group,' he still had unprotected sex with one of them (Antonia, who did not inject drugs). However, he did not want anybody to know this; she went to his house in another part of town.

> I'm telling you because I don't mind telling you, but I don't want you telling other people we know locally that I've told you I go with Antonia.... If I go with a woman, I don't need to go and do it in the *barrio* and let tongues wag. I prefer to do things privately. People love to talk although it doesn't bother me, I've got my business and I'm doing well. But I've got my status to think about and I don't want tongues wagging about me.

I knew many customers like Joaquin who, although aware of HIV, still had unprotected sex with the *barrio* prostitutes, even though they saw them as part of an extremely 'high-risk group.' They also had unprotected intercourse with other sexual partners. Thus many of them were able to accommodate the relationship with the particular prostitute with whom they had sex. They defined themselves to be not at risk because they went only with 'clean' prostitutes or with prostitutes who were their 'friends.' For example, Alfonso, a 63-year-old retired carpenter, appealed to the efficacy of his relationship with one of the prostitutes in relation to HIV prevention. 'That's one reason why I only really go with Rita. I've known her a long time.' These examples are significant in terms of a discussion of 'high-risk groups' or 'behaviour,' as this group of men saw themselves as belonging to a 'low-risk group' by virtue of the particular relationship that they had with a prostitute, even if, in some senses, they perceived her as part of a 'risk group.'

WHOSE RESPONSIBILITY?

The reader may have noticed that in my above discussion of Joaquin, the issue of his responsibility to protect others did not arise. This is because, in common with most other clients, Joaquin never expressed the view that he might potentially be HIV-positive himself. He consistently put the emphasis on the prostitutes, even though he divided them into different groups.

Earlier in this chapter, I discussed issues of HIV and responsibility in relation to prostitution. In the light of this discussion, it is not surprising that what most of my male informants in Spain — ex-customers and customers alike — had in common was that they rarely saw themselves as a locus of possible transmission. They all talked about 'the other' (defined by countless hegemonic discourses as a negative other) potentially transmitting the virus to them. Only one customer ever spoke to me about wishing to protect his partner — in this particular case, his wife — but significantly not the sex worker with whom he had unprotected intercourse.

Much of this silence on the part of customers with regard to responsibility is connected to their historical role in prostitution. Socio-economic and cultural prescriptions do not encourage them to think of themselves as responsible. Indeed, they are not encouraged to think of themselves as members of a client group at all; they are 'simply men doing what men do' (Jöhncke 1993, personal communication).

The Uses and Abuses of Condoms

Textual discourses on condom use in prostitution in a number of different genres including those of academic writing and of health education, are often articulated through discourses on responsibility. They are usually couched in the language of responsibility or lack of it on the part of prostitutes. This language is now shifting, with the recognition of many researchers and health educationists of the roles of clients in the condom negotiation process.

In the *barrio*, few customers volunteered unsolicited information about condom use. However, when asked, most of them talked freely about condoms. None of the clients I spoke to admitted that they had had to negotiate condom use with prostitutes. All of them presented condom use as a matter of their own personal choice.

Many of them told me that they did not use condoms, despite the fact that they recognized them as a form of protection against *el sida*. Just because they generally did not want to wear condoms did not mean that protection was not an issue for them. However, as I suggested above, clients were rarely concerned about protecting other people; they were generally concerned about protecting themselves. One of their greatest forms of protection appeared to be connected to complex ideas about the link between the perceived male sex drive and the notion of 'natural' sex. Many customers saw themselves as controlled by natural sexual urges. 'I was driven to it' was a popular conception.

Customers have a number of different reasons for not using condoms. Their complaints were often based on the 'fact' that condoms led to sex that was not sensitive. This is no doubt partly because many of these men had experienced sexual intercourse with condoms in the past that had greatly affected the enjoyment of intercourse, and were unable to accept that technology had moved on. In addition, a considerable number of customers complained that they had difficulty maintaining an erection during sex. For some customers, this can be attributed to the consumption of alcohol. Using a condom often exacerbated this; they felt under pressure to have quick sex. (Very often they were allotted 20 minutes for the entire transaction.) Thus customers felt a great deal of pressure to perform. And for them, performance meant a 'natural' sex act with a hard penis. No wonder condoms did not figure in this ideal.

Thus the notion of 'natural sex' acted as a potent prophylactic, as the men saw themselves as doing what came naturally to them. The notion of 'naturalness' has great semantic weight. It conjures up ideas of something that is '(morally and physiologically) correct.' It does not conjure up ideas of a condom. It would be possible to expand this, suggesting that customers who held this philosophy saw themselves, on some level, as both belonging to a 'non-risk group' ('men with a natural sex drive') and engaging in 'non-risk behaviour' ('natural sex'). Thus, although many customers were concerned about the risks of HIV, and to some extent knowledgeable about possible transmission, this other 'knowledge' took greater precedence.

The following extracts from my fieldnotes illustrate how men articulated worries about condom sensitivity, 'natural' sex, and HIV protection. The first relates to a married client in his 50s. He told me that he did not have 'enough' sex with his wife. He had unprotected sex with a number of different prostitutes in the *barrio*, both IDUs and non-IDUs.

> I'm afraid of AIDS much more than you think. No, I never use condoms, but I try to go with women who look O.K. I've tried to use condoms with my wife, but they're no good, they spoil my pleasure. I often pray to God, asking him to stop me getting AIDS. I'm a religious man, but the trouble is, my body told me to come here and have sex. I need it a lot. If I don't get it I feel physically sick, go mad and can hardly see straight.

In this case, the man's sexual 'need' was tied up with ideas about 'natural sex' as discussed above.

The second example is that of a client who was 78 years old at the time of my fieldwork. He had been going to the *barrio* for many years. In the past, he had had sex with a number of different prostitute women, but he did not have sex with them much any more because he considered himself too old. He said that his wife could not have sex because she had heart problems:

> But I'm very scared of getting AIDS. Especially because of my wife. I don't want to give it to her. I hope God will keep me safe. I don't use condoms because I'm not used to them. At my age once you've got it up, you have to take advantage of it and put the condom on quick. Otherwise my 'little friend' will flop. It's all right for young men who get hard-ons quickly but I take ages.

Another client, a man who lived alone and who was in his 40s, was a regular client of an IDU prostitute. (Both she and her partner have since died of HIV-related diseases.) He was slightly worried about *el sida* but would never use a condom with her. Nor had he ever been for an HIV test, because he said that he felt fine. 'I take risks, I know, but the pleasure's not the same.' He had been lucky and had never had any STDs, 'but I know it's a risk, especially as she injects.'

A minority of clients insisted that they were not at all concerned about HIV. One of these was a chef in his late 30s. He was a regular client of one of the *barrio*'s non-IDU prostitutes. To my knowledge, he did not have any other sexual partners. His reasons for not being worried about HIV were connected to this issue of friendship and trust. However, they were also connected to his perception that he was not a member of a 'risk group.'

> Spanish men need lots of sex. AIDS doesn't worry me. I don't like condoms and I prefer to do it naturally. I never use condoms. I'm not scared because I always go with a woman I know well and whom I can trust. They'd tell me if they had anything. The condom campaign on at the moment is good but it isn't aimed at me. I don't need them, they're good for people who don't want to get pregnant and for homosexuals.

RISKY BUSINESS?

My discussion of prostitutes' clients in the *barrio* reveals how men who buy sex employ HIV prevention strategies. Many trust their own eyes and also put their lives into the hands of others. For many clients, the most potent prophylactic that they have is the notion of trust. Many of the sexual contracts took place within the seemingly contradictory context of, on the one hand, romantic friendship — love, even — and trust, and on the other hand, payment up front, lack of credit, and lies from both parties amounting to a lack of trust. Although it appears to be a positive notion, trust is a word that covers a variety of sins. In purporting to 'trust' prostitutes, clients conveniently put the entire responsibility for HIV prevention into their hands. And their ideas about HIV prevention do not wholly concur with those of health educators. It was not that, as might be expected, clients 'trusted' prostitutes to practise safer sex with other sexual partners. It was rather that they expected prostitutes to tell them if they had *el sida*, thereby not simply 'trusting their own eyes,' but also trusting those of other people.

In the *barrio*, misconceptions about the biological construction of the virus and HIV-related diseases no doubt contributed to the lack of safer sex practices. Even so, most customers perceived themselves to be at risk. However, they conceptually minimized their risks through the employment of 'prophylactics' such as trust, friendship, and abdicated responsibility. These factors relate to the manner in which individuals use the information that they have to construct their own ideas about 'high-risk behaviour' and 'high-risk groups' — in short, how they construct hierarchies of knowledge (see Young 1981).

Thus the data on clients presented above reveal the many different ways in which different clients *themselves* constructed their identities and behaviours in relation to 'groups,' 'behaviours,' and HIV. It shows how some of them might respond well to a 'behaviours' campaign, but how others actually manipulated notions of 'groups' and 'behaviours' in order to accommodate their own (risky) behaviour.

Hence the sheer complexity of the 'groups vs. behaviours' controversy is further illustrated. It is complex not only at the level of research design — how do we go about targeting a group? — but also in relation to the emic context — actors use these categories themselves. My ethnography has shown that actors are not passive recipients of health education messages. They have ways of manipulating categories to suit themselves. Hence concentrating on 'behaviours' rather than 'groups' may still not have the positive effect that we think.

The manner in which individuals construct their own notions of 'high-risk behaviour' and 'high-risk groups' is informed by, and in turn reconstructs, their own (hierarchies of) 'knowledge' of HIV. Thus the debate about the efficacy of terms such as 'high-risk behaviour' or 'high-risk groups' must include a consideration of what kinds of things people know or believe and what they do with their knowledge or beliefs. People manipulate the things they know in order to create a space in which they allow themselves to do what they want to do.

Thus, to recap an example from my own data, although Joaquin 'knew' that prostitutes in the *barrio* were a 'high-risk group,' he accommodated his sexual partnership with Antonia alongside this 'knowledge.' His 'knowledge' that Antonia was a 'trustworthy friend' took precedence over the 'knowledge' that she was in a 'high-risk group.' These kinds of examples point to the elasticity of the human mind to be creative with the information that it receives.

The stories of other clients discussed above point to the fact that clients did not necessarily see HIV in a vacuum from other risks. They also suggest that some clients took risks self-consciously. Perhaps some of these clients were not quite as blind as Beck would have it. It might simply be the case that they chose to arrange the knowledge they had in a particular hierarchy, positioning the taking of risks above the possibility that they might suffer from a potentially fatal disease at an indiscriminate time in the future. And it may also be the case that some clients derived pleasure from the potential danger of short-sightedness, rather than accepting the implications of blindness.

Finally, let us return to Arturo, the client who told me that he didn't worry about HIV: life was full of risks, even if you weren't always aware of them. I wasn't persuaded, as the following extract from my fieldnotes makes clear:

> Arturo made me really angry with all that stuff about risk. It makes me sick. I respect his right to take risks for himself, but he's like so many other clients. He seems blind to the fact that he could potentially infect someone else. What will it take to make him realize that he should take some responsibility?

I once thought that researchers needed to make a self-conscious political decision to target male clients, a (relatively invisible and unstigmatized) 'group.' and encourage them to accept some responsibility for their roles in prostitution. I now realize that this is not nearly as easy as it might seem. Research that has done this has, in my opinion, sought only further to stigmatize prostitution in general.

Nevertheless, in relation to HIV, I would tentatively suggest that health educators working in Spain do need to go beyond the dissemination of basic knowledge about safer sex 'behaviour,' towards disarming the (ab)use of those potent myths of 'natural sex,' 'friendship' and 'trust' to manipulate and/or to buy 'AIDS-free sex.' Perhaps this is best achieved at a local level, highlighting risk contexts and working with *all* the individuals involved. Still, whilst this may produce better health education and HIV prevention, it will not necessarily reduce stigmatization. Socio-geographical contexts can carry stigmatization of individuals who frequent them in much the same way that the particular identities of individuals in 'groups' do.

ACKNOWLEDGEMENTS

I should like to thank the Economic and Social Research Council for financially supporting the research upon which this chapter is based. I must also acknowledge the help of Alison Field and Steffen Jöhncke in organizing my thoughts. My argument has benefited from discussions with my colleagues at Keele University, although any remaining errors are my responsibility. All translations are my own. My most considerable debt is of course to my informants.

NOTES

1. Ronald Frankenberg is one amongst many anthropologists who have pointed this out (1992). He argues that 'groups' singled out for anthropological HIV research are ideologically constructed — they are invariably not the white, heterosexual majority. Hence HIV research has been conducted In relation to stigmatized marginals: gay men, prostitutes, and intravenous drug users (IDUs).

2. Nevertheless, one reason why it is problematic for anthropologists to completely abandon talk of 'risk groups' has to do with issues of power and funding. For example, in some North American cities, HIV and AIDS is increasingly prevalent in poor black and Hispanic neighbourhoods. In this sense the emphasis on 'risk groups' (or, possibly less controversially, 'risk contexts') should highlight social, economic and political inequalities. Talking about 'risk behaviours' in relation to these 'communities' (outside educational messages) depoliticizes the social, economic and cultural context of HIV infection. My discussion of GMFA concurs with this. They have chosen to reconstruct themselves as a 'risk group,' possibly as a strategy to gain funding.

3. Note the contradiction in maintaining a commitment to discussing 'high-risk behaviours' and yet singling out 'high-risk groups' for re-

search. This might be put down to sloppy linguistics; authors (including myself) discuss prostitutes (or sex workers) and (sometimes) clients, rather than the buying and selling of high-risk sex. However, it is difficult to see how one could find out about selling and buying high-risk sex without starting from the 'group.' Perhaps this could be approached less controversially by examining socio-geographical networks (see Wallace 1991). Nevertheless, this would do little to help health education tackle the 'groups vs. behaviours' issue.

4. In all, I spoke to over 100 clients, a small number of whom were not strictly *barrio* clients. I conversed with many of these men on more than one occasion, and tape-recorded interviews with 15 clients. Most of them were Spanish men from a low-income bracket and were between the ages of 35 and 85. Few clients had received formal education beyond the age of 12. Approximately half of them were married; a number were widowed or divorced. A minority were single or living with a female partner. Many consumed a large quantity of alcohol before having sex with a sex worker. Some were alcoholics, and a few were IDUs. Although I have no space to explore this here, the role of customers' consumption of alcohol with regard to HIV is an important part of the issue of responsibility.

5. When I returned to my fieldsite in 1992, the number of IDUs appeared to have risen, although it is hard to state precisely by how many. The prostitute population of the *barrio* was constantly changing. A number of the prostitutes supported unemployed male or female partners. However, these partners generally had a very low profile in the *barrio*.

6. I know of at least three drug-injecting prostitute women who have died of HIV-related illnesses. Thus far, I have no knowledge of any clients in my immediate research area having received an HIV-positive diagnosis. This may be because none are thus far infected. It is more likely that none have thus far seen themselves as likely to be infected; hence few have had an HIV test. Given the context of prostitution in the *barrio*, one can only assume that men who buy unprotected penetrative sex are to some extent at risk of being infected with HIV, or just as important, of infecting someone else with it.

REFERENCES

Alexander, P. 1989. A Chronology, of Sorts. In: *Matters of Life and Death: Women speak about AIDS*, edited by I. Rieder and P. Ruppelt. London: Virago.

Ardener, E. 1975. Belief and the Problem of Women. In: *Perceiving Women*, edited by S. Ardener. London: Dent.

Beck, U. 1987. The Anthropological Shock: Chernobyl and the Contours of the Risk Society. *Berkeley Journal of Sociology* 33:153–165.

Day, S. 1993. Dealing with Marginality: Anthropological Perspectives on HIV Risk Reduction Among Prostitute Women. Paper presented at the conference on HIV/AIDS in Europe: The Challenge for Anthropology. Southbank University, London.

Douglas, M., and M. Calvez. 1990. The Self as Risk Taker: A Cultural Theory of Contagion in Relation to AIDS. *Sociological Review* 38(3):445–464.

English Collective of Prostitutes. 1988. *Prostitute Women and AIDS: Resisting the Virus of Repression*. U.S. Prostitutes Collective.

Frankenberg, R. 1992. What Identity's At Risk? Anthropologists and AIDS. *Anthropology in Action* 12:6–9.

Giddens, A. 1990. *The Consequences of Modernity*. Cambridge: Polity Press.

Glick-Schiller, N., D. Lewellen, and S. Crystal. 1991. Culture or Politics? An Examination of the Culturological Analysis of AIDS Risk. Unpublished paper.

Higard, C., and L. Finstad. 1992. *Backstreets: Prostitution, Money and Love*. Cambridge: Polity Press.

Krimsky, S., and D. Golding, eds. 1992. *Theories of Risk*. New York: Praeger Press.

Wallace, R. 1991. Social Disintegration and the Spread of AIDS: Thresholds for Propagation Along 'Sociogeographic' Networks. *Social Science and Medicine* 33:1155–1162.

Young, A. 1981. The Creation of Medical Knowledge: Some Problems in Interpretation. *Social Science and Medicine* 15B:379–386.

Part III

Sexual Risk Among
Western Gay Men

Chapter

EIGHT

Sexual Negotiations: An Ethnographic Study of Men Who Have Sex with Men

*Benny Henriksson and
Sven Axel Månsson*

The findings of research on sexuality and risk behaviour seem often contradictory. On the one hand gay and bisexual men are reported to have changed drastically their sexual behaviour through the adoption of *safer sex* strategies, which combine an affirmation of sexual choice with rational disease prevention.[1] On the other hand, men who have sex with men are still found to continue to have unprotected sex. Ten years after Berkowitz and Callen published *How to Have Sex in an Epidemic*, Ekstrand et al. (1992) detected that almost 60 per cent of the gay and bisexual men in their sample had taken part, once or more, in unprotected anal intercourse over a period of four years. The number of *new* infections among gay and bisexual men is approximately 10 per month in Sweden. This may not sound alarming in an international context, but it suffices to cause us to ask ourselves what weaknesses are still to be found in a safer sex strategy.

The traditional approaches of social and epidemiological research have persistently focused on those individual characteristics that are assumed to explain why certain people continue to take risks. This has led to the assumption that a person who continues to engage in risk behaviour is disturbed. This, in turn, favoured the adoption of preventive strategies that sanction social control, treatment, and even quarantine. In the last few years the term 'relapse' has been introduced, suggesting parallels with drug abuse and dependency. Another popular and deep-rooted theory considers *promiscuity* as the main cause of HIV transmission among gay and bisexual men.[2]

Underlying most strategies for the prevention of HIV infection (regardless of whether or not these are organized by gay organizations or public authorities) is the belief that risk behaviour is the result of insufficient knowledge. According to others, prominence should be given to the role of alcohol. Both views have proven rather weak in explaining risk behaviour among men who have sex with men because of their failure to take account of the social and cultural context in which sexuality and risk behaviour occur (Bolton 1992b). An essential element of this context is the *sexual encounter* and its negotiated order (Davies and Weatherburn 1988).

MAIN ISSUES AND METHOD

The key focus of our study was on how the process of sexual negotiation is carried out at places where men have sex with men and on how men make sense of the sexual encounters they have in such places. As a setting for our study we chose the *erotic oases* in present-day Swedish gay culture; in this case, three video clubs. Other erotic oases are public toilets, parks, nude beaches, sauna clubs, bar backrooms, etc. — places that are part of the gay and bisexual subculture found all over the Western world (Delph 1978; Haff 1991).

Our main questions were: What are the patterns of social and sexual interaction between men who have sex with men in such places? How do they negotiate about sex? How do they present themselves on stage (Goffman 1959)? How do they announce sexual availability and sexual preferences? We were also interested in strategies used to alienate (or 'cool out') sexually unattractive visitors

(Goffman 1952). Finally, we were interested in what kind of sexual techniques the men used and if, and how, safer sexual practice was included in the negotiation process.[3]

Our main research method was *participant observation*. Five male observers with different social and educational backgrounds were trained to make observations and collect field notes in the video clubs investigated. Each observer made approximately 20 visits to the clubs, each visit lasting four to five hours. The observers were recruited from the gay community and were all regular and experienced visitors to different gay subcultural scenes. In short, they were true insiders (Adler and Adler 1987) and had considerable knowledge of the field.

Since it was considered extremely valuable to obtain as much detailed information as possible concerning all types of sexual negotiations taking place in the milieu, our observers were instructed to act just as they normally did when they visited these places. As regular visitors, they easily passed as members and they did not have to 'become the phenomenon.' Since they usually did participate in sexual encounters, and since the context in which these took place was what we were most interested in, we did not apply any restrictions on their participation. The only restriction the observers themselves agreed upon beforehand was to accept and engage only in *safer sex* practices *if* they were involved in sexual encounters. Undoubtedly some of the most valuable field notes are derived from those occasions where the observers themselves engaged in sexual negotiations and sexual practices. The notes from these episodes display, in great detail, each step of the negotiation procedure. Especially valuable here are the observers' own narrative reflections about what they were experiencing in different situations.[4]

Within the team, there has been continued scientific debate about what degree of participation in the life and activities to be studied was most adequate. The only thing we can say for certain is that total participation and total passivity both have their advantages and disadvantages. Outsider as well as insider roles cause bias (Styles 1979).[5]

STOCKHOLM'S GAY SCENE

Anyone who believes that sex at public toilets is a new invention should listen to the stories that some of our oldest informants can tell about the 'glory holes' at some of the city's numerous wooden outhouses in the 1940s.[6] The ideal type of homosexual man who entered the scene in those days was rather effeminate. The gay clubs were members-only clubs, carefully hidden behind locked doors and curtained windows. There was a considerable amount of male prostitution, especially during the Second World War.[7]

With the coming of the end of the 1960s and during the 1970s a different scene took over. Venues such as discos, bars, etc., came into existence which, while still underground, but more easy to find, were either openly gay or more or less exclusively visited by gay men and lesbians. During the 1970s at least 20 gay clubs and bars existed in Stockholm, among them three gay saunas. The image of Swedish Erotica was known all over the world, although most of this pornography was actually produced in the US. The ideal type of gay male in Stockholm in the 1970s was a mixture of queen, the androgynous type of the then dominant youth culture, and the emerging San Francisco 'wannabee butch man.'

In Sweden, like elsewhere, the coming of the 1980s meant a drastic change to the more hedonistic gay lifestyle of the 1970s. Approximately 50 per cent of those who tested HIV positive appeared to be gay or bisexual men. During the 1980s two major discourses of HIV prevention developed, the safer sex strategy of the gay community, and the more social control-oriented strategy of the responsible authorities. These two discourses have not always found agreement on the right way to handle the HIV problem. In 1985 the (then social democratic) government introduced a new law on infectious diseases which actually allowed the authorities to isolate HIV-positive persons who 'did not behave' (Henriksson 1988; Henriksson and Ytterberg 1992).[8]

In 1987, the government introduced a special law forbidding gay saunas. The law was criticized mainly for being a shot in the dark, since men continued to have sex at other erotic oases. It was also criticized for being counterproductive, since it hindered gay organizations in their attempts to implement counselling or HIV prevention at places that could be defined as 'allowing sex on its premises.' The law was more a symbolic act of the government than a contribution to real prevention (Brox 1986).

At the same time the government gave financial support to the Swedish Federation for Gay and Lesbian Rights'(RFSL) new house in the centre of Stockholm. When this — 'Europe's Largest Gay House' — was opened in 1988, it symbolized the shift from the earlier 'closeted' gay scene to a more open and proud one. The house has no curtains in its windows. It even advertises itself with neon signs and a bookshop. At the opening ceremony the appearance of prominent cultural and political personalities showed that this part of the gay culture had become widely accepted. Furthermore, a parliamentary committee was instructed to investigate the possibility of introducing a law on registered partnership for gay and lesbian couples.[9]

The rationale behind this — well-intended but contradictory — policy of both support and prohibition probably lay in an attempt by the government to encourage stable relationships among gay men through the establishment of meeting places far away from the erotic oases, which were considered to be foci of infection. In this way public concern was very much directed towards supporting and accepting the 'well behaved' gay men and lesbians while educating the 'badly behaved.' This attitude is very much in line with the old tradition of the Welfare State as a Good Father, who sets life in order for his children (Hirdman 1989). This Father was surprised that some of his children wanted to solve their problems in their own way. The Father wanted to change the HIV prevention strategy of the gay organizations (i.e., safer sex) into a strategy that emphasized testing and contact tracing, and through a large media campaign he attempted to raise the awareness of the general population. HIV had to be 'dehomosexualized' in order to fit into the public discourse (Henriksson and Bjurström 1988; Patton 1988).

Many gay and bisexual men indeed left the scene because of AIDS. Others visited the oases less frequently; but for quite a few, both younger and older men, occasional sexual encounters still play an important role. Nowadays, however, a drastic change has taken place. Gay and bisexual men generally practise safer sex techniques — but obviously not all of them, and not all of the time.

THE STAGE

In its role as an erotic oasis the gay sauna has been replaced by, among other places, the video club. It is this scene that we will examine more closely in this chapter. In what follows we will present a description of the cruising patterns at some of these video clubs. Here Erving Goffman's (1959) metaphors for social interaction are particularly relevant. There is a striking resemblance between the social interaction that takes place here and a stage play as performed in a theatre. We perceive actors and an audience, backstage and on-stage behaviour, scripts and prompters, stage directions and stagehands.

The observations for this study were conducted in a number of these clubs, each with its own distinctly different characteristics. One of the clubs describes itself as 'Europe's largest porno house.' It is run by a large porno and sex club company that normally addresses a heterosexual audience. In this video club you can either watch a movie on three big screens upstairs or you can go downstairs to watch any of the over 60 different pornographic videos that are shown simultaneously in small cabins. The films attract people with diverse sexual tastes; heterosexual, gay, lesbian, bisexual, animal, sadomasochistic, etc. There are about 30 small cabins in the hall and in all of them you can zap between the 60 video channels. The sound, coming simultaneously from all the cabins, is sometimes a total cacophony.

Another club has been rebuilt since the law on sauna clubs was introduced in 1987. Previously it had numerous lockable cabins, but now there are more open salons where different porno movies are shown. In the first room the visitor can watch heterosexual films, in the one farther down bisexual films, and gay films are shown nearest the rear of the premises. This organization of the movies is important. At this video club a more insecure man can start by watching heterosexual films just inside the entrance, then advance to the next room, where he can watch bisexual films, and eventually graduate to watching gay films in the rooms farther down.

Yet another video club is situated on the outskirts of the city. This was a regular gay sauna before 1987, but after the law was introduced it was rebuilt as a video club. Here too, the supply of films can suit both heterosexual and homosexual men's interest, but the audience is obviously mainly gay or bisexual.

The visitors to the video clubs have to learn how to use the premises. They have to know whether or not the staff are 'friendly and well disposed.' They have to learn how to find their way once inside the premises. They have to discover what is allowed and what is a 'no, no!' It takes a while for a novice to comprehend all these things. One important part of this game is to be able to distinguish between the *hot* and the *protected* areas.

Hot Areas

Some parts of the premises are especially *hot*. Here you are expected and allowed to approach someone sexually. To be present in a certain area of the premises announces one's sexual availability. There are many strategies for responding to different approaches from other actors. And, to make matters more complicated, some of the performances taking place in these hot places are either 'open' to the audience or 'closed.'

One of the video clubs is divided into smaller salons where different types of movies are shown (straight, bisexual, gay). This means that there are some dark corridors or passages between the salons. Certain passages here are very hot. To lean against the wall in one of these passages signals that you are open for suggestions. Several video clubs have small cabins for private viewing. These, of course, are also perfect for sexual encounters. If you sit in one of the small cabins with the door slightly open, you are probably putting out a sexual invitation.

Some of the video clubs are furnished with two-seater sofas, rather than the normal circles of movie seats. A considerable degree of cultural competence is required to know how to sit on these sofas in order to show either availability or lack of interest. To sit on one of the two seats with the legs slightly spread is often a sign of availability. To sit in the middle of the sofa 'occupying' both seats is, of course, a sign of inaccessibility.

In some video clubs back-rooms have developed behind suitably hung curtains in front of emergency exits or some other corners of the premises. These corners may be very hot. At yet another video club the foyer between the movie rooms and the toilets is regarded as a suitable place for 'asking for a dance,' with a long row of men walking to and from the toilets while eyeing the 'wallflowers' on the sofa. Now and then the men's eyes meet and the man sitting on the sofa strolls after the first man into the toilet.

The toilets are hot places. One of the toilets has two rooms and the inner room has a 'glory hole' in the door, probably constructed by a visitor. This place is very popular. Some men hold court there for hours. This is predominantly a place for oral sex. In other places the owners themselves have deliberately built in such services.

Protected Areas

Other areas are *protected*: sexual contacts are not expected there, and not allowed. Protected areas function as a refuge for straight men or men who simply want to take a rest. Others use these protected areas more artfully. Sometimes they are occupied by men who seem to be 'straight' but who, with this 'disguise,' may actually intend to make themselves even more attractive. After a while such a person may move over to the hot places, where he gets some extra attention. Straight men are often highly valued.

Persons who close the cabin door at video clubs — if there are cabins, of course — want to be left free of attention, at least for the time being. Men who place themselves in one of the rows closest to the screen in the heterosexual salon will probably also be left alone, but may, in exceptional circumstances, be approached by some of the more tenacious hunters. The back rows closest to the aisle are not protected at all against advances from men who are standing behind them trying to catch other men's attention. A certain armchair in the gay film room in one of the video clubs is protected, while a similar armchair farther back closer to the entrance is fairly hot. The type of film shown is generally irrelevant. A room with straight films may be as hot as one showing gay movies.

The Actors

Men of all ages, from 17 to 90, are visitors to the clubs. It is somewhat surprising that so many young men find them attractive. Some clubs are obvious 'after hours' places, where you can go after the gay discos have closed. A couple are actually open 24 hours a day. The clubs seem to fulfil a need for initiation — or *rites-de-passage* — into gay sexuality for some young men (Herdt 1992). The gay discos, the organizational gatherings, the bars, are all important places for social activities, and maybe even for searching for Mr. Right. However, some young men seek more uncomplicated ways of having sex in order to 'get it over with.'

Most of the visitors to the gay video clubs identify themselves as gay men, but some have told us that they consider themselves to be straight or bisexual; some are married. Why do straight men visit gay video clubs, and why do they sometimes take part in a sexual act with another man? Are they 'closet gays'? Maybe, but not necessarily. Some heterosexual men do not seem to react negatively to erotic attention from other men or to the erotic excitement that often exists in these places. The video clubs are first and foremost homo-social milieus. At times some of these men, maybe on their way home after work, or at lunch, cross the border of their sexual identity and engage in an anonymous sexual encounter with another man. This in fact bears many resemblances to male sexual patterns that we can witness in many other cultures (Schmitt and Sofer 1992).

Some of the clubs are more gay than others. In some video clubs it is assumed that you are interested in having sex with other men until you have demonstrated otherwise. You are expected to be gay or bisexual. In others it is far more hazardous to make this assumption.

Outsiders often ask themselves what attracts men from such different backgrounds to hang around for hours at places where pornographic videos are shown. Pornographic videos, both heterosexual, bisexual, and gay, can be rented for approximately the same price as the entrance fee to the video clubs, and you can keep the movies in your home for 24 hours. The films, of course, are one of the attractions, but they seem to play an astonishingly small role. It isn't even necessary to show gay films. Sometimes places that show almost exclusively straight films are just as attractive as those showing predominantly gay or bisexual movies. It is something else that attracts: the opportunities these places, and other erotic oases, provide for homo-social intercourse and sexual encounters between men. Even if by no means all male visitors fulfil their sexual fantasies with other men, the homoerotic atmosphere seems to be the most important part of the video clubs' inner life. For some men the clubs serve as a safe place for cruising and for others they also offer a reasonably safe place for quick and often anonymous sexual encounters.

It is not only the visitors who participate in the performance. Sometimes it is very difficult to know whether the owners are really aware of what's happening on the premises or not. At one level both the owners and the visitors have a mutual interest in disguising the fact that sexual acts are taking place. But at the same time it is in the interest of the owners to let the visitors know in a circuitous manner that they are allowed. Due to the law on gay saunas this is a carefully constructed scene, created by the visitors and the owners of the clubs in co-operation. The aim is to provide space on the premises where sexual acts can take place without revealing this to outsiders (such as plain clothes policemen).

In certain clubs this deception seems to occur without participation of the owner, but in others the whole thing looks much more like an ingeniously and skillfully rehearsed play where owner, staff, and visitors all perform on the same stage. However, the video clubs usually do not show the same 'membrane' phenomenon as the public toilets. There is no need to adjust your dress and position each time someone walks through the door, as Humphreys (1970), Delph (1978), and Haff (1991) have described. One of the problems involved in this deception is that the owners are reluctant to display safer sex messages and to distribute condoms on the premises, as this would indicate that sexual acts are actually occurring.

Script and Choreography

A special cruising script, with its own choreography, has emerged at the video clubs. It is important to note that the performances bear a greater resemblance to a pantomime than to a normal play. The main form of communication consists of nonverbal expressions and movements (Eibl-Eibesfeldt 1979). If we ignore a few whispers, and some moaning and whimpering, the only sound heard comes from the somewhat exhausting soundtracks of numerous acts of sexual intercourse on the screen. Apart from this, the video clubs are a very good example of Delph's 'silent community.' Not many words were either spoken or overheard during several hundred hours of observation. This is quite different from the pattern common at heterosexual cruising places, like singles bars, where the spoken word is a part of both the cruising and the cooling out strategies (McCall et al. 1991).

The script tells the visitors how to approach each other in a proper way and the appropriate way of showing interest, or lack of it. The visitors must use a special language in order to present themselves to their co-actors and perhaps also to an audience.

> I decide to answer his signals. I choose to meet his eyes when he passes by, and we both turn towards each other when we have passed. Another way to confirm the contact is to watch the same movie in the same cabin as the one you are interested in, which I do. After approximately ten minutes, after having met several times, we are both standing in the door to two cabins beside each other. After several mutual eye contacts and a quick smile — which is responded to — he invites me into his cabin with a nod. (Observer's field notes, Sunday morning, 3 a.m.)

The pantomimic dance performed at the video clubs involves following the person in whom you are interested all around the locality, until you get him where you want him, i.e., where you can have sex, or at least where you can negotiate the possibilities in more detail. A man sits on one of the sofas. Another man sits down on the sofa, beside the first man. The first man 'asks for a dance' with a glance, followed by a gentle touch of his crotch. If the glance is met, the man rises and starts walking around in the club to other rooms, watching other films. The second man, if he is interested, follows. The second man may be leaning against the wall close to the first one. The first one moves again with the other, clinging to the first man's 'skirt.' Finally they end up near the toilets or one of them drifts behind the curtain to the back-room, with the other following. When inside, new dance steps follow. Now the negotiation is more concerned with the way the two will have sex. Standing in one of the corners of the back-room with your back towards the others and glancing through the tiny slot of the curtain most probably signals that you are interested in passive anal sex, while leaning against the wall most probably signals that you like oral sex or active anal sex. A man who squats on his bended knees is ready to give a 'blow job.'[10] Another strategy, mostly seen in the corridors of video club two, is to stand so close to another visitor that you actually rub your own body against the other man's body.

> If the response is positive there are different alternatives for continuation. A walks over to another room to find out if B is interested. If he is, he follows, not immediately but after a minute. This is repeated a couple of times and in a while the two end up at a place where the sexual act can take place. (Observer's field notes, Wednesday, 11 p.m.)

> One man is leaning against the wall in one of the rather narrow passages, at least pretending to watch the movie in the room in front of him. Another man approaches, passing the first man a couple of times to see if he gets any eye contact. The man who is standing still answers the glance and maybe reinforces the sign of interest by placing his hand on his crotch. Then, finally, depending on his sexual preferences, the second man places himself behind the first man or in front of him, squeezing either his penis against the other man's bum or vice versa. (Observer's field notes, Friday night, 1 a.m.)

Cooling out

Sophisticated strategies have also developed to avoid intimate contacts or to 'turn down' or 'cool out' (Goffman 1952) attentive admirers. Sometimes the fact that someone is actually speaking is a clear indication that there is no point in continuing the complimentary call. To keep close to a friend is another strategy used mainly by the younger men visiting the clubs late at night. Their giggling and whispering keeps admirers at a safe distance.

The way one sits in the two-seat sofas is a clear indication. A man sitting in the middle of the sofa covering his crotch with his jacket is probably not very open to sexual invitations. On the other hand this can also be the starting point of something. The best way to find out is to sit down beside him, trying to make eye contact, and to show your own availability. Maybe he is masturbating furtively inside his trousers. So far this looks like a match. He is open to sexual attentions, but maybe not from the person sitting beside him. One cool out strategy would be to stop masturbating and fold one's arms demonstratively. If that is not enough, and the other man remains, or even worse, starts to send more obvious signals, the first man may rise from his seat with an audible sigh and walk away.

Some men sit on the sofas showing their 'weapons.' This is often, of course, a clear invitation and also a 'presentation of the self' and one's phallic merits. But it does not necessarily indicate an invitation. The display of an erect penis while sitting 'on post' can also be an avoiding — or even aggressive — act, a marker of space and territory (cf. Eibl-Eibesfeldt 1979). The observers many times witnessed a great hesitation among the men to approach someone in this position.

Why Bother About Dancing?

In most gay video clubs you do not risk being caught by anyone on the staff. At least two of the clubs are run by gay staff and they do not seem to mind what goes on. So why bother about all those advanced pirouettes, like birds in a courtship dance? Maybe the dance is the main attraction. Or maybe the dance is a necessary part in the complicated process of sexual negotiation between people who are, in most cases, total strangers. The worst thing that can happen at places like this is rejection. If you approach each other step by step and very carefully put your offers and demands on the negotiation table, you will discover at an early stage whether the other person (a) is interested, (b) suits you, (c) is interested in what you are interested in, (d) is willing to have sex here, (e) is interested in having sex the way you prefer it, etc.

But the dancing is also a reflection of the long history of repression of same-sex behaviour which has forced gay and bisexual men to conceal and disguise their sexual acts both from the authorities and from a hostile environment. This has also forced the men to concentrate on sophisticated rituals for negotiating the act, rather than on the rites of attendance (Foucault 1982).

The Act

The aim of the performances is in most cases the sexual act, even though we also see quite a number of 'cock teasers'[11] who obviously enjoy the dance more than the sexual act itself. What kind of sexual techniques are used at the video clubs, and can they be considered to be safer?

Most of the sexual encounters that take place in the video clubs involve masturbation and mutual masturbation: approximately 60 per cent of all sexual acts.[12] The second most popular way of having sex here is undoubtedly oral sex. Like masturbation, it can be performed concealed, in the toilet, or more publicly, behind the curtain, in the aisles, or even in the sofas and seats. We estimate that approximately 35 per cent of all sexual acts in the video clubs consist of oral sex.

In comparison with mutual masturbation and oral sex, anal sex is rarely practised in the video clubs. Our estimate is that this makes up only a few per cent of all sexual acts. There are very practical reasons for not participating in anal sex in these clubs. Furthermore, there are still many taboos surrounding it, even among men who have sex with men. Since unprotected anal intercourse is the most risky sexual technique for transmitting HIV, anal sex may also have come to be considered even more shameful in recent years, at least if done publicly.[13] For that reason it is most often practised behind closed doors, for example, in the toilets or in the home of one of the persons involved. However, our observers did witness some acts of anal sex in at least one of the video clubs.

Is the sex taking place in the video clubs safer or unsafe, and what factors make the sexual encounter safer/unsafe? Since most of the sexual acts are masturbation, they are in the majority of instances safe.[14] The observers witnessed a number of oral acts, which may arguably be labelled safer sex. The most problematic observation, of course, is the amount of unsafe sex that occurs at places like the video clubs, i.e., predominantly unprotected anal sex. When the observers witnessed anal sex a condom was used in most of the cases. This is considered to be safer sex.[15] But we also observed cases where persons let themselves be anally penetrated without any protection, which of course is unsafe sex.

NEGOTIATIONS ABOUT SAFER SEX

One very important question is whether safer sex has been included in the video club 'dance,' and whether a fusion is possible between the quick and silent act and the rules for safer sex. A good deal of the men had obviously already prepared for the negotiation at home. Some carried condoms and some had small packages of lubricants in their pockets. Others seemed to be much less prepared for safer sex. This, of course, is one of the reasons why it is so important that safer sex accessories to be available on the premises.

We found many different strategies for the inclusion of communication about safer sex practices in this dance. Some stopped in the middle of an act when their partner tended to go over the limit, for example, trying to penetrate or be penetrated by the other person. Some handed over a condom to the other partner. Others just put a condom on themselves. There is no need for verbal speech in this manner of communicating, but sometimes a few words were overheard, such as, 'Put this on and fuck me.'

In most of the cases it was the passive partner who introduced a condom into the negotiation procedure around anal sexual encounters. If the passive partner did not put the condom on the negotiation table, the act was usually an unsafe one. If one partner demanded a condom, the other partner most often accepted this as a fact of life. No one walked away or interrupted an anal sex act if a condom was introduced. But this did occur in oral sex sessions. The passive partner, in particular — the one that sucked — sometimes avoided this if the partner introduced a condom. There is obviously a common consent about the use of condoms in anal sex, but not in oral sex. We also noted that when a younger and older man were involved in sexual activities, the younger man often relied on the older to direct the negotiations. We will use two concrete examples of sexual negotiations to illustrate our reasoning.

Negotiation Position 1

A tall, slim man in his 30s is standing to the right behind the curtain gazing out over the room through the tiny slot between the curtain and the wall. A couple of older men are also loitering behind the curtain. A man enters the back-room and places himself behind the first man. After a while he places his hand on the first man's behind. The first man stands still and pulls out his penis and starts masturbating. The second man works the first man's jogging pants down to his knees and continues with rather advanced finger exercises. The first man is standing still and picks up what I later realised was a tube of lubricant, squeezing out some of the contents into his hand (you could hear it) and rubs his ass with the lubricant. The second man has now pulled out his prick, but instead of fucking the first man he penetrates him with his fingers. After a while I can observe that the younger man pulls out a condom, unwraps it and, without even turning around, with his hands behind his back he threads the condom on the other man's cock. After that the younger man takes from his pocket what must have been a bottle of poppers and inhales a couple of times, and finally leans forward, after which the second man fucks him, for a long time. Several people have gathered around the two, since the younger man is having difficulties keeping his mouth shut, and is groaning quite loudly. Everybody tries, in one way or the other, to take part and masturbate him, suck him or stick their fingers up his ass while he is being fucked. He tries to keep most of those attempts away. (Observer's field note, Saturday night, 02:30 a.m.)

Negotiation Position 2

There are approximately five or six persons behind the curtain. A very attractive young person, around 18 to 20, is standing there without moving for a long time. Nobody seems to dare to court him. He reminds me of the beautiful princess who never got the prince because no prince believed that he was good-looking enough. He wears worn-out jeans and a white tank top. He leans towards the wall, but takes no initiatives of his own. A man in his 40s, with leather jacket, jeans, and leather boots, finally places himself in front of the young man and soon touches his crotch. He meets with no resistance and his hands continue to touch the young man's body, especially his nipples. The older man is very rough and now and then he slaps the younger man's buttocks. The older man pulls out his penis, pressing the younger man onto his knees, after which the younger starts to suck him. After a while the younger man rises again and starts to kiss the older man. The young one unbuttons his jeans and lets them fall to the floor, turns his back to the older man and more or less 'threads on' to him. The older man cannot possibly have had the time to put on a condom. In any case the young man didn't do anything to assure himself that his partner was wearing a condom. (Observer's field notes, Friday evening, approximately 00:30 a.m.)

The above stories are both examples of sophisticated sexual negotiations, but there is one important difference between the two. In the first, the consequence of the negotiation is safer sex, in the second, the outcome of the negotiation is unsafe sex.

TOWARDS RETHINKING HIV PREVENTION: COMPETENCE VERSUS OBSTACLES

One important finding in our study is that most sexual activities occurring at video clubs can be labelled 'safer.' Other studies, for example by Bolton et al. (1994) on gay saunas in Belgium and by

Koegh et al. (1992) on public toilets in London have shown similar results.

Another important finding, which the first example above shows (the man who puts on the condom behind his back), is that some of the men have developed a great deal of competence in safer sex negotiations. These conclusions are important because they contradict the popular misapprehension among the authorities and mass media of the video clubs (and other erotic oases) as foci of infection.

On the other hand, our study also shows that some of the men obviously have not developed the same competence, as the second example above shows. In order to be able to understand the obstacles to safer sex we must not fall back on theories that indicate only individual shortcomings; rather, we must deepen our efforts to understand what it is in the social interaction and in the context where this interaction takes place that affects the outcome of the negotiation.

The architectonic structure of the premises can support or counteract safer sex negotiations. If erotic oases like the video clubs offered a safe environment that encourages safer sex, by for instance exhibiting eroticized safer sex messages, this would naturally encourage the men to include safer sex techniques in their sexual negotiations. We saw very few signs of such messages during our field work.

Another contextual aspect is the extent to which the pornography shown at video clubs exhibits safer or unsafe sexual encounters. We can only speculate on their effect, but we have noted that there were very few safer sex messages in the pornography shown at the clubs investigated.

One important factor influencing safer sex negotiation is what we would like to call the *symbolic value* of sexuality, which refers to the meaning and value the men attach to certain sexual techniques or to having sex in a certain context.

Problems may arise when rules about safer sex techniques do not fit into this symbolic economy. Many men tell us how important it is to them to feel their partner's sperm inside them when they have anal sex. For these men the use of condoms can be experienced as an artificial barrier to the intimacy they seek. For many the erotic oasis itself has become loaded with symbolic values that are sometimes in conflict with safer sex practices.

CONCLUSIONS

Gay and bisexual men have created their own cultural meanings around sexuality. Gay men have not only managed to counteract the repression of their sexuality by constructing new ways and unorthodox places where it is possible to have sex; they have also managed to eroticize having sex in the places where they have been forced to meet. Representatives of the authorities and the moral elite have always looked on these erotic oases with great suspicion. AIDS has provided new arguments and become a 'good enemy,' legitimizing legal restrictions on, for example, gay saunas.

Our study has shown that these erotic oases are important to many gay and bisexual men. It also shows that a sophisticated system of communication has developed to facilitate the negotiation of sexuality in these places. One example of this is the 'dance' at the video clubs which we have described in this chapter. Another example is the handkerchief codes which were common signs of sexual preference in the male bar culture of the larger American cities in the 1970s (Patton 1989b). Our study has also revealed that many visitors to video clubs are competent sexual negotiators and that it is possible to include rules for safer sex in their sexual script.

Gay and bisexual men, however, are quite understandably less experienced in safer sex negotiation than in 'normal' sexual negotiation (Richardson 1987; Patton 1989a, 1989b; Davies and Weatherburn 1991). Safer sex competence has a social history of only 10 years. The problem is that gay men are expected to be able to manage to negotiate in every sexual situation: when newly in love, when finding someone for a one-night stand, when standing in the bushes of the Bois de Bologne in Paris, in the steam sauna of the Thermos in Amsterdam, or at the video clubs in Stockholm. In all these situations gay men are supposed to use signals for what they like and for the demands they make on the sexual encounter, and they are assumed to be able to manage in a practical way the accessories needed for safer sex practices.

Sexual conduct is the result of an order which is negotiated in social interaction. Sexuality is in this sense a social construct which can be changed over time. But such changes may be difficult to achieve, since such a negotiated order may also be apprehended as an essential part of a person's or a group's life. There is an important element of tenacity in all social structures, including sexuality.

Our observations and interviews have shown that some sexual preferences are often experienced as fixed or essential parts of human identity, and are therefore perceived as very difficult to change. We believe that current HIV prevention policies, whether organized by gay organizations or public authorities, have not taken this symbolic economy of sexuality fully into consideration. Instead, it has been believed that risky sexual behaviour can be changed either by propaganda in favour of stable relations or through traditional education and information.

HIV prevention is indeed in one sense a question of education and we believe that it is very important to continue the safer sex educational programmes involving most gay organizations. In this form of education, it seems most important to give participants the possibility of discussing their sexual preferences and experiences in relation to safer sex negotiations. The dramaturgical approach developed by some gay organizations is promising (Taylor and Lourea 1992; Eriksson and Knutsson 1991).

But traditional education is not enough if we want people to really minimize risky behaviour. It might be a good idea for organizations working on HIV prevention to ask themselves how the competence of the men we have described has been achieved, how it can be better used in future preventive work, and what the major obstacles to this competence are. To be able to be a competent safer sex practitioner and to develop negotiation skills, one has to have sex. It is a logical, but at the same time, a challenging conclusion, especially for those who believe that the only solution to the HIV problem is steady partners and monogamy. If we take our findings seriously we should rather tend to recommend that people be more promiscuous. There is a large grain of truth in the pedagogical thesis that nothing is so effective as learning by doing, especially if the 'mentor' is a very competent person. Why should we feel uncomfortable about using this knowledge in safer sex education?

The reason why the moral elite finds ideas like these too challenging is probably because gay men's sexuality has been labelled as either consumerist or the result of repression, which does not fit into the politically correct idea of how to have sex. This viewpoint is not only becoming rampant among the authorities; it is also gaining ground among groups of AIDS activists and gay politicians (Henriksson 1990; Nichols 1989). To be able to develop a new ethic around safer sex we have to get rid of such 'closet moralism' (Patton 1989a). The 'dances' at the video clubs are important parts of a sexual negotiation which can include safer sex rules and norms. What we have to achieve is an eroticization of safer sex practices and the incorporation of safer sex rules into these negotiations. We also believe that the role of HIV prevention is not to interfere with where people meet, where they have sex, or how they have sex — with one exception, and that is to advise people how to have safer sex. Almost any sexual preference can be made safer, very often with relatively small changes to a person's sexual life.

NOTES

1. Several studies confirm that the *safer sex* strategy is more effective than the traditional control and prohibition policies (e.g., Brandt 1987).

2. There is no simple relationship between having multiple partners and HIV infection (Bolton 1992a). Swedish physicians have recently noted that the vast majority of newly infected gay men contracted HIV within a stable relationship (RFSL 1992).

3. This study of video clubs forms part of an extensive, ongoing research project which also includes other places, such as public toilets, parks, public bathhouses, and nude beaches.

4. Our rationale for not asking the observers to restrict their participation in sexual encounters is similar to the arguments in favour of the 'complete observation role' listed in social science textbooks as one of many different observer roles valuable in observation studies (Emerson 1981; Jorgensen 1989; Patton 1980). It is no different from Becker's (1963) reasons for participation as a jazz musician and marijuana smoker; Milner's (Milner and Milner 1973) mingling with black pimps in a Californian bar; Jules-Rosette's (1975) strategy of 'becoming' a member of a native African fundamentalist Christian group; Buford's (1991) participation in football hooliganism; Sanders's (1988) way of hanging out at tattoo shops, observing, and being tattooed; Douglas's (1977) way of becoming a nude bather; Wolf's (1990) involvement in a motorcycle club; Gallmeiers (1991) participation in the life of a hockey club; Corzine and Kirby's (1977) participant observations of gay sexual encounters in a highway rest area; Styles's (1979) observations at gay baths in Los Angeles; Delph's (1978) observations at different American erotic oases; or Haff's (1991) participant observations of sex between men in Copenhagen public toilets.

5. Warnings have been sounded about attempts to play a complete insider role (for instance, in the first years of the Chicago School), which entail the risk of going native. Later scholars (Denzin 1962, 1978; Douglas 1976) have defended complete participation with less reservation, and one can easily interpret Erving Goffman's speech during the 1974 Pacific Sociological Association Meeting (Goffman 1974/1989) to mean that acting as a total insider is a desirable goal of all fieldwork, albeit one that is difficult to achieve. This, of course, in no way dis-

claims the fieldworker's responsibility to discuss and reflect upon the way the researcher himself or herself influences the activities being studied, and the ethical dilemmas involved. Some researchers of sexuality argue for and actually take part in sexual acts. Others have used more restrictive strategies. For example, the way Ponte (1974) chose to observe, from his car, encounters between men at public parking lots, without even going into the toilet where the sexual encounters took place, prevented him from making any real ethnographic descriptions. Laud Humphreys' role as a watchqueen of the tearooms is an example of more direct participation, even though he did explicitly point out that he was not involved in sexual activities (Humphreys 1970). Delph (1978) states that there are many different ways and degrees of obtaining insider status, and that he used them all. Haff (1991) agrees fully with this and claims that he tried both a total involvement and a more passive observing role, and Bolton (1992c) argues in favour of using one's own sexual encounters as the most important field material. Most studies of erotic oases have been conducted in gay subcultural milieus (Humphreys 1970; Delph 1978; Ponte 1974; Haff 1991). At straight cruising places it is less usual to have sex on the premises, but participant observation studies have shown that cruising does occur. See, for example, Cloyd's study (1976) of heterosexual encounters within a bar-room environment; Holter's (1981) observations of the cruising patterns at Norwegian ballrooms; McCall et al. (1991) on the 'cooling out' strategies of women at American singles bars who react to excessively importunate male suitors; and McNeil's (1992) detailed description of heterosexual and bisexual swingers clubs in contemporary New York. Only a few ethnographic studies have been conducted on sex shops and pornographic movie or video clubs. For example, in 1973 Karp and Sundholm each published studies on pornographic bookstores in the Time Square area of New York and pornographic arcades in downtown San Francisco. Donnelly also studied the moral order of pornographic movie theatres (Donnelly 1981), and Perkins and Skipper (1981) studied gay pornographic and sex paraphernalia shops. These studies describe, among other things, the social risks, including the risk of being seen and labelled as a social deviant, that follow the visit to such shops. Donnelly speaks of 'running the gauntlet.'

6. In the male gay subculture a 'glory hole' means a hole, big enough to insert your penis, in the wall between two toilet cabins or in the door of the cabin, to facilitate oral sex.

7. Sweden took no part in World War II because of its 'neutrality,' but the country was of course prepared for war. Those young men who did compulsory military service during this period, called the 'recruits,' usually stayed away from home and girlfriends for very long periods.

8. There was a political shift in 1991. A coalition of four parties took over the task of government: Liberals, Conservatives, Christian democrats, and the Centre party. The new government has not changed any of the laws criticized here. In 1994 there was a new shift back to a social democratic government.

9. The new Partnership Act was finally approved by the Parliament in 1994.

10. Giving a 'blow job' denotes a passive role in oral sex, that is the man who sucks the other's penis is giving a blow job.

11. 'Cock teaser,' in the gay subculture, refers to someone who likes to flirt and to sexually arouse another man, but who almost never completes the sexual encounter. He just likes to tease.

12. An estimate from field notes.

13. At the same time there are many indications that anal sex continues to play an important role in gay and bisexual men's sexual fantasies and practices. For example, much of the sex talk on the Swedish telephone company's gay chat line is about 'getting fucked,' i.e., the sexual technique which, from an HIV transmission point of view, is the most risky one if practised without a condom. It is noteworthy that most of these wishes are expressed by younger men. One can only speculate on the reasons behind these tendencies. Maybe the warnings against anal sex in connection with HIV information have in fact increased the wishes among gay and bisexual men to practise it, even if only on a fantasy level. Maybe the attraction lies in the forbidden and the risky. Or maybe it is another example of what Michel Foucault and others have described as an effect of the increased talk about it during recent years. The simple fact that anal sex has been much more discussed, even if in connection with such connotations as shame, danger, something one should avoid, perversion, etc., may actually have constructed an attraction to the phenomenon, or rather legitimized the development of one's inner fantasies around anal sex.

14. There is some conceptual confusion around the concept of safer sex. Early on in the AIDS epidemic representatives of gay organizations more or less 'invented' the concept of safe sex as a constructive strategy to minimize the risk of HIV transmission between men who have sex with men. This was long before governments around the world had even formulated any plans to combat the disease. Patton (1989b) and others have pointed out that the focus in HIV prevention was twisted away from safer sex to promoting testing and more moral recommendations, such as 'stick to one partner,' when governments did get involved. The concept of safe sex was never fully acknowledged by governments and medical researchers.

At the same time, many felt uneasy with the concept of safe sex, because it is almost impossible to guarantee that a certain sexual act or technique is 100 per cent safe. But it is still important to distinguish between risky behaviour and behaviour that is fairly safe. Therefore the concept of safer sex was understood as a better concept than that of safe sex. But the problem is that the concept of safer sex is not very clear and often leads to misinterpretations.

There is a worldwide debate about what can be agreed upon as safer sex, and the scientific judgments are far from unanimous. If we can trust many epidemiological studies, oral sex can be said to be safer sex, even if it is not 100 per cent safe. That is, it is safer, but not safe (Calzavara and Coates 1988; Coates et al. 1988).

There are one or two cases documented in Sweden where oral sex without a condom seems to be the most probable route of transmission. But compared with the vast majority of cases where a clear connection between unprotected anal sex and HIV transmission has been demonstrated, such cases are very few.

In the public debate around safer sex, medical experts and representatives of the media constantly, whether consciously or unconsciously, mix up the two concepts of safe and safer sex. Suggestions are consistently being made by medical experts, for example, that the gay organizations are irresponsible since they state that oral sex is safe sex, when they in fact have claimed that oral sex is safer sex, but *not* safe sex.

15. Please note: safer, but not safe sex, because a condom may break.

REFERENCES

Adler, P.A., and P. Adler. 1987. Membership Roles in Field Research. *Qualitative Research Methods* 6.

Becker, H.S. 1963. *Outsiders, Studies in the Sociology of Deviance*. London: Collier-MacMillan.

Berkowitz, R., and M. Callen. 1983. *How to Have Sex in an Epidemic*. New York.

Bolton, R. 1992a. AIDS and Promiscuity: Muddles in the Models of HIV Prevention. In: *Rethinking AIDS Prevention. Cultural Approaches*, edited by R. Bolton and M. Singer. Philadelphia: Gordon and Breach Science publishers.

Bolton, R. 1992b. Alcohol and Risky Sex: In Search of an Elusive Connection. In: *Rethinking AIDS Prevention. Cultural Approaches*, edited by R. Bolton and M. Singer. Philadelphia: Gordon and Breach Science publishers.

Bolton, R. 1992c. Mapping Terra Incognita: Sex Research for AIDS Prevention. An Urgent agenda for the 1990s. In: *The Time of AIDS: Social Analysis, Theory, and Method*, edited by G. Herdt and S. Lindenbaum. London: Sage.

Bolton, R., J. Vincke, and R. Mak. 1994. Gay Baths Revisited. An Empirical Analysis. *GLQ* 1:255-273.

Brandt, A.M. 1987. *No Magic Bullet. A Social History of Veneral Diseases in the United States, since 1980*. New York: Oxford University Press, expanded edition.

Brox, O. 1986. Den store stygge björnen. Norsk Sovjet-politikk som politisk symbolspill (The Big Bad Wolf. Norwegian/Soviet Policy as Political Symbolic Play). *Samtiden* 3:37–41.

Buford, B. 1991. *Among the Thugs*. London: Secker & Warburg.

Calzavara, L., and T. Coates. 1988. Risk Factors for HIV Infection in Male Sexual Contacts of Men with AIDS or AIDS-Related Conditions. *Journal of Epidemiology* 128.

Cloyd, J.W. 1976. The Market-Place Bar: The Interrelation Between Sex, Situation, and Strategies in the Pairing Ritual of Homo Ludens. *Urban Life* 5(3):293–312.

Coates, T., C. Hoff, and R. Stall, eds. 1988. Changes in Sexual Behaviour of Gay and Bisexual Men Since the Beginning of the AIDS Epidemic. Manuscript prepared for Centers for Disease Control, USA.

Corzine, J., and R. Kirby. 1977. Cruising the Truckers: Sexual Encounters in Highway Rest Area. *Urban Life* 6(2):171–192.

Davies, P.M., and P. Weatherburn. 1991. Towards a General Model of Sexual Negotiation. In: *AIDS. Responses, Interventions and Care*, edited by P. Aggleton, G. Hart, and P.M. Davies. London: The Falmer Press.

Delph, E.W. 1978. *The Silent Community. Public Homosexual Encounters*. Beverly Hills: Sage.

Denzin, N.K. 1962. On the Ethics of Disguised Observation: An Exchange Between Norman Denzin and Kai Erikson. *Social Problems* 15:502–506.

Denzin, N.K. 1978. *The Research Act. A Theoretical Introduction to Sociological Methods*. New York: McGraw-Hill.

Donnelly, P. 1981. Running the Gauntlet: The Moral Order of Pornographic Movie Theaters. *Urban Life* 10(3):239–264.

Douglas, J.D. 1976. *Investigative Social Research: Individual and Team Field Research*. Beverly Hills: Sage.

Douglas, J.D., P.K. Rasmussen, and C.A. Flanagan. 1977. *The Nude Beach*. Beverly Hills: Sage.

Eibl-Eibesfeldt, I. 1979. Similarities and Differences Between Cultures in Expressive Movements. In: *Non-Verbal Communication. Readings with Commentary*, edited by S. Weitz. New York: Oxford University Press.

Ekstrand, M. 1992. Safer Sex Maintenance Among Gay Men: Are We Making Any Progress? *AIDS* 6:875–877.

Emerson, R. 1981. Observational Field Work. *Annual Review of Sociology* 7:351–378.

Eriksson, N., and S. Knutsson. 1991. *Ett förebyggande projekt i Malmö om säkrare sex bland män som har sex med män.* Rubber ware (A Prevention Project in Malmö About Safer Sex Among Men Who Have Sex with Men. Rubber Ware). Malmö: RFSL-Rådgivningen.

Foucault, M. 1982. Sexual Choice, Sexual Act: An Interview with Michel Foucault. *Salmaguni* Fall 1982/Winter 1983:10–24.

Gallmeier, C.P. 1991. Leaving, Revisiting, and Staying in Touch. In: *Experiencing Fieldwork. An Inside View of Qualitative Research*, edited by W.B. Shaffir and R.A. Stebbins. London: Sage.

Goffman, E. 1952. On Cooling the Mark Out: Some Aspects of Adaptation to Failure. *Psychiatry* 15:451–463.

Goffman, E. 1959. *The Presentation of Self in Everyday Life.* New York: Doubleday.

Goffman, E. 1974/1989. On Fieldwork. Transcribed and edited by Lyn H. Lofland. *Journal of Contemprary Ethnography* 18(2):123–132.

Haff, J. 1991. Byens erotiske oaser. *Sex mellem maend på offentlige steder* (The Erotic Oases of the City: Sex Between Men at Public Places). Copenhagen: Institutet for Kultursociologi, Köpenhamns universitet.

Henriksson, B. 1988. *Social Democracy or Societal Control. A Critical Analysis of the Swedish AIDS Policy.* Stockholm: Glacio.

Henriksson, B. 1990. Sexual Identity, AIDS and the Moral Left. Paper presented at the International Conference on Homosexuality and HIV, Copenhagen.

Henriksson, B., and E. Bjurström. 1988. Heterosexualiseringen av HIV/AIDS-diskursen (The Heterosexualization of the HIV/AIDS Discourse). *Sociologisk Forskning* 25(2–3):29–46.

Henriksson, B., and H. Ytterberg. 1992. Sweden: The Power of the Moral(istic) Left. In: *AIDS In The Industrialized Democracies. Passions, Politics and Policies*, edited by D.L. Kirp and R. Bayer. New Brunswick: Rutgers University Press.

Herdt, G. 1992. 'Coming Out' As Rite de Passage: A Chicago Study. In: *Gay Culture in Amercia. Essays From the Field*, edited by G. Herdt. Boston: Beacon Press.

Hirdman, Y. 1989. *Att lägga livet till rätta* (To Put Life in Order). Stockholm: Carlssons.

Holter, Ø.G. 1981. Sjekking. *Kjærlighet of kjønnsmarked* (Cruising. About the Love and Gender Market). Oslo: Pax.

Humphreys, L. 1970. *Tearoom Trade. Impersonal Sex in Public Places.* New York: Aldine Publishing Company.

Jorgensen, D.L. 1989. *Participant Observation. A Methodology for Human Studies.* London: Sage.

Jules-Rosette, B. 1975. *African Apostles*. Ithaca, NY: Cornell University Press.

Karp, D. 1973. Hiding in Pornographic Bookstores. *Urban Life and Culture* 1:427–451.

Keogh, P., J. Church, S. Vearnals, and J. Green. 1992. Investigation of Motivational and Behavioural Factors Influencing Men Who Have Sex with Men in Public Toilets (Cottaging). VIIIth International Conference on AIDS/IIIrd STD World Congress. Amsterdam, July 19–24.

McCall, P., C. Robinson, and D.A. Snow. 1991. 'Cooling Out' Men in Single Bars and Nightclubs. Observations on the Interpersonal Suvival Strategies of Women in Public Places. *Journal of Contemporary Ethnography* 19:423–449.

McNeil, L. 1992. Love Among the Ruins. *Details* March:32–40.

Milner, R., and C. Milner. 1973. *Black Players. The Secret World of Black Pimps*. New York: Bantam Books.

Nichols, M. 1989. Lesbian Sexuality. *Lambda Nordica* 3–4.

Patton, C. 1988. De-Homosexualization of AIDS, Testing Instead of Safer Sex. Paper presented at the conference: Homosexuality, Before, During and After HIV, Stockholm. Institute for Social Policy.

Patton, C. 1989a. Cindy Patton on Safer Sex, Community and Porn. *Rites* (April):10–12.

Patton, C. 1989b. Test kontra säkrare sex (Tests Versus Safer Sex). *Lambda Nordica* 1(1):10–12.

Patton, M.Q. 1980. *Qualitative Evaluation and Research Methods*. London: Sage.

Perkins, K., and J. Skipper. 1981. Gay Pornographic and Sex Paraphernalia Shops: An Ethnography of Expressive Work Settings. *Deviant Behavior* 2(2):187–199.

Ponte, M.R. 1974. Life in a Parking Lot: An Ethnography of a Homosexual Drive-In. In: *Deviance. Field Studies and Self-Disclosures*, edited by J. Jacobs. Palo Alto, CA: National Press Books.

RFSL (Swedish Federation for Gay and Lesbian Rights). 1992. Mannen bakom statistiken. Sexuell identitet hos män som hivsmittats vid sex med andra män, Hearing i Stockholm, 5 mars 1992. (The Man Behind the Statistics. Sexual Identity Among Men Who Have Been Infected with HIV Through Sex with Other Men, Hearing, 1992).

Richardson, D. 1987. *Women and the AIDS Crisis*. London: Pandora.

Sanders, C.R. 1988. Marks of Mischief: Becoming and Being Tattooed. *Journal of Contemporary Ethnography* 16(4):395–432.

Schmitt, A., and J. Sofer. 1992. *Sexuality and Eroticism Among Males in Moslem Societies*. Binghamton, NY: Haworth Press.

Styles, J. 1979. Outsiders/Insiders. Researching Gay Baths. *Urban Life* 8(2): 135–152.

Sundholm, C. 1973. The Pornographic Arcade. *Urban Life and Culture* 2(April):85–104.

Taylor, C., and D. Lourea. 1992. HIV Prevention: A Dramaturgical Analysis and Practical Guide to Creating Safer Sex Interventions. In: *Rethinking AIDS Prevention. Cultural Approaches,* edited by R. Bolton and M. Singer. Philadelphia: Gordon and Breach Science publishers.

Wolf, D.R. 1990. *The Rebels: A Brotherhood of Outlaw Bikers.* Toronto: University of Toronto Press.

Chapter NINE

Social Stress and Risky Sex Among Gay Men: An Additional Explanation for the Persistence of Unsafe Sex

John Vincke and Ralph Bolton

The thesis of this study is that, in some instances, the risky sexual behaviour of gay men can be viewed as an outward stress reaction due to social oppression and rejection. In this paper we first review studies of current levels of risky sex among gay men. Second, we situate the practice of unsafe sex within the context of social stress theory and then, after delineating this theoretical domain, we summarize the empirical findings that support the thesis. Finally, we test our thesis.

THE CURRENT LEVEL OF RISKY SEXUAL
BEHAVIOUR AMONG GAY MEN

Although gay men have changed their sexual behaviour substantially since the advent of AIDS (Becker and Joseph 1988; Stall, Coates,
and Hoff 1988; Catania et al. 1989; Bolton et al. 1992), the level of
risky sex remains seriously problematic within gay male populations. Dubois-Arber et al. (1991) reported that in Switzerland 23 per
cent of their research subjects practise unprotected anal sex. In Italy
the percentage is 50 (Sasse et al. 1991). An even more recent study
from the same country showed that, of a sample of 1393 homosexual
and bisexual men, 83.1 per cent reported having sex with non-steady
or with both steady and non-steady partners. This substantial subgroup accounts for even more than 80 per cent of reported unprotected anal intercourse (Sasse et al. 1992). In England and Wales
the percentage having unprotective insertive or receptive anal sex is
27 (Weatherburn et al. 1991). In Belgium in 1989, 21.4 per cent and
27.7 per cent of those having sex with non-regular partners reported
unprotected insertive and receptive anal sex, respectively (Mak et al.
1990). Kelly et al. (1990) report on research in three small cities in the
southern United States. In the two months prior to the study, 25 per
cent and 23 per cent of the respondents practised unprotected insertive and receptive anal sex, respectively. These cross-sectional findings are corroborated by longitudinal data from the Netherlands,
where a group of 365 men was followed over the period 1986–1989.
Before the first data collection 14 per cent of that group practised
safer sex and continued to do so through 1989. In 1987 an additional
8 per cent joined this group. In 1988, this increased by 9 per cent and
by 8 per cent in 1989. However, by 1989 35 per cent of the group still
had not initiated safe sex (de Vroome, Sandfort, and Tielman 1991).
Additional data from a national sample of gay men ($n = 206$) in the
Netherlands show that 44 per cent engaged in insertive anal intercourse. Only 16 per cent of the men engaging in insertive anal intercourse always used condoms. The same study also reports that of the
39 per cent that practised receptive anal intercourse only 20 per cent
protected themselves consistently (Houweling et al. 1992). Research
in England for the period January 1988 to July 1989 found that 58 per
cent practised only safe sex; 10 per cent began safe sex; 15 per cent
reverted to unsafe practices; and 17 per cent persisted in unsafe
behaviour. An additional 16 per cent who were playing safely in
January 1988 and in July 1989, reported instances of unsafe sex within that period (Hart et al. 1991). The Chicago cohort of the MACS

project reported the following trends for 1986–1989. After one year of observation 53 per cent of the participants remained safe, 6 per cent became unsafe, and 31 per cent were inconsistent about risk taking. The authors of this study conclude that the augmented practice of safe sex goes along with an alarming 'backsliding to unsafe sex' (Adib et al. 1991). An additional study by these authors concludes that occasional episodes of unsafe sex, rather than continuous unsafe behaviour, account for the majority of recent potential exposures to HIV among the Chicago MACS/CSS subjects (Adib, Ostrow, and Joseph 1992). Ekstrand and Coates (1990) report on data from the San Francisco Men's Health Study. Within their cohort 686 gay men were followed from 1984 to 1988. Twelve per cent reported that they had unsafe sex after a period of safe sex. Fully 10 per cent had unprotected receptive anal sex during each year of the period studied. Also in San Francisco, 258 young men, 17–25 years of age, were surveyed. The practice of unprotected anal sex among them was as follows: 42.9 per cent for the men 17–19 years old, 24.7 per cent for the men 20–22 years old and 29.9 per cent for those 23–25 years old. The overall prevalence of HIV infection for these young men was 12 per cent (Nieri et al. 1992). In Ireland of a total of 454 homo/bisexual men 58 per cent had had anal sex in the year preceding the interview. Only 48 per cent of these men always used condoms, while 20 per cent of those engaging in anal sex never used condoms (Wyse et al. 1992). Considering the cited levels of unsafe sex in different gay male populations, in combination with the high prevalence of HIV infection within these populations, we can conclude that risky sex still is an actual and urgent problem.

The second report of the Committee on AIDS Research and the Behavioral, Social, and Statistical Sciences of the National Academy of Science in the US (Miller, Turner, and Moses 1990) came to a similar conclusion. It noted that, after almost a decade of monitoring behavioural changes among gay men, there is evidence of 'relapse' in the gay population. The following factors are mentioned as contributing to the 'backsliding' to risky sex: a preference for unprotected anal intercourse; social support for high-risk behaviour; being in love with the sexual partner; 'knowing' that a partner is seronegative; receiving a request from the partner for unprotected sex; using alcohol and drugs; not having condoms available; having higher levels of unsafe behaviour at the baseline; and the perception that behavioural change would not offer protection from infection. It also stated that maintaining safer sex behaviour over time is particularly problematic if people do not enjoy the physical result produced by the safer methods or find the psychological costs associated with change too great. The fact that these factors emerge as explanations for persistence of or 'relapse' into unsafe sex results from the theoretical perspectives guiding the research. Most of the work to date has drawn heavily on theoretical paradigms formulated before the AIDS epidemic and is derived from the sociology and psychology of health behaviour. These theoretical approaches use several social-psychological variables to explain why people exhibit different levels of behaviour change. In these models behaviour change is seen as the product of a complex interplay among variables such as AIDS knowledge, perceived susceptibility, social network norms, self-efficacy, locus of control, AIDS anxiety, denial, and AIDS visibility (Baum and Nesselhof 1988; Catania, Kegeles, and Coates 1990; Coates, Temoshok, and Mandel 1984; Mays, Albee, and Schneider 1989; Morin 1988). Besides these variables, the use of various mind-altering drugs, including alcohol, is hypothesized to be a major impediment to comprehensive and consistent behaviour change (Hingson et al. 1990; Leigh 1990; McCusker et al. 1990; McKirnan and Peterson 1989a, 1989b; Molgaard, Nakamura, and Elder 1988; Morgan Thomas, Plant, and Plant 1990; Plant 1990a, 1990b; Robertson and Plant 1988; Stall 1988; Stall et al. 1986; Stall and Wiley 1988; cf. Bolton et al. 1992).

With the exception of one factor (social network norms for high-risk behaviour) one gains the impression from this literature that sexual behaviour in general and unsafe sex in particular is a purely psychological phenomenon operating within a social void. It cannot be doubted that psychological factors contribute to unsafe sex. However, neither can it be doubted that sexual behaviour takes places within a social space. To identify that space, we need only turn to the epidemiological characteristics of AIDS. Although AIDS in the US and Europe is still most prevalent among homosexual and bisexual men and in large metropolitan areas, the epidemic is spreading rapidly among users of intravenous drugs and their sexual partners, minority individuals whose behaviour places them at risk, women and children (Institute of Medicine 1991).

Generally, the Western social space of AIDS is related to some kind of discrimination and some material, cultural, or social disadvantages. The social space of seropositive people and people with AIDS in the Western industrialized world needs to be considered in connection with the psychological explanations given for the persistence and reoccurrence of unsafe sex (see above). Can insights into the characteristics of this space provide additional, even crucial, explanations for why a substantial percentage of gay men still practises risky sex?

SOCIAL STRESS THEORY

McGrath (1970) proposed considering stress as a series of phenomena that occur over time and that include environmental stimulation, perception, and interpretation of the stimulus by the person as well as the person's responses to the perceived stimulus. Pearlin et al. (1981) defined social stress as consisting of sources of stress, mediators, and stress outcomes. Two general sources of stress are mentioned in the literature. The first covers the impact of life events on people's subjective and objective well-being (Avison and Turner 1988; Ensel and Lin 1991; Lin and Ensel 1989; McLeod and Kessler 1990; Mirowsky and Ross 1986; Pearlin et al. 1981; Pearlin 1989; Sandler and Robert 1985; Tausig 1982). The second source involves chronic stress situations (Kessler, Price, and Wortman 1985; Klitzman et al. 1990; Pearlin et al. 1981). Both psychological and physical health indicators have been used as stress outcomes (Berkman 1986; House, Liandis, and Umberson 1988; Kessler et al. 1987; Lin and Ensel 1989). Finally, the study of mediators concentrates on those social and personal resources that can alter the impact of the stressors on the stress outcome. Cassel (1976) postulated that the environment contained not only 'stressors' but also factors that could contribute to host resistance. Considerable effort has gone into identifying the forces that contribute to host resistance. The study of social support and coping strategies is central here (Bachrach and Zautra 1985; Billings and Moos 1984; Coyne, Aldwin, and Lazarus 1981; Folkman and Lazarus 1980; Folkman et al. 1986; Folkman and Lazarus 1986; Holahan and Moos 1986; Mattlin, Wethinghton, and Kessler 1990; McCrae and Costa 1986). The technical study consists of identifying how social support and/or coping strategies add to host resistance. A distinction is drawn between intervening, suppressing (counteracting-buffering), and interacting (interaction buffering) effects (Alloway and Bebbington 1987; Barrera 1986; Lin, Woelfel and Light 1985; Wheaton 1985). Social stress theory applied to the study of AIDS sexual risk behaviour among gay men implies that one considers risky sexual practices as the stress outcome. Accordingly, one has to identify the specific stressors, stress mediators, and mediating mechanisms to explain why a substantial group of gay men continuously or occasionally practise unsafe sex.

RESEARCH FINDINGS

The idea of applying social stress theory to the study of sexual risk behaviour arises partly from our own research on the factors determining the well-being of gay men. Central to this approach is the process of 'coming out.' Coming out is the disclosure in one's social environment of one's same-sex emotional and sexual orientation (Cass 1979; Coleman 1982; Lee 1977; Ponse 1978; Schafer 1976; Troiden 1979, 1988, 1989; Weinberg 1978). The process involves a restructuring of self and of one's social relationships following the reaction of one's significant others to one's same-sex erotic orientation. Therefore, coming out is not merely an individual phenomenon but rather a transactional process in which responses of one's social environment, especially social support, are of crucial importance.

Social support provides members of society with a sense of identity and continuity of meaning. Social support is a key aspect of social control within this framework. Through the manipulation of social support, societies provide or withdraw respect, evaluative appraisal, emotional assistance, and the assurance that someone will be there when things go wrong. Accordingly, societies elicit socially expected behaviour through the manipulation of emotions and sense of identity.

When gay men bond with other men for emotional and erotic gratification, they violate the social expectations of the heterosexual male role. Frequently their social environment reacts negatively and tries to get them to conform to social norms by the threat of effective withdrawal of social support. Some gay men find psychosocial support within peer groups or in an accepting familial environment. Others, however, continue to live in a chronic conflict situation, struggling for a sense of identity that is congruent with their inner feelings and desires.

Our previously reported research findings revealed how the social oppression of gay men results in high levels of reported symptoms of depression (Vincke, Bolton, and Mak 1990; Vincke, Mak, and Bolton 1991). The effects of oppression, however, were mediated by social support. Our analysis of the determinants of unprotected insertive and receptive anal sex suggests a connection between the experience of oppression and the taking of sexual risks (Vincke et al. 1992). In this study, the perception of control over one's life course suppressed the effects of withdrawal of social support. Analyzing this more thoroughly, we found that, especially among subjects with high control, the experience of low social support resulted in increased sexual risk taking. This was clearly an instance of counteractive buffering. In a third analysis we tested the hypothesis that perception of control also functions as an interactive buffering agent between oppression and depression and sexual risk taking (Vincke, Bolton, and Mak 1992). Taken together, our analyses suggested that the social oppression of gay men, experienced as the withdrawal of social support, created considerable distress, leading to depression and sexual risk behaviour. Additional research findings relevant to the formulation of our thesis come from Stiffman, Cunningham, and Dore (1992), who identified the forces leading to an increase of risk behaviour among inner city young adults. Increases in risk behaviour were predicted by stressors (1 per cent); estimates of personal risk (3 per cent); and mental health problems (suicide symptoms, 6 per cent; substance abuse, 5 per cent). Nichols (1989) also reports research showing that socio-economic factors associated with high rates of intravenous drug use among minority populations, such as poverty, unemployment, and inadequate education, are also associated with higher rates of HIV infection in major urban centres of the northeast in the US. Clearly a substantial part of these socio-economic strains are experienced either as stressful life events or as chronic stress situations.

An additional building block comes from research showing that there are different ways of dealing with stress: in particular outward and inward reactions. Horwitz and White (1987), for example, stated that females tend to internalize distress, resulting in depression, whereas males tend to externalize distress, which can lead to problem drinking; but the male/female dichotomy is rather crude as a classification. However, males and females exhibit different levels of instrumentality, emotionality and attributional styles, such as the perception of control. (For a review of the relevant literature see Giele 1988.) Still, the idea of different reactions to stress is stimulating and has been incorporated in our hypothesis.

SOCIAL STRESS AND SEXUAL RISK
TAKING AMONG GAY MEN

The thesis of the present study is that the risky sexual behaviour of gay men is sometimes an outward stress reaction following social oppression. Social oppression is seen as the source of stress, while depression and sexual risk behaviour are the stress outcomes. In our previous analyses we showed that the perception of being in control, in combination with low social support resulting from high oppression, was associated with high levels of risk behaviour. In this study we will concentrate on the perception of control as a mediating factor, leading to either an inward or an outward stress reaction.

The perception of control is an attribution about the causal order of the processes in which one participates. Through attributional processes, people seek to understand their social world. They do this primarily by attributing various characteristics and intentions to the actors within it, including themselves (Eiser 1988). These attributions are grounded in experience and anticipate future actions. Therefore, learning provides the basis of the perception of control as an attributional style. Subjects with a perception of high control try actively to solve problems they encounter. They cope outwardly with those stressors they encounter. Subjects with a perception of low control react passively or inwardly. Therefore, we hypothesize that gay men experiencing high levels of social oppression, perceiving themselves as having low control, will report a high level of depressive symptoms and low frequencies of unprotected anal sex. Gay men with a perception of high control, and confronted with social oppression, will report lower depressive symptoms and higher frequencies of unprotected insertive and receptive anal sex. In this formulation, the effects of social oppression depend on the level of control one attributes to oneself. Therefore, the perception of control functions as an interaction variable.

In testing our hypothesis we introduced competing variables to explain depression and unprotected anal sex, such as age and relationship status. Steady relationships have a documented negative relationship with depression (Mirowsky and Ross 1986). Age, too, appears to be negatively associated with risky sexual behaviour, while partnership has a positive effect (see Miller, Turner, and Moses 1990). Finally, we introduced AIDS knowledge as an additional control variable. Interaction terms measure not only interaction effects, but also the main effects of the component variables. We also used 'perception of control' and 'level of social oppression' as independent variables.

METHODS

Participants

The present study is part of a wide-ranging investigation of gay life in Flanders (Belgium) entitled the 'Gay Services Research Project' (GSRP), begun in 1989 (Mak et al. 1990; Vincke, Mak, and Bolton

Table 1. Demographic Characteristics of the GSRP
(Gay Services Research Project) Cohort

	n	%
Age (years)		
<21	7	1.8
21–30	151	39.9
31–40	159	42.0
41–50	35	9.2
51–60	17	4.5
>60	10	2.6
Education		
Legal minimum (to age 15)	14	3.7
Years above legal minimum:		
1–3	43	11.3
4–6	99	26.1
7–9	128	33.8
>9	95	25.1
Marital status		
Single	322	85.1
Married	20	5.2
Married, but separated	5	1.3
Divorced	27	7.1
Widowed	5	1.3
Gay relationship status		
Steady partner	237	62.5
No steady partner	142	37.5
Religion		
Catholic	134	35.4
Protestant	3	0.8
Jewish	2	0.5
Humanist	74	19.5
Atheist	87	23.0
Other	31	8.2
Non-religious	48	12.6

1991). Participants in the study, recruited by key persons (network sampling) in the spring of 1989 throughout the Flemish region of the country, were guaranteed confidentiality; for those recruited by key persons, anonymity was also guaranteed since only the key persons knew the identities of the men they recruited. Table 1 contains the demographic characteristics of the sample. The men ranged in age from 17 to 78 years, with just over 80 per cent aged 21–40 (mean age

= 33.8 years, standard deviation = 9.9). Teenagers as well as men over 50 are undoubtedly somewhat under-represented in this cohort. As in most research on gay men, the cohort is more highly educated than the general population, with over 50 per cent having some education beyond secondary school (university or non-university professional training).

The Interview

Interviewing in this study was done by computer using an interactive program designed for use on personal computers. The research setting was a large classroom with 18 personal computers arranged on desks in rows. All questions were closed-ended, and a participant could not review and change answers once entered. Participants were given brief instructions on how to enter their responses — experience with computers was not necessary, since the design of the instrument mirrored the use of ATMs, with which all informants were familiar.

Operationalisation

To measure depression we retained the first factor from a factor analysis of thirty-six items of the Hopkins Symptom Checklist (Derogatis et al. 1974). Respondents rated the items (e.g., wanting to be alone, feeling hopeless about the future, feeling fearful) on a five-point scale. The retained factor corresponded to the depression subscale. This dimension explained 40 per cent of the total variance (Cronbach's alpha = 0.920).

Perception of control was measured with seven items. Subjects expressed their agreement or disagreement (five-point scale) with the following items: many people suffer through no fault of their own; I feel that I'm being pushed around in my life; others always run away with the rewards; I feel helpless in dealing with the problems I encounter; I have little control over the things that happen to me; there is little I can do to change the things that happen to me; at times I feel I get a raw deal out of life. The average interitem correlation was 0.371, with a standardized alpha of 0.803.

We measured insertive and receptive anal intercourse without a condom as follows. We first posed the question: 'When you have sex with someone, do you fuck/get fucked without a condom?' Possible answers were: (1) I used to, but not any more; (2) no, not now nor in the past; (3) sometimes; (4) regularly; (5) always. To obtain a linear scale for the frequency of anal intercourse, we collapsed categories 1 and 2.

Partnership status was measured as a dummy variable with (0) no steady partner and (1) steady partner. The respondent's perception of the acceptance of his sexual orientation by others was measured as follows. An index was constructed by summing the level of acceptance expressed for the sexual orientation of the respondent on a three-point scale by father, mother, brothers/sisters, heterosexual friends, boss and co-workers. Parents where given a weight coefficient of 3, siblings of 2, and the others of 1. The final index was constructed by summing these weighted scores. To create an AIDS knowledge index we used three questions dealing with safe sex and a correct interpretation of HIV antibody tests.

ANALYSIS

All analyses reported here were performed using CSS 3/Statistica from Statsoft. The first step of the analysis consisted of dichotomizing perception of control and social oppression. We chose the mean scores as cutting points because these two variables approximated the normal distribution. This procedure classified 217 subjects with high control and 162 with low control; 189 men with high oppression, and 190 with low oppression. We then cross-classified these two dichotomies. In our hypothesis it is essential that oppression is actually experienced. Therefore, for the remainder of the analysis we use only the combination of high oppression (above the mean score) with a perception of low control ($n = 95$), and high oppression with a perception of high control ($n = 94$). These two combinations were integrated into one dummy variable, which we called control/oppression.

In the last step of the analysis, the dummy variable control/oppression was entered in a discriminant analysis. The outcome variable consists of two groups. We used the k-means clustering procedure to assign respondents to two groups on the basis of their depression scores and frequency of unprotected anal sex. An analysis of variance was performed on these groups to assure that they differed significantly on the key variables. Group 1 ($n = 119$) and group 2 ($n = 260$) differed significantly (ANOVA $p < 0.000$) on all three variables (Table 2). This dichotomy became the outcome variable of this study. However, this dichotomy cannot simply be identified as a classification of inward stress reactors versus outward stress reactors. Men having low depressive symptoms and high levels of unpro-

Table 2. Analysis of Variance: Results from
k-Means Cluster Analysis

Crossprd. variable	Between SS	df	Within SS	df	F	Signif. p
Depression	231.8618	1	112.5310	377	776.7803	0.000000
Anal receptive	6.5486	1	222.7442	377	11.0836	0.000957
Anal insertive	17.3169	1	259.4009	377	25.1675	0.000001

tected anal sex could just as well be men in a steady relationship, rather than men with outward stress reactions. Therefore we introduced the control variables age, partnership status, AIDS knowledge, perception of control, and level of oppression as competing explanations for membership in the outcome categories. If our hypothesis that oppression in combination with perception of control leads to different stress reactions is correct, then our control/oppression variable should contribute significantly to the discriminant function explaining group memberships when checking statistically for the competing variables.

RESULTS

The multivariate Box M test, which checks the homogeneity of variance and covariance of the variables across groups, is not significant ($p = 0.07$). Since this test is sensitive to deviations from multivariate normality, and given the insignificant result, we can apply discriminant analysis with confidence. Overall, Wilks' lambda for the discriminant function is 0.535 ($p < 0.000$) (see Table 3). An additional indicator for evaluating the 'goodness' of the discriminant function is the eigenvalue. This measure can be interpreted as the ratio of the between-groups to the within-groups sums of squares of the discriminant scores. High eigenvalues suggest high discriminating power. With an eigenvalue equal to 0.867, we can conclude that the discriminating ability of the derived function is very high.

The results can be interpreted using the factor structure matrix and the standardized coefficients for the canonical variables (see Table 4) (Stevens 1986). The latter do not necessarily give the same results as the factor structure matrix. One major difference between the two measures is that the standardized coefficients are partial coefficients, with the effects of the other variables removed. They also have a

Table 3. Discriminant Analysis: *df* for all *F*-Tests: 1,183

Variable	Wilks' lambda	Partial lambda	F to remove	p-level	Toler.	1-Toler. (R-sqr.)
Control	0.569976	0.939706	11.74174	0.000755	0.475128	0.524872
Aidsknow	0.538876	0.993939	1.11596	0.292182	0.969194	0.030806
Age	0.561476	0.953932	8.83764	0.003348	0.955262	0.044738
Steady	0.636101	0.842019	34.33469	0.000000	0.978056	0.021944
Oppress	0.535733	0.999770	0.04217	0.837526	0.972772	0.027228
ContOppr	0.553241	0.968131	6.02397	0.015048	0.471354	0.528646

Discriminant function analysis results. Number of variables in the model = 6. Wilks' lambda: 0.5356095; approx. *F* (6,183) = 26.44447; *p* < 0.00000.

Table 4. Factor Structure Matrix

Variable	Standardized coefficients for canonical variables	Factor structure matrix correlations variables - canonical roots (pooled-within-groups correlations)
	Root 1	Root 1
Control	−0.522745	−0.727217
AIDS knowledge	−0.116046	−0.063509
Age	0.322254	0.142085
Steady partner	0.589764	0.549398
Oppression	−0.022580	0.114106
Control/oppression	−0.381564	−0.642762

different interpretation. The factor structure matrix contains the correlations between the variables and the discriminant score. For each case, and for each outcome group separately, the Pearson correlation coefficient is computed between the discriminant score and the variable, and then combined across groups. These correlations are used to interpret the dimensions. The standardized coefficients indicate which variables are redundant and which are not. The largest correlation is with perception of control (−0.727) and with the interaction between control and high oppression (−0.624). Bearing in mind the coding procedure of the variables, the first correlation indicates that high controllers belong to the group of low depression with high frequencies of risky sex. The second correlation suggests that subjects experiencing high oppression and having high control also belong to the second group. The correlation between relationship status and the discriminant score is 0.549. This suggests that men with a steady partner show lower levels of depression and higher levels of un-protected anal sex. The remaining variables have a zero correlation with the discriminant scores. Taken together, these results imply that the underlying dimension discriminating between the two groups most importantly reflects the perception of control in combination with social oppression, and as a main effect. Although age does not correlate highly with the discriminant scores, it is a non-redundant variable. Older men belong to the group having lower depression and higher frequencies of unprotected anal sex.

We can use the results of the discriminant analysis to classify the subjects into groups containing the inward or outward stress reac-tors. Using group sizes as a priori probabilities, we arrive at a global-ly correct classification of 90.5 per cent. The success rate for the group of the outward reactors is 95.7 per cent. Using equal a priori prob-abilities (0.5) results in a success rate of 81.5 per cent and 80.1 per cent as total and outward reactor group classification, respectively.

The outcome variable we used in this discriminant analysis is a mixed variable of depression scores and reported frequencies of risky sex. Therefore it is no surprise that age and partnership status are significant. These results reflect the reported associations with depression and risky sex. Yet the results of the discriminant analysis support our hypothesis. After testing for the main effects of control and oppression, the interaction between high oppression and a per-ception of being in control contributes to the discrimination between the two groups.

DISCUSSION

This study is based on a critique of the almost exclusive use of psychological variables in the study of AIDS sexual risk behaviour. The use of psychological variables need not be abandoned, but our approach combines psychological characteristics, such as the percep-tion of control, with one specific characteristic of the social space of AIDS, namely social oppression.

Social conditions shape the space in which individuals function psychologically. Individuals with different psychological character-istics handle social conditions differently. It was our contention that gay men who perceive themselves to be in control, when confronted with social oppression, will show an outward stress reaction consisting of low depression and high frequencies of unprotected anal sex. The results of our analysis support this hypothesis.

How can we interpret this finding? Gay men who experience oppression and who have high levels of control do not accept the rejection of their genuine inner feelings. The acting out of their stress through intensive sexual contacts is their way of maintaining control over their personal life space, despite the negative attitude of their social environment. They reaffirm their sexual identity through these contacts, thereby taking a stand against prevailing negative social attitudes. This acting out *is not* a deliberate, planned reaction. Therefore they do not anticipate the risk associated with their sexual activity, and anal sexual contacts become unprotected.

The perception of control holds a prominent place within the health behaviour literature: different theoretical approaches incorporate this concept. There is a firmly developed research tradition on locus of control (Rotter 1966, 1990) and on the mastery concept (Pearlin et al. 1981). Together with challenge and commitment, control is also an integral part of the psychological construct of hardiness (Kobasa, Maddi, and Kahn 1982). These research approaches agree on the beneficial effect of control on the maintenance of health and on the instigation of health behaviour. Yet in this study we ultimately arrived at the conclusion that the perception of high control can have detrimental effects on the practice of safe sexual behaviour. One major reason for this deviation from the mainstream findings is that we incorporated two different stress outcomes in one outcome variable. Therefore our results cannot simply be interpreted as an interactive buffering effect. Buffering means that the buffering variable protects against the negative impact of stress. The idea, put forward in the literature, that multiple stress reactions are possible, should make us guard against too hasty an acceptance of a unique beneficial effect of some buffering agent when only one stress outcome is studied.

This study, based on cross-sectional data, bears all the deficiencies associated with cross-sectional research when trying to establish causal explanations. We are currently preparing longitudinal research to analyze more thoroughly sexual risk taking within the theoretical context of social stress theory. This theoretical approach will not furnish a complete answer to the question of why some gay men continue to practise sexually risky behaviour, despite AIDS. As stated in our review of current levels of risky sex, a substantial proportion of gay men did change their behaviour. We have to look for additional explanations for those who did not initiate or maintain safe sex. Several forces are probably at work here. Social stress might be one of them.

REFERENCES

Adib, M.S., Adib, S., J. G. Joseph, D.G. Ostrow, M. Tal, and S.A. Schwartz. 1991. Relapse in Sexual Behaviour Among Homosexual Men: A 2-Year Follow-Up from the Chicago MACS/CSS. *AIDS* 5:757–760.

Adib, M.S., D.G. Ostrow, and J.G. Joseph. 1992. Longitudinal Patterns of Sexual Behaviour Change and Relapse in the Chicago Macs/CCS Cohort. Paper presented at the VIII International Conference on AIDS, Amsterdam, July 19–24.

Alloway, R., and P. Bebbington. 1987. The Buffer Theory of Social Support. A review of the Literature. *Psychological Medicine* 17:91–108.

Avison, W.R., and R.J. Turner. 1988. Stressful Life Events and Depressive Symptoms: Disaggregating the Effects of Acute Stressors and Chronic Strains. *Journal of Health and Social Behaviour* 29:253–264.

Bachrach, K.M., and A.J. Zautra. 1985. Coping with a Community Stressor: The Threat of a Hazardous Waste Facility. *Journal of Health and Social Behaviour* 26:127–141.

Barrera, M. 1986. Distinctions Between Social Support Concepts, Measures, and Models. *American Journal of Community Psychology* 14:413–445.

Baum, A., and S.E. Nesselhof. 1988. Psychological Research and the Prevention, Etiology and Treatment of AIDS. *American Psychologist* 43:900–906.

Becker, M.H., and J.G. Joseph. 1988. Aids and Behavioral Change to Reduce Risk: A Review. *American Journal of Public Health* 78:394–410.

Berkman, L.F. 1986. Social Networks, Support, and Health: Taking the Next Step Forward. *American Journal of Epidemiology* 123:559–562.

Billings, A.G., and R.H. Moos. 1984. Coping, Stress, and Social Resources Among Adults with Unipolar Depression. *Journal of Personality and Social Psychology* 46:877–91.

Bolton, R., J. Vincke, G. Mak, and E. Dennehy. 1992. Alcohol and Risky Sex: In Search of an Elusive Connection. In: *Rethinking AIDS Prevention*, edited by R. Bolton and M. Singer. Philadelphia: Gordon and Breach Science Publishers.

Cass, V. 1979. Homosexual Identity Formation: A Theoretical Model. *Journal of Homosexuality* 4:219–35.

Cassel, J.C. 1976. The Contribution of the Social Environment to Host Resistance. *American Journal of Epidemiology* 104:107–123.

Catania, J.A., T. Coates, S.M. Kegeles, M. Ekstrand, J.R. Guydish, and L.L. Bye. 1989. Implications of the AIDS Risk Reduction Model for the Gay Community: The Importance of Perceived Sexual Enjoyment and Help-Seeking Behaviors. In: *Primary Prevention of AIDS: Psychological Approaches*, edited by V.M. Mays, G.W. Albee, and S.F. Schneider. Newbury Park, CA: Sage Publications.

Catania, J.A., S.M. Kegeles, and T.J. Coates. 1990. Towards an Understanding of Risk Behaviour: An AIDS Risk Reduction Model (ARRM). *Health Education Quarterly* 17:53–72.

Coates, T., L. Temoshok, and J. Mandel. 1984. Psychosocial Research Is Essential to Understanding and Treating AIDS. *American Psychologist* 39:1309–1314.

Coleman, E. 1982. Developmental Stages of the Coming-Out Process. *Journal of Homosexuality* 11:31–43.

Coyne, J.C., C. Aldwin, and R.S. Lazarus. 1981. Depression and Coping in Stressful Episodes. *Journal of Abnormal Psychology* 90:439–47.

Dubois-Arber, F., J.B. Masur, D. Hausser, and E. Zimmermann. 1991. Evaluation of AIDS Prevention Among Gay Men in Switzerland. Paper presented at the VII International Conference on AIDS, Florence, June 16–21.

Eiser, J.R. 1988. *Social Psychology. Attitudes, Cognition and Social Behaviour*. Cambridge: Cambridge University Press.

Ekstrand, M.L., and T.J. Coates. 1990. Maintenance of Safer Sexual Behaviors and Predictors of Risky Sex: The San Francisco Men's Health Study. *American Journal of Public Health* 80:973–977.

Ensel, W.M., and Lin Nan. 1991. The Life Stress Paradigm and Psychological Distress. *Journal of Health and Social Behaviour* 32:321–341.

Folkman, S., and R.S. Lazarus. 1980. An Analysis of Coping in a Middle-Aged Community Sample. *Journal of Health and Social Behaviour* 21:219–39.

Folkman, S., and R.S. Lazarus. 1986. Stress Processes and Depressive Symptomatology. *Journal of Abnormal Psychology* 95:107–13.

Folkman, S., R.S. Lazarus, C. Dunkel-Schetter, A. Delongis, and R.J. Gruen. 1986. The Dynamics of a Stressful Encounter: Cognitive Appraisal, Coping and Encounter Outcomes. *Journal of Personality and Social Psychology* 50:922–1003.

Giele, J.Z. 1988. Gender and Sex Roles. In: *Handbook of Sociology*, edited by N. Smelser. Newbury Park, CA: Sage Publications.

Hart, G.L., J. McClean, M.Boulton, J. Dawson, and R. Fitzpatrick. 1991. Maintenance and Change in Safer Sex Behaviours in a Cohort of Gay Men in England. Paper presented at the VII International Conference on AIDS, Florence, June 16–21.

Hingson, R.W., L. Strunin, B.M. Berlin, and T. Heeren. 1990. Beliefs About AIDS, Use of Alcohol and Drugs, and Unprotected Sex Among Massachusetts Adolescents. *American Journal of Public Health* 80:295–299.

Holahan, C.J., and R.H. Moos. 1986. Personality, Coping, and Family Resources in Stress Resistance: A Longitudinal Analysis. *Journal of Personality and Social Psychology* 51:389–95.

Horwitz, A., and H.R. White. 1987. Gender Role Orientations and Styles of Pathology Among Adolescents. *Journal of Health and Social Behaviour* 28: 158–170.

House, J.S., K.R. Liandis, and D. Umberson. 1988. Social Relationships and Health. *Science* 241:540–45.

Houweling, H., T. Sandfort, L. Wiessing, M. Bosga, W. Schop, and R. van den Akker. 1992. Prevalence of HIV Infections and Risk Factors Among Homosexual Men in the Netherlands. Paper presented at the VIII International Conference on AIDS, Amsterdam, July 19–24.

Institute of Medicine. 1991. *The AIDS Research Program of the National Institutes of Health. Report of a Study*. Washington, DC: National Academy Press.

Kelly, J.A., J. St. Lawrence, T.L. Braasfield, Y. Stevenson, Y. Diaz, and A.C. Hauth. 1990. AIDS Risk Behaviour Patterns Among Gay Men in Small Southern Cities. *American Journal of Public Health* 80:416–418.

Kessler, R.C., R.H. Price, and C.B. Wortman. 1985. Social Factors in Psychopathology: Stress, Social Support and Coping Processes. *Annual Review of Psychology* 36:531–72.

Kessler, R.C., J.S. House, J. Turner, and J. Blake. 1987. Unemployment and Health in a Community Sample. *Journal of Health and Social Behaviour* 28:51–59.

Klitzman, S., J.S. House, B.A. Israel, and P.R. Mero. 1990. Work Stress, Nonwork Stress, and Health. *Journal of Behavioral Medicine* 13:221–243.

Kobasa, S.C., S.R. Maddi, and S. Kahn. 1982. Hardiness and Health: A Prospective Study. *Journal of Personality and Social Psychology* 42:168–177.

Lee, J.A. 1977. Going Public: A Study in the Sociology of Homosexual Liberation. *Journal of Homosexuality* 3:49–78.

Leigh, B.C. 1990. The Relationship of Substance Use During Sex to High-Risk Sexual Behaviour. *Journal of Sex Research* 27:199–213.

Lin Nan, and W.M. Ensel. 1989. Life Stress and Health: Stressors and Resources. *American Sociological Review* 54:382–399.

Lin Nan, M.W. Woelfel, and S.C. Light. 1985. The Buffering Effect of Social Support Subsequent to an Important Life Event. *Journal of Health and Social Behaviour* 26:247–263.

Mak, R., R. Bolton, J. Vincke, J. Plum, and L. Van Renterghem. 1990. Prevalence of HIV and Other STD Infections and Risky Sexual Behaviour Among Gay Men in Belgium. *Archives of Public Health* 87–98.

Mattlin, J.A., E. Wethington, and R.C. Kessler. 1990. Situational Determinants of Coping and Coping Effectiveness. *Journal of Health and Social Behaviour* 31:103–122.

Mays, V., G.W. Albee, and S.F. Schneider, eds. 1989. *Primary Prevention of AIDS. Psychological Approaches*. Newbury Park, CA: Sage Publications.

McCrae, R.R., and P.T. Costa. 1986. Personality, Coping and Coping Effectiveness in an Adult Sample. *Journal of Personality* 54:385–405.

McCusker, J.J., J. Westenhouse, A.M. Stoddard, J.G. Zapka, M.W. Zorn, and K.H. Mayer. 1990. Use of Drugs and Alcohol by Homosexually Active Men in Relation to Sexual Practices. *Journal of Acquired Immune Deficiency Syndromes* 3:729–736.

McGrath, J.E. 1970. A Conceptual Formulation for Research on Stress. In: *Social and Psychological Factors in Stress*, edited by J.E. McGrath. New York: Holt, Rinehart, and Winston.

McKirnan, D.J., and P.L. Peterson. 1989a. Alcohol and Drug Use Among Homosexual Men and Women: Epidemiology and Population Characteristics. *Addictive Behaviour* 14:545–553.

McKirnan, D.J., and P.L. Peterson. 1989b. Psychosocial and Cultural Factors in Alcohol and Drug Abuse: An Analysis of a Homosexual Community. *Addictive Behaviour* 14:555–563.

McLeod, J.D., and R.C. Kessler. 1990. Socioeconomic Status Differences in Vulnerability to Undesirable Life Events. *Journal of Health and Social Behaviour* 31:162–172.

Miller, H.G., C.F. Turner, and L.E. Moses. 1990. *AIDS. The Second Decade*. Washington, DC: National Academy Press.

Mirowsky, J., and C.E. Ross. 1986. Social Patterns of Distress. *Annual Review of Sociology* 12:23–45.

Molgaard, C.A., C.H. Nakamura, and J.P. Elder. 1988. Assessing Alcoholism as a Risk Factor for Acquired Immunodeficiency Syndrome (AIDS). *Social Science and Medicine* 27:1147–1152.

Morgan Thomas, R., M.A. Plant, and M.L. Plant. 1990. Alcohol, AIDS Risks and Sex Industry Clients: Results from a Scottish Study. *Drug and Alcohol Dependence* 26:265–269.

Morin, S.F. 1988. AIDS: The Challenge to Psychology. *American Psychologist* 43:838–842.

Nichols, E. 1989. *Mobilizing Against AIDS*. Cambridge: Harvard University Press.

Nieri, G., G.F. Lemp, R.P. Watson, S. Nguyen, M.K. Parisi, and A.C. Clevenger. 1992. HIV-1 Seroprevalence and Risk Behaviors Among Young Gay Men in San Francisco. Paper presented at the VIII International Conference on AIDS, Amsterdam, July 19–24.

Pearlin, L.I. 1989. The Sociological Study of Stress. *Journal of Health and Social Behaviour* 30:241–256.

Pearlin, L.I., M.A. Lieberman, E.G. Menaghan, and J. Mullan. 1981. The Stress Process. *Journal of Health and Social Behaviour* 22:337–356.

Plant, M.A. 1990a. Sex Work, Alcohol, Drugs, and AIDS. In: *AIDS, Drugs, and Prostution*, edited by M. Plant. London: Tavistock/Routledge.

Plant, M.A. 1990b. Alcohol, Sex and AIDS. *Alcohol and Alcoholism* 25:293–301.

Ponse, B. 1978. *Identities in the Lesbian World: The Social Construction of Self.* Westport, CT: Greenwood Press.

Robertson, J.A., and M.A. Plant. 1988. Alcohol, Sex and Risks of HIV Infection. *Drug and Alcohol Dependence* 22:75–78.

Rotter, J.B. 1966. Some Problems and Misconceptions Related to the Construct of Internal and External Locus of Control of Reinforcement. *Journal of Consulting and Clinical Psychology* 45:489–493.

Rotter, J.B. 1990. Internal Versus External Control of Reinforcement. A Case History of a Variable. *American Psychologist* 45:489–493.

Sandler, I.N., and G.T. Robert. 1985. Assessment of Life Stress Events. In: *Measurement Strategies in Health Psychology,* edited by P. Karoly. New York: John Wiley and Sons.

Sasse, H., A. Bigagli, F. Chiarotti, P. Martucci, D. Greco, and F. Grillini. 1991. Homosexual Practices with Steady and Non-Steady Partners Among Men Frequenting Public Gay Meeting Places in Italy. Paper presented at the VII Conference on AIDS, Florence, June 16–21.

Sasse, H., A. Bigagli, F. Chiarotti, F. Farchi, D. Greco, and F. Grillini. 1992. The Potential of HIV Transmission Through 'Unprotected' Anal Intercourse with Non-Steady Partners Among Homo/Bisexual Males Living in an Open Couple. Paper presented at the VIII Conference on AIDS, Amsterdam, July 19–24.

Schafer, S. 1976. Sexual and Social Problems of Lesbians. *Journal of Sex Research* 12:50–69.

Stall, R. 1988. The Prevention of HIV Infection Associated with Drug and Alcohol Use During Sexual Activity. In: *AIDS and Substance Abuse,* edited by L. Siegel. New York: Harrington Park Press.

Stall, R., L. McKusick, J. Wiley, T.J. Coates, and D.G. Ostrow. 1986. Alcohol and Drug Use During Sexual Activity and Compliance with Safe Sex Guidelines for AIDS: The AIDS Behavioral Research Project. *Health Education Quarterly* 13:359–371.

Stall, R.D., Th.J. Coates, and C. Hoff. 1988. Behavioral Risk Reduction for HIV Infection Among Gay and Bisexual Men: A Review of Results from the United States. *American Psychologist* 43:878–885.

Stall, R., and J. Wiley. 1988. A Comparison of Drug and Alcohol Use Habits in Heterosexual and Homosexual Men. *Drug and Alcohol Dependence* 22:63–74.

Stevens, J. 1986. *Applied Multivariate Statistics for the Social Sciences.* Hillsdale New Jersey: Lawrence Erlbaum Associates.

Stiffman, A.R.R., R. Cunningham, and P. Dore. 1992. Change in AIDS Risk Behaviors from Adolescence to Adulthood. In: *Science Challenging AIDS,* edited by G.B. Rossi, E. Beth-Giraldo, L. Chieco-Bianchi, F. Dianzani, G. Giraldo, and P. Verani. Basel: Karger.

Tausig, M. 1982. Measuring Life Events. *Journal of Health and Social Behaviour* 23:52–64.

Troiden, R.R. 1979. Androgyny: A Neglected Dimension of Homosexuality. *Humanity and Society* 3:122–35.

Troiden, R.R. 1988. Homosexual Identity Development. *Journal of Adolescent Health Care* 9:105–13.

Troiden, R.R. 1989. The Formation of Homosexual Identities. *Journal of Homosexuality* 17:43–74.

Vincke, J., R. Bolton, R. Mak, and S. Blank. 1993. Coming-Out and AIDS-Related High-Risk Behaviour. *Archives of Sexual Behaviour.* 22:559–86.

Vincke, J., R. Bolton, and R. Mak. 1990. Stress, Physical Complaints, Role Impairment and the Coming-Out Process. Paper presented at the annual meeting of the American Sociological Association, Washington, DC.

Vincke, J., R. Bolton, and R. Mak. 1992. Minority Status: The Perception of Control and AIDS-Related Sexual Risk Behaviour. Paper presented at the Annual Meeting of the American Sociological Association, Pittsburgh.

Vincke, J., R. Mak, and R. Bolton. 1991. *Mannen met Mannen. Welzijn, Relaties en Seksualiteit.* Gent: CGSO/AIDS Referentie Centrum.

Vroome, E. de, T. Sandfort, and R. Tielman. 1991. Sources of Information Used and the Adoption of Safer Sex Among Gay Men. Paper presented at the VII International Conference on AIDS, Florence, June 16–21.

Weatherburn, P., A.J. Hunt, P.M. Davies, F. Hickson, T.J. McManus, and A.P. Coxon. 1991. Incidence of Anal Intercourse: Changes in a Cohort of Gay Men in England and Wales 1987–1990. Paper presented at the VII International Conference on AIDS, Florence, June 16–21.

Weinberg, T.S. 1978. On 'Doing' and 'Being' Gay: Sexual Behaviour and Homosexual Male Self-Identity. *Journal of Homosexuality* 4:143–56.

Wheaton, B. 1985. Models for the Stress-Buffering Functions of Coping Resources. *Journal of Health and Social Behaviour* 26:352–364.

Wyse, D., M. Quinlan, M. Scully, J. Barry, and L. Pomeroy. 1992. Sexual and HIV Behaviour Amongst Homosexual/Bisexual Men in Dublin. Paper presented at the VIII International Conference on AIDS, Amsterdam, July 19–24.

Chapter
TEN

Risk in Context: The Use of Sexual Diary Data to Analyse Homosexual Risk Behaviour

Anthony P.M. Coxon and N.H. Coxon

This is a study of gay men's sexual behaviour under the impact of AIDS which uses the method of diaries. It is an integral part of the work of Project SIGMA (Socio-Sexual Investigations of Gay Men and AIDS), which is a longitudinal study of the sexual and social lifestyle of gay and bisexual men in England and Wales (and also part of the English study under the auspices of WHO Global Programme on AIDS Homosexual Response Studies). SIGMA is one of the largest cohort studies in Europe and the only study in the UK to have emerged from the gay community. Initial work began in 1983, and funding followed in 1987. To date, the Project has interviewed over 1000 men, half of whom have been interviewed four times at (median) intervals of 10 months. The main aims of the study are to describe the sexual behaviour and lifestyles of gay and bisexual men; to monitor changes in sexual behaviour in relation to

HIV/AIDS; to examine attitudes to different sexual behaviours and relationships; to investigate reactions to safer sex practices; and to estimate prevalence of HIV and other viral infections in a non-clinic group of gay and bisexual men.

Project SIGMA uses several complementary methods of obtaining information, including: the *detailed structured interview* in which each respondent is asked for detailed information on sexual history and current practices (centred upon the Index of Sexual Behaviour, Coxon et al. 1992), numbers of sexual partners, health, and attitudes towards HIV and safer sex; the *sexual diaries*, a daily record of sexual activity kept by respondents for a month after each interview (see Coxon 1988b; so far we have collected information on about 30,000 sexual encounters which allows a unique analysis of their structure); *blood and/or saliva samples* collected at the interview by trained staff and tested for HIV-1 antibodies and other viral markers (results are available to respondents through trained counsellors); and the *postal survey of sexual behaviour*, a self-completion questionnaire which appears in the gay press periodically. In this chapter we concentrate primarily upon the method of sexual diaries.[1]

METHODS FOR COLLECTING SEXUAL DATA

There are various methods for collecting data for analysis of sexual behaviour, and their merits depend on what is needed from the data. Retrospective interviews and questionnaires are useful for obtaining general and 'memorable' aspects of behaviour (such as whether a given sexual behaviour has ever been experienced), but they are not efficient means of obtaining detailed data (such as accurate estimates of the frequency, or sequences of behaviour) that can more appropriately be obtained from the method of sexual diaries. The main reason for this is that accurate retrospective recall of detailed sexual behaviour is rarely reliable or accurate beyond a few days.[2]

On the other hand, selection bias is higher in the use of diaries than in survey techniques, simply because keeping a monthly diary on a daily basis involves a more prolonged commitment, and it is unlikely to be undertaken by those with a very inactive sex life, thus biasing estimates upward. A further possible drawback is that volunteers may record their behaviour in a way which they expect it *should* be (perhaps modifying the account to be more in accord with safer sex). On investigation, these drawbacks seem not to appear, and many results agree with one's intuition and with the data obtained by different methods. Preliminary research evidence suggests that

SIGMA sexual diary form   (Version: 11/92)

ID Number   :   *XY*   /   *00123*   /   *5*

Week beginning: *Sun 3*   /   *May*   /   1992
                    (day)   (month)   (year)

Remember, each session should include:
— The Time, The Place, The Partners (from partner list)
— Then, the session in your own words (or the code if you are confident).
— If you 'come' (ejaculate) in the session, remember to be explicit about
where it goes and *always* to record the use of condoms.
— List any accompaniments you use (poppers, lubricants, drugs, sex toys, ...)

SUN DAY 3rd	9 am My flat, P1 We deep kissed, and moved into a '69.' Whilst doing it I began to finger him. Then he wanked me (both using poppers) and I came. Following that I wanked him till he came.
MON DAY 4th	7.30 am I woke up to find P1 wanking me. Then he sucked me off, and I came in his mouth. We began using poppers and I sucked him, carrying on to fuck him (with condom), whilst he wanked himself. He came, I didn't.

Figure 1. Part of a SIGMA diary.

counts of sexual behaviours based upon self-reports in the interview
are systematic distortions of the more reliable counts derived from
the diaries.[3]

COLLECTING DIARY DATA IN PROJECT SIGMA

At each wave of the investigation, the subject produces a (retrospective) diary of the last week's sexual behaviour in the presence of the
interviewer in the context of the ordinary interview. This ensures that
the diarist understands what needs to go into the diary, and also
provides indirect evidence of the ability to recall detailed information. At the end, he is given a month diary kit (SIGMA 1993), and he
returns the completed diary after the month period. The diary form
is completed each day, and explicit instructions are given for its
completion. The diary is filled out in ordinary language, within the
framework specified, and respondents are encouraged to use 'street
language' if they wish to. An example of part of a completed week
form is given in Figure 1.

When the completed diary is received back, it is encoded according to a scheme described in Coxon et al. 1992, summarised, and then entered into a database for subsequent analysis.

The chief *methodological advantages* of the diary method are its ease and flexibility: (a) it is naturalistic (some respondents are accustomed to keeping some sort of sexual diary anyway); (b) it is easily adapted to record sexual data from those of any sexual orientation (or, indeed, to domains other than sex); (c) it can be augmented to obtain other concurrent information (such as alcohol and other substance consumption in a sexual context; see Weatherburn et al. 1993); and (d) it can be expanded to take into account such aspects as coital position.

There are a number of more *substantive advantages* of the diary method: (a) it allows the detail of sexual behaviour to be recorded and analysed, and to be encoded intact, since the researcher knows the context of any sexual act — location (time, place), the actors (sexual partners), the adjuncts to sex (such as condoms, lubricants, toys, 'poppers'[4]), and is able to place their use in the correct context; (b) uniquely, it permits the analysis not only of individual behaviour (such as, 'What is the average number of times a gay man engages in oral intercourse in a month?') but of the 'volume' (or 'outlet' to use Kinsey's phrase) of behaviour, where the denominator is all the sexual *acts* involved (as in, 'What proportion of young gay men's sexual activity in a month consists of oral intercourse?'); (c) it allows *sequences* of sexual activity to be analysed. Sometimes this can be crucial, for we need to know whether unsafe behaviour tends to occur at the start, middle, or end of a sexual session, and the meaning of acts such as anal intercourse can be substantially different when it occurs as an end-marker rather than as an incidental activity; and (d) it allows issues of power or dominance in sexual behaviour to be investigated by systematically encoding the modality of the act (which partner does what to whom) and thus allowing gendered distinctions to be made between reciprocated and dominance sessions — the former where the other partner tends to do the same thing in return to his partner, the latter where one partner is repeatedly the submissive, the other the dominant partner (Davies 1990).

In this chapter, these claims are illustrated with respect to the analysis of two aspects of sexual behaviour, and especially anal intercourse: the *effect of relationship type on sexual behaviour* and *behavioural progression in a sexual act* (answering the questions: where is anal intercourse located in a sexual session, and what difference does it make?)

BACKGROUND

Before proceeding further, it is important that the reader understand the basics of the system of encoding the structure of sexual behaviour that we have developed, since the results in the tables make use of it (Coxon 1988a; Coxon et al. 1992). Essentially, every diary is encoded into a database from which application programs may analyse the results. The encoding process simply translates the respondent's description of sexual behaviour into a structured formal language that readily lends itself to computer representation.

Every diary pack has a preliminary face-sheet eliciting information on HIV status, relationship type, geographic location, etc., in the form of a few preliminary questions, together with a table for the respondent to list sexual partners (with their characteristics) who are involved in their sexual transactions. The characteristics include demographic and descriptive information about each partner,[5] and the list is built up as the diary progresses.[6]

The remainder of the diary looks similar to a normal diary, giving space for every day in which the diarists may write what they have done. They are instructed to enter the time and date, then to describe in normal ('street') language precisely what they did, according to a provided set of criteria.[7] Each such spatially and time-limited sexual encounter is referred to as a *session* and may involve one or more persons. Each session forms a separate record in the database. The sexual session is subdivided into sexual *acts*, each of which is finally described by the *behaviour* and its *modality* and by its *outcome* — basically whether and how and where ejaculation occurs.[8]

To aid understanding, take the following simple example of a sexual session:

Session: = { PW AS AF }

This *session* consists of three *acts* (a session may contain many acts, but must contain at least one). The first character of each act is the *modality*, and any remaining characters are the *behaviour*. (The encoding process is far more complex than this, but it is not necessary to go into depth for the results at this stage.)

The behaviour describes *what (sexual act)* is done, and the modality describes *who does it*. There are five modalities, which define *who does what* and *to whom* from the diarist's (also referred to as *Ego's*) point of view. Ego's partner is referred to as *Alter* (see Table 1).

A comment is in order about the 'H' modality. Although Ego is not involved directly in this modality, what his partner does by himself

Table 1. Modalities of Sexual Acts

[S]	Self:	Behaviour performed by Ego on himself
[A]	Active:	Behaviour performed by Ego on his partner
[P]	Passive:	Behaviour performed by his partner on himself

The other modalities are:

[M]	Mutual:	Behaviour performed simultaneously by both partners to each other
[H]	Him:	(Opposite of 'S'). Ego's partner does it to himself

may have possible consequences for HIV transmission (the original stimulus for our development of the method), such as when Alter masturbates himself and ejaculates over Ego.

In the example above, 'PW' means that the behaviour here is 'W' (masturbation), and the modality is Passive, i.e., Ego is masturbated by Alter. The whole sexual session quoted would be read as:

Ego is passively masturbated (PW)
then Ego actively performs fellatio on Alter (AS)
then Ego actively engages in anal intercourse with Alter (AF)

In the actual diary this may well have been written as:

He wanked me, then I sucked him off, then I fucked him.

The diary thus preserves the *sequence* or *progression* of behaviour, which is an important aspect of many types of analysis. Table 2 lists the current set of recognized behaviours (sexual acts).[9]

A GENERAL VIEW OF BEHAVIOUR

At the simplest level, information can be obtained from respondents' diaries to match commonly used interview-based variables such as information referring to the prevalence and incidence of various sexual activities. In interviews, this is obtained by asking the respondent him/herself to estimate how often (or whether) a given sexual act has been engaged in during a specified period.[10] In the sexual diaries such information is derived *post factum* by the researcher by counting how often a given activity occurs in the diary script.

Table 2. List of Sexual Behaviours

Code letter(s)	Sexual behaviour	'Street' term
W	Masturbation	'Wanking'
F	Anal intercourse	'Fucking'
S	Fellatio	'Sucking'
DK	Deep kiss	
V	Vaginal intercourse	
CN	Cunnilingus	
RI	Anilingus	'Rimming'
TF	Inter-femoral frottage	'Thigh fuck'
FG	Ano-digital insertion	'Fingering'
FI	Ano-brachial insertion	'Fisting'
BR	Body rubbing/frottage	
MA	Massage	
CP	Corporal punishment	
TT	Nipple play	'Tit torture'
WS	Lindinism	'Water sports'

The first area of interest is to see how figures derived from sexual diaries compare at the aggregate level to interview responses.[11] Table 3 deals with incidence of sexual behaviour by modality, i.e., the percentage of those (in a month) who had *ever* in the course of their diaries done each of several given sexual behaviours (rows) in the given modality (columns). Thus, 24 per cent of the 610 diarists had engaged in active anal intercourse ('fucked a guy') and 25 per cent had engaged in passive anal intercourse ('been fucked by a guy') in the last month.

The percentages for Self and Him modalities are generally small or not relevant for our present purposes, due to their physical difficulty or impossibility or irrelevance. There are some exceptions: *Solo Masturbation* is important because it is the most prevalent sexual behaviour, and *His Masturbation* indicates that a quarter of the diarists experienced their partner's solo masturbation in a sexual session.

The more interesting point concerns active and passive variants of sexual behaviours. In a stable and closed population, the figures for active and passive variants of a sexual behaviour should be identical. In fact, the figures are surprisingly close to equality, and there is no

Table 3. Percentage Incidence of Persons Ever Engaging in
Specified Sexual Acts by Modality: Data from One-Month Diaries

Behaviour	Modality				
	Self	Active	Passive	Mutual	His
Anal intercourse	NP	#24	#25	NP	NP
Fellatio	NP	#45	#43	#23	NP
Masturbation	#87	#46	#47	#39	25
Anilingus	NP	#11	#10	#4	NP
Ano-brachial insertion	*	2	2	*	*
Vaginal intercourse	NP	3	NP	NP	NP
Inter-femoral frottage	*	#8	#7	2	*
Ano-digital insertion	3	13	11	4	*
Body rub	1	#16	#13	#19	*
Massage	*	13	11	6	*

Percentage of diarists in data set who have exhibited tabulated behaviour in the last
month. Total diarists = 610. '#' indicates comparison with ISB data. '*' indicates less
than 1%. NP indicates not possible or extremely rare due to physical limitations.

tendency for there to be more active diarists than passive diarists, as
one might expect.[12] For sexual diary data the differences are smaller
than the data from any other method, indicating their greater validity.

How similar are these diary data to aggregated self-report data
obtained by the interview method?[13] At first sight and looking at the
actual percentages, they are rather different, with some major dis-
crepancies: the rank-order correlation is modest ($\tau = 0.77$). More
interestingly, the Pearsonian (linear) correlation is much higher ($r = 0.95$), and the regression equation

Y (estimated interview percentage) $= 15.82 + 0.94X$ (diary percentage)

reveals that the relationship is close to absolute, but with an added
constant of about 16. That is, if the diary data are more reliable, then
the interview method systematically overestimates the incidence figures but keeps a virtually identical profile. One possibility is that in
the interview respondents actually use an interval greater than one
month and correctly remember having done X, but have done it in a
longer period. There is one notable exception: the figures for anal

intercourse (active: 29 vs. 24 and passive: 28 vs. 25) are markedly similar, which may indicate that gay men are able to recall with unusual accuracy whether or not they have engaged in this most implicated behaviour.

ANALYSIS OF 'VOLUME': BEHAVIOURAL TRENDS

In a report on an earlier diary sample (Coxon and Carballo 1989) it has been said that 'the vast majority of gay men's sexual activity is taken up by the three main behaviours of masturbation, fellatio and anal intercourse.' The justification for this statement is clearly seen in diary analysis, where the act (as opposed to the person) can be used as the unit of counting. This is termed 'analysis of volume' in our account and is a mode of analysis only feasible using the diary method. It makes it possible to ask not only how many men did X, or how often they did it, but also: 'What proportion (as a fraction of all sexual acts performed) of a person's (or a group's) total outlet consisted of X?' Table 4 illustrates the proportions (of the total number of sexual acts in this data set) which various sexual behaviours occupy.

In fact, over 80 per cent of all behaviour in the sample consists of these three main activities: masturbation, fellatio, and anal intercourse. Masturbation is by far the most common activity and accounts for three-fifths of the total outlet, with Solo Masturbation accounting for over one-third of all sexual acts. The low figure for DK (deep kissing) is simply a reflection of the fact that most diarists don't consider it to be a sexual act, and therefore don't record it consistently.[14] The next 16 per cent of sexual outlet is distributed between BR (frottage), DK (deep kissing), FG (digital-anal insertion), MA (massage) and RI (anilingus).

Expressed in terms of the total sexual outlet for the group, heterosexual activity (vaginal intercourse (VF) and cunnilingus (CN)) is very low indeed. Table 3 shows that 3 per cent of the individuals in the last month had a heterosexual encounter, but this represents merely 0.4 per cent of the total sexual outlet. It would seem that Britain is peculiar in this respect compared to other WHO Homosexual Response Studies sites (see Coxon 1992: §3.2), showing the lowest figures out of all the seven nations.

BEHAVIOUR AND RELATIONSHIPS

Within the diaries, sexual relationship types are defined, following the SIGMA conventions, as: (a) one exclusive regular partner

Table 4. Sexual Behaviours as Proportion of Total Sexual Acts

Behaviour	Frequency of acts	Percentage of total
Masturbation (W)	20,976	58.3
Fellatio (S)	5,990	16.7
Anal int. (F)	2,017	5.6
Frottage (BR)	1,683	4.4
Deep kissing	1,346	3.7
Ano-digital insertion (FG)	1,057	2.9
Massage	921	2.6
Anilingus (RI)	813	2.3
Inter-femoral frottage (TF)	460	1.3
Corporal punishment	269	0.8
Nipple play (TT)	148	0.4
Ano-brachial insertion (FI)	133	0.4
Vaginal intercourse (VF)	126	0.4
Lindinism (WS)	39	0.1
Cunnilingus	7	0.02
Total acts	35,981	100%

Table 5. SIGMA Typology: Relationship by Age Types

	Age		
Relationship	Under 21	21 to 39	Above 39
One regular partner	I	II	III
Regular partner(s) and others	IV	V	VI
No regular partner	VII	VIII	IX

('closed'); (b) one or more regular partners and others ('open'); and
(c) no regular partner. Each of these relationship types is subdivided
into three age ranges. Each cell of the resulting nine-fold design is
given a label, in the form of a roman numeral, as shown in Table 5.

Patterns of sexual behaviour can then be studied by looking at
how the sexual outlet of each of these nine types differs. This is done

by treating that type's total sexual outlet as 100 per cent, and then looking at how it is divided between the three most common sexual behaviours and their associated modalities. (This is termed unconditional or volume analysis, as opposed to conditional analysis, where the individual is the unit of analysis.)

An exhaustive analysis of the whole data set by type was performed and gave the results presented in Table 6. They are worthy of considerable attention, since once again, these are data which are unobtainable by any other method. Each section of the table represents a separate modality, which is then in turn divided by sexual activity.[15] For example, Table 6.1 indicates that 22.2 per cent of the total 694 (Table 6.5) sexual acts done by type I individuals (those aged 21 and under and in a closed relationship) consist of solitary masturbation, compared to 54.1 per cent of type VII (those aged 21 and under with no regular relationship). This suggests that having no regular partner has the effect of doubling the reliance on masturbation for these young men (see Davies et al. 1992).

The behavioural characteristics for each type are well defined:

Masturbation. Those with no regular partner (VII, VIII, IX) show a very high incidence of solo-masturbation, whereas those in closed relationships (I, II, III) have a very low incidence.

Anal intercourse. Those with no regular partner (VII, VIII, IX) show the lowest incidence of any form of anal intercourse, with most of their values being significantly less than the 'average' figure indicated in the ALL column. Those in closed relationships show a consistently higher level of both active and passive anal intercourse. Active anal intercourse is significantly higher for type III (the older partners in a regular relationship), and this is shown in Table 7.[16] But there is no significant variation in the passive form (see Coxon et al. 1993 for further treatment of this question).

Fellatio. Fellatio seems to transcend the relationship limits, and does not show any consistent relationship pattern. Types IV, V, and VI have the highest figures for fellatio, but we should bear in mind that type IV is by far the smallest set, and so we cannot treat the result as reliable.

No other form of behaviour exhibits a significant relationship type or age dependency.

BEHAVIOURAL PROGRESSION WITHIN THE SESSION

Anal intercourse is recognized as the form of sexual behaviour that is implicated most significantly in the transmission of HIV. From a

Table 6. 'Volume' Analysis of Sexual Behaviour by Modality
and Type of Relationship (the following percentages are
expressed as a proportion of the total sexual outlet of
the indicated type of sexual behaviour:
W = masturbation; F = anal intercourse; S = fellatio)

6.1: Modality = self: solo activity by act (masturbation) and type

	ALL	I	II	III	VI	V	VI	VII	VIII	IX
W	34%	22.5	22.8	19.7	15.3	31.0	21.4	54.1	53.7	44.6

6.2 Modality = active: active (Ego to Alter) by acts and type

	ALL	I	II	III	IV	V	VI	VII	VIII	IX
W	6.9	10.0	7.5	7.7	2.4	7.2	9.9	4.2	4.8	6.3
F	2.6	4.0	2.8	10.5	2.4	2.4	3.5	1.4	1.2	2.6
S	7.5	7.2	7.0	7.5	12.9	8.0	10.3	6.4	5.8	6.6

6.3 Modality = passive: (Alter to Ego) by acts and type

	ALL	I	II	III	IV	V	VI	VII	VIII	IX
W	6.7	8.5	7.5	5.2	7.0	7.1	8.4	5.0	4.1	5.0
F	2.4	3.0	4.0	3.8	4.7	2.2	2.2	1.5	1.5	2.2
S	6.2	7.5	7.0	3.6	9.4	7.3	5.2	4.8	5.0	4.2

6.4 Modality = mutual: (Alter and Ego simultaneously) by act and type

	ALL	I	II	III	IV	V	VI	VII	VIII	IX
W	7.4	7.2	6.0	3.6	11.8	6.8	10.4	6.8	5.6	11.0
F	–	–	–	–	–	–	–	–	–	–
S	2.8	2.6	3.2	4.8	4.7	2.4	4.5	2.0	1.9	1.9

6.5 Total sexual outlet by type (frequency of acts)

	ALL	I	II	III	IV	V	VI	VII	VIII	IX
	194155	694	2748	478	85	1136	2792	1368	2545	5800

Table 7. Sexual Outlet for Active Anal Intercourse (AI)
(number of acts of active AI per month)

Relationship	Under 21	21 to 39	Over 39
One partner	4.0	2.8	10.6
Regular partners and others	2.4	2.4	3.6
No regular partner	1.4	1.2	2.7

behavioural point of view, it would be interesting to see what types of behaviour are most likely to precede and lead on to anal intercourse of some form. We already know that anal intercourse is most typically the end-marker of a session, and the sequence in a sexual session may be so constrained that anal intercourse becomes virtually inevitable. Moreover, different behaviours may precede the active as opposed to the passive variant. Is this true?

In a preliminary analysis of the *co-occurrence* of sexual acts it was found that the two acts most likely to occur *in the same sexual session* as anal intercourse are masturbation and fellatio. Starting with this, precedence analysis was then applied to the sessions to see what behaviour is most likely to lead on to anal intercourse.

'Precedence analysis' is essentially a frequency count of how many times a given act precedes another in a sexual session. The analysis uses a 'sensitivity' parameter called 'width' which defines how many acts are taken into consideration by the analysis as preceding the reference act. For example, consider the following session:

Session 1:= { AW PW PF AS }

Let us use PF as the reference base; the AS is ignored in a precedence analysis, since it follows the reference. If the width is one, then only PW is counted as the precedent, but if the width is 2, then both PW and AW count as precedents. Thus the width value defines how many acts are visible to the analysis previous to the reference base. But the same act can occur more than once in a session, and this has to be allowed for. Consider the following example:

Session 2:= { AFI AS PW AS AF }

If AF is the reference base, then the three (distinct) precedent acts are: AFI, AS, and PW. But AS occurs twice, and is therefore given a higher

Table 8. Precedence Analysis for Anal Intercourse

[1] Precedent reference base: active anal intercourse (AF)

		Width	
Act	1	2	3
AS	49	89	126
PS	85	118	146
AW	31	61	73
PW	31	51	64

[2] Precedent base: passive anal intercourse (PF)

		Width	
Act	1	2	3
AS	50	89	123
PS	42	80	101
AW	26	38	52
PW	33	51	61

precedence value. In the above example, the precedence value of AS (with AF as the reference) has a value of 2 *if the width is* 3, but a value of 1 *if the width is* 2, the reason being that the second AS is out of the range of width visibility when the width is 2. (Width does not include the reference act itself.)

Let us turn now to the diary data (see Table 8). Looking at both the Active and Passive tables, the rank order of likely precedence is the same, independent of the width of the precedence. Active/insertive anal intercourse is most likely to be preceded (in order) by:

(Passive Sucking/Receptive Fellatio)
(Active Sucking/Insertive Fellatio)
(Active Wanking/Masturbation), and
(Passive Wanking/Masturbation)

In brief, this can be expressed as a rule: *'If I fuck a guy, sucking is most likely to precede it (rather than wanking), and I'm most likely to be sucked by him first.'*

Passive/receptive anal intercourse, by contrast, is most likely to be preceded (in order) by:

(Active Sucking/Insertive Fellatio)
(Passive Sucking/Receptive Fellatio)
(Passive Wanking/Masturbation), and
(Active Wanking/Masturbation)

In brief: *'If I am fucked by a guy, sucking is, again, most likely to precede it, and I'm most likely to suck him first.'* (This accords with gay received wisdom and underwrites once again the symbolic dominance/subservience role of anal intercourse.)

In many ways these are the two sides of the same coin — seen from Ego's and Alter's perspective. A 'successor analysis' of active and passive fellatio would reveal the similar point: 'If you suck your partner, you're likely to go on to be fucked by him,' and 'If you are sucked by your partner, you are likely to be expected to go on to fuck him.'

If anal intercourse occurs in a sexual session, then it is most commonly the end-marker, and is very likely indeed to result in ejaculation, so this is where attention needs to be focused for a more accurate knowledge of how risk occurs (or is prevented). But this is another story (see Coxon and Coxon 1993).

USEFULNESS OF DIARY ANALYSIS

The results given by the diary analysis are very reliable and conclusive when studying the behaviour of individuals at the session level. Because of the short duration of the diaries (usually about a month or so), it is not so effective for time-generalized analysis (such as genuine 'ever' figures). It does, however, give a good idea of relative proportions of sexual behaviour, since total sexual outlet sets may be analysed by various independent variables (such as type, status, geographic location).

The greatest strengths of diary analysis, and areas in which it is worth particular further study, are in the analysis of the volume of sexual behaviour, of sexual role segregation, and co-occurrence, precedence, and successor analyses. These are all methods used to study behaviour at the session or individual level. The use of condoms during sessions is also an important part of the study, and one area in which diary analysis can, in principle, perform well.

Perhaps the most striking difference is that data are *derived* in the case of diaries, whereas data represent subjects' accounts (or estimates) in the case of interviews. There is no warrant for believing that the two will necessarily give rise to the same conclusions (indeed, the comparison of the two is an important component of our validation studies). But it is clearly seen from this analysis that sexual diaries are capable of providing unique data which is also uniquely adapted to answering problems of considerable epidemiological and policy relevance.

USE OF DIARIES IN ANTHROPOLOGICAL SETTINGS

In the research reported here, sexual diaries have been used as an auxiliary method of data collection and validation within a Western European context. The reliability and utility of diaries in other contexts depends on a number of factors:

Whether diary-keeping is an accepted procedure in the culture. For gay men, and for sexual and romantic activity in general, diary-keeping is a popular, though often a private, pastime, and is often written in code to ensure confidentiality (McCormick 1980). The social science use (see also Pomeroy, Flax, and Wheeler 1982) consists primarily in persuading respondents to do so for scientific purposes.

Anonymity must be guaranteeable. Whilst some diarists care not who knows their secrets, for others the diary records what no one else knows, and somehow the social scientist has to safeguard this secrecy, especially if the matters being recorded are illegal, deviant, or even simply private. At least one SIGMA diarist was expelled from his lodgings because his landlady 'found' his sexual diary.

The diary does not depend on a written format. Although diaries are most conveniently kept in writing in literate cultures, there is no reason why they must be. We have used both tape recorders and electronic pocket memos to record (and have diarists record) their diaries.

The diary does not depend on a long period. Although we have found that a month is the minimum period for reliable data, some diarists can be persuaded to keep it for much longer. (However, we believe that persons who keep the diary longer may differ in important ways from our other respondents.) Also, card versions of day entries can be devised which allow an encrypted version of events to be sent through the mail on a daily basis, thus avoiding problems of partial-completion and loss; it also helps avoid contamination due to recognition of trends by the diarist, if this is felt to be a problem.

The diary can be completed at leisure. Communicating about sexual behaviour (and especially uncommon behaviour) is often not feasible or is subject to systematic bias if elicited in the presence of others. Diaries can be completed at any time convenient to the respondent.

Diary information can as well be based on observation as on the subject's report. Although not always feasible, the structure of sexual behaviour underlying the diary code makes it possible to use it as a rapid shorthand for situations such as immediate re-interview, and our current studies of competent encoders' encodings of a common video stimulus (gay male pornographic sequences) show that high agreement on 'chunking' and description of sexual activity can be achieved.

* * *

The sexual diary is a robust, easy-to-use method for collecting reports (and/or observations) on detailed and sequential aspects of sexual behaviour. So long as common meanings are established before its use, respondents find them straightforward and even interesting to complete, and the data can be used to answer questions which interviews based on retrospective recall are ill-adapted to answer. Probably the most telling shortcoming is that volunteer (selection) bias is likely to be strong — including the earlier point about the difference in diary-keepers. This can be minimized by careful strategies to improve participation (Rosenthal and Rosnow 1975).

Because of the inherent detail of the diary account, it lends itself to serendipitous discovery and since it provides a general trace of behaviour it can provide well-adapted information if new foci of research become imperative. With the rapid increase in our understanding of HIV transmission, this cannot but be for the best.

NOTES

1. This research is supported by grants from the Department of Health (UK), the Medical Research Council, and the World Health Organization to Project SIGMA (Essex). These bodies are in no way responsible for the views expressed in this chapter.
2. This, and other issues of reliability and validity of SIGMA sexual diary data are currently under investigation by the senior author, with funding from the Department of Health. For discussion of relevant experimental and theoretical findings see Linton (1986) and Brewer (1988).

3. Interview estimates tend to be 'chunked' aggregates of week estimates (e.g., a respondent will mentally estimate the last week's frequency and then multiply up by four for a month estimate), be reported in rounded quantities (e.g., multiples of 5 or 10), and be subject to an individual distortion factor. Current research centres on the comparison of estimates provided by the subject *after* the return of the diary with those calculated from the diary of the same period (Coxon 1988b).

4. 'Poppers' refer to amyl or butyl nitrite sniffed to give a quick 'high' by cardiovascular dilation.

5. The respondent is asked to provide the following information about each sexual partner: [1] Whether he is *regular/occasional/'one-off'*; [2] His *age* (if you know it, or your guess); [3] How long you have been having sex with him; [4] Where you met him; [5] His HIV status (one of: Negative, Positive, or Don't Know), together with the partner's sex, if it is not male.

6. For reasons of confidentiality we did not ask the respondent to give the actual name of his contacts and in the case contacts, this was never known. Systematic network tracing is thus precluded by our adoption of this self-denying ordinance.

7. Instructions are contained in 'Instructions for Completing a Sexual Diary,' SIGMA 1990.

8. Since the SIGMA system was developed explicitly with HIV transmission in mind, it is necessary to distinguish *which* partner ejaculates, and where the ejaculate goes — in/on the partner, in a condom, etc. This is encoded in the SIGMA coding system but is not discussed further here (see Coxon et al. 1992).

9. Such a list is of its very nature open; sexual adventurousness and inventiveness, together with shifting labels for acts, make it so. Taking the respondents' terminology as definitive does introduce methodological problems of overlapping categories, such as occur for essentially the same activities as 'NN' ('nipple nibbling') and 'TT' ('tit torture'), and of apparently equivalent categories which reverse the modality — compare 'sucking' and 'mouth-fucking').

10. The diaries of this study are all completed by men (hence the use of male gender throughout), but there is no reason why this should be so.

11. The sexual diaries are held in DbaseIV and CARDBOX-PLUS format. The programs for subsequent analysis are contained in the software package SDA [Sexual Diary Analysis] written in TOPSPEED C by Huw Coxon with funding from the Department of Health, whose help is gratefully acknowledged. Copies of the programs, selected data, and documentation are available at cost from Project SIGMA (attn: N.H. Coxon), University of Essex.

12. Because in general receptive anal intercourse has lower prestige or is deemed more submissive than the insertive variant.

13. Reported in SIGMA 1990 (Table 5.5, pp. 129–130). Because these data are obtained using the ISB, which has the same structure as the Diary codes, direct comparison is possible. The 17 cells entering the comparison are marked with '#' in Table 3. The values, in order, are: 24 (AF), 28, 61, 58, 39, 90 (SW), 65, 63, 61, 23, 23, 10, 26, 23, 42, 38, 40 (MBR).

14. And also because it was only recently re-introduced into the list of behaviours. It was initially excluded on the grounds that it could not be implicated in HIV transmission, and was re-introduced as a marker for tracking CMV (cytomegalovirus) sero-conversion.

15. Each row of the table is better represented as an Age × Relationship table, whose entries are the relevant percentages. In previous analyses (Coxon 1987), each table is then analysed using an ANOVA or resistant analysis such as Median Polish (see note 16).

16. To illustrate the additive analysis mentioned in note 15, when the data of Table 6.2 (F) (i.e., active anal intercourse; also shown in Table 7) are analysed using Tukey's Median Polish, the results table is as follows:

| | AGE | | | Effect of |
REL	<21	21–39	>39	REL
Closed	0	–1.0	5.3	1.6
Open	0	0.2	–0.1	0
No reg.	0	0	0	–1.0
Effect of age:	0	–0.2	1.3	Total: 2.4

The overall (total) value is 2.4 per cent, and compared to this the effects of age and relationship are small — being in a closed relationship raises the percentage by 1.6 per cent; being over 39 raises it by a further 1.3 per cent, whilst having no regular relationship decreases it by 1 per cent. The entries in the body of the table are the 'interaction' or residual/joint effects, so the *combined* effect of being in a closed relationship and between 21 and 39 decreases it by 1 per cent. By far the greatest effect of all is being in a closed relationship and over 39: this adds an effect more than twice the size of the overall effect. (Adding the total, row, column, and interaction effect (necessarily) yields the original data. Thus the 'closed relationship/age less than 21' cell comprises:

Total + Closed + Age < 21 + Closed-and-age < 21

i.e.,

 2.4 1.6 0 0 = 4.0%,

as in Table 6, 6.2 (F) cell I).

REFERENCES

Brewer, W.F. 1988. Memory for Randomly Sampled Autobiographical Events. In: *Remembering Reconsidered: Ecological and Traditional Approaches to the Study of Memory*, edited by U. Neisser and E. Winograd. Cambridge: Cambridge University Press.

Coxon, A.P.M. 1987. The Effect of Age and Relationship on Gay Men's Sexual Behaviour: A Preliminary Analysis of Sexual Diary Data. Cardiff: SRU Working Paper.

Coxon, A.P.M. 1988a. 'Something Sensational…' the Sexual Diary as a Tool for Mapping Detailed Sexual Behaviour. *Sociological Review* 36(2):353–367.

Coxon, A.P.M. 1988b. The Numbers Game: Gay Lifestyles, Epidemiology of AIDS and Social Science. In: *Social Aspects of AIDS*, edited by P. Aggleton and H. Homans. London: Falmer Press

Coxon, A.P.M. 1992. England and Wales Report: WHO Homosexual Response Studies. Essex: Project SIGMA.

Coxon, A.P.M., and M. Carballo. 1989. Research on AIDS: Behavioural Perspectives. Editorial Review. *AIDS* 3(4):191–197.

Coxon, A.P.M., with P. Weatherburn, A.J. Hunt, and, P.M. Davies. 1992. The Structure of Sexual Behaviour, *Journal of Sex Research* 29(1):61–83.

Coxon, A.P.M., N.H. Coxon, with P. Weatherburn, A.J. Hunt, F. Hickson, P.M. Davies, and T.J. McManus. 1993. Sex Role Separation in Sexual Diaries of Homosexual Men. *AIDS* 7(6): 877–882.

Davies, P.M. 1990. Patterns in Homosexual Behaviour: Use of the Diary Method. In: *Sexual Behaviour and Risks of HIV Infection*, edited by M. Hubert. Bruxelles: Facultés Universitaires Saint Louis, pp. 59–78.

Davies, P.M., P. Weatherburn, A.J. Hunt, F.C.I. Hickson, T.J. McManus, and A.P.M.Coxon. 1992. Young Gay Men in England and Wales: Sexual Behaviour and Implications for the Spread of HIV. *AIDS Care* 4(3):259–272.

Linton, M. 1986. Ways of Searching and the Contents of Memory. In: *Autobiographical Memory*, edited by D.C. Rubin. Cambridge: Cambridge University Press, pp. 50–67.

McCormick, D. 1980. *Love in Code, or How to Keep Your Secrets*. London: Eyre Methuen.

Pomeroy, W.B., C.C. Flax, and C.C. Wheeler. 1982. *Taking a Sex History: Interviewing and Recording*. London: Collier Macmillan.

Rosenthal, R., and R.L. Rosnow. 1975. *The Volunteer Subject*. New York: Wiley.

SIGMA. 1990. Longitudinal Study of the Sexual behaviour of Homosexual Males Under the Impact of AIDS. Final Report to Department of Health, Project SIGMA.

SIGMA. 1993. *Notes on Keeping a Sexual Diary*. Colchester: Project SIGMA.

Weatherburn, P., P.M. Davies, F.C.I. Hickson, A.J. Hunt, T.J. McManus, and A.P.M.Coxon. 1993. No Connection Between Alcohol Use and Unsafe Sex Among Gay and Bisexual Men. *AIDS* 7(1):115–119.

Chapter ELEVEN

Talking About AIDS: Linguistic Perspectives on Non-Neutral Discourse

William L. Leap

Speakers of English use language in special ways when they talk about the AIDS pandemic and its effects on their lives. They draw on code words and phrases when identifying HIV illnesses, describing symptoms, and assessing treatment strategies. They adjust word order, disguise subject reference, and make other changes in sentence and paragraph form when discussing high-risk behaviour or commenting on the social conditions which encourage risk-taking. Sometimes, when AIDS is the topic under discussion, people explore their thoughts and feelings in great verbal detail; other times, they make their thoughts and feelings known by saying nothing at all.

All discussions of AIDS are rule-governed speech events. What speakers understand about the pandemic and its effects on their lives helps them choose the features of grammar and discourse which are relevant to the messages they want to convey in such settings. Frequently, such closely meshed relationships between language and experience create formidable barriers to AIDS education and outreach efforts. In this chapter, I examine language use from two such speech events, and I show how text-oriented linguistic research can help practitioners (1) identify social meanings which speakers have assigned to AIDS and (2) develop intervention strategies appropriate to those domains.

BACKGROUND

As a linguist, my entry point in this research is text-specific instances of conversation, narration, question asking and answering, or other forms of situated discourse. Texts are not arbitrary linguistic phenomena. Text form (e.g., sentence syntax, paragraph organization), as well as text content (the issues, topics, and themes which the text explores), reflect speaker decisions regarding what should (and should not) be said on the issues being addressed within that speech setting. In other words, texts can be studied as intentional constructions, and as context-specific products of choice-making. The evidence of intention and choice displayed within each text provides access to the speaker's construction of context-specific messages and to the larger discourse of which those messages are a part.

Frequently, text-centred research confirms claims about AIDS discourse which ethnographers have developed through analysis of other types of social data. And in the process, such research often shows how widely attested features of discourse take on particular significance within the speaker's presentation of message and meaning in specific social domains. In some cases, text-centred research provides a basis for criticizing and working claims about AIDS discourse developed from non-linguistic data sources (or developed in spite of them). I discuss each of these conditions in greater detail in the following sections.

AIDS AS A DISEASE OF 'THE OTHER'

During the earliest years of the AIDS pandemic, the biomedical characteristics of what were later to be termed HIV illnesses were puzzling to many people and the social implications of these ill-nesses were frightening. Intensifying these conditions was the absence of agreement regarding the appropriate name for these phenomena. In the main, practitioners favoured terms like gay related immune deficiency (GRID), community acquired immune deficiency syndrome (CAIDS), or gay bowel syndrome, labels which 'identified the disease by whom it hit rather than what it did' (Shilts 1987: 158). Acquired immune deficiency syndrome (AIDS) came into use in 1982 and quickly replaced these older, more targeted references (see Example I and associated discussion in Murray and Payne 1989). But as AIDS became an accepted reference for the medical condition, so did the notion of risk groups and the identification of forms of behaviour (promiscuity, male co-sexual erotics, intravenous drug use) which were most likely to place persons within situations of risk. As Clatts and Mutchler have noted, such designations draw explicit connections between AIDS and the 'dangerous and anti-social 'other,'" connections which become problematic for AIDS research and education because they 'fix our attention on a relatively small range of possible vectors of this disease ... and direct our attention away from other possible factors of (its) aetiology and spread' (1989:14, 19–20).

These connections between AIDS, danger, anti-social behaviour, and the other have real implications for the grounding of AIDS discourse in context-specific text construction. The terms risk and at-risk are anything but neutral in their suggestion of deliberately unobserved restraint. The term AIDS itself is heavily marked for irregular reference (Leap 1990:139–140), given the connotation of its headword (syndrome), the ambiguity of its key modifier (deficiency indicates absence, not presence), and the length of the unabbreviated construction. The use of the abbreviation intensifies this sense of irregularity by obscuring the presence of these meanings within sentence structure. Other vocabulary used in AIDS-related text-making — whether they come from the medical discourse on sexually transmitted diseases (STDs) or are derived through analogy or metaphor from other sources (e.g., American English labels like 'the plague,' or the deliberately context-specific '(s)he's lost a lot of weight') — underscore the differences between AIDS discourse and reference-making in everyday life and reinforce AIDS-related messages of distance and danger. The same is true in American Indian and other language-minority speech communities, where sources outside of the community's language tradition, rather than the community's own linguistic resources, become the base for the socially appropriate AIDS vocabulary.

Paraphrasing Clatts and Mutchler (1989), all of these terms have the potential for fixing attention on a small range of possible references (i.e., the dangerous, anti-social other) and direct(ing) attention away from other, equally possible references. Speakers may not have such outcomes in mind when they use these words and phrases to express references to AIDS. But these are the messages established when speakers use such expressions in text-making, and their use of these expressions coincides with messages about AIDS established by features of sentence syntax, by question-answering strategies, and elements of narrative style which they also employ in those settings.

Example I

(P = Physician/Anthropologist. R = Respondent)

```
 1  P:  Where do you think you got the HIV?
 2  R:  The person I was living with.
 3  P:  Where did he get it?
 4  R:  His travels.
 5  P:  Was he, did he have many partners?
 6  R:  I really couldn't say; I believe so.
 7  P:  Did you have many partners?
 8  R:  No. Uh, none.
 9  P:  Do you have any friends with HIV?
10  R:  Not to my knowledge.
11  P:  Do you know people with AIDS?
12  R:  No, not that I know of.
13  P:  How about friends, do they treat you—
14  R:  I have not told my friends.
15  P:  You've kept this secret?
16  R:  Yes.
17  R:  (Pause) As far as the disease itself, it is not worth what I
18      have to go through.
19  P:  Say that again.
20  R:  The severity of the illness. If I knew this was what it
21      was all about, I would not have gotten involved.
22  P:  ... When you say if you knew what you had to go through you
23      wouldn't have done this, what would you have done? What
24      could you have done to protect yourself?
25  R:  I would not have gotten involved in the gay lifestyle.
26  P:  Do you feel that people have a choice between a gay
27      lifestyle and a straight lifestyle?
28  R:  I did, since I was primarily a bisexual.
29  P:  Were you ever married?
30  R:  Yeah, seven years.
```

```
31  P:  Can you tell me about your ideas when you switched from
32      primarily heterosexual to primarily homosexual?
33  R:  Oh, this is a new experience, let me try this out, let
34      me try this also.
```
                        Source: Leap 1991:278–279

Consider, in this regard, the dialogue in Example I, a bedside interview between a 50-year-old HIV positive, symptomatic gay man and a physician/anthropologist visiting the hospital ward to which the respondent had recently been assigned.[1] The physician had spoken with the respondent several times prior to this interview. Their familiarity helps explain the respondent's willingness to answer candidly to the physician's abruptly worded questions about his private life.

At the beginning of this discussion, the physician asked the respondent to explain how he contracted his illness. His reply cited another, specifically the person he was living with (line 2), who, the respondent believed, had many sex partners during his travels (lines 4, 6). The respondent, on the other hand, had not had many partners (line 8), and added that he did not know anyone with AIDS and had not told any of his friends about his own illness (lines 9–16).

In the second segment of the discussion (lines 17–25), the respondent looks critically at his illness — 'it is not worth what I have to go through' (lines 17–18); and at his life as a gay man — 'if I knew that was what it was all about, I would not have gotten involved' (lines 20–21). Contextually, the referent of the 'it' pronoun in line 20 could be either the disease/illness (as was the case for it in line 17) or the gay lifestyle, the implied object of the sentence verb in line 21, the stated reference in line 25, and the focus for discussion in the remainder (lines 26–34) of this text.

The comments on gay lifestyle actually centred around the respondent's description of his gender career. He specified that he was primarily a bisexual (line 28), that he was married for a period of time (line 30), and that he chose to switch from a heterosexual to a gay lifestyle (lines 30 ff.). Importantly, he claims to have responded enthusiastically to opportunities which became available to him once he began to define himself as primarily homosexual: 'Oh, this is a new experience, let me try this out, let me try this also' (lines 33–34).

Several features characterize the speakers' use of language in this dialogue. First of all, AIDS is clearly the central theme in this discussion, and concerns about AIDS are implicit in all of the speakers' statements; however, the term 'AIDS' never occurs in the respondent's comments. When references to AIDS are unavoidable (lines 17,

20), he uses more neutral, highly context-dependent synonyms (illness, disease); otherwise, he lets the wording of the physician's questions establish the frame of reference for a concise, and usually unelaborated, reply.

Concise, unelaborated responses were especially evident in the opening section of the dialogue. Here the respondent's statements contain noun constructions, but only rarely are they accompanied by verbs. In other words, he identifies persons or states of activity as appropriate to the discussion, but he leaves the details of the action undescribed.

Hence, the respondent notes that his roommate travelled, though he does not explain why he travelled or where he went and denies knowing anything about the roommate's sexual activity while away from home. He indicates that he has friends, though he says nothing about them nor does he explain why, if they are his friends, he has not told them about his illness. What little he does say on these themes is presented in sentences dominated by negative markers ('never,' 'not,' 'no'). The one sentence in this section which does not fit that syntactic pattern (line 16) contains a single-word, unelaborated comment ('yes') — which serves to bring this line of questioning to a close.

Even when the physician's questions probed for greater detail, the respondent's replies continued to be succinct and cryptic, obligating the physician — and the linguist — to interpret sentence meanings in terms of their own sources of data. For example, the respondent's expression 'the person I was living with' (line 2) could describe several types of domestic relationships in gay culture. The linkage between the respondent's illness and the roommate's adventurousness while away from home provides the only clue that the living arrangement was personal and intimate, yet that connection has to be inferred from multiple comments of physician and respondent, and is not explicitly indicated in the text on its own.

Respondent comments continued to be tersely constructed during the final section of the interview and, as before, the comments offer only glimpses into the issues under discussion (his gender career). This time, however, the glimpses are much more richly detailed. Instead of presenting himself as a shadow-figure with only vaguely detailed social connections to those around him, the respondent positions himself as the central actor in the events he identifies. That is, he made the choice to become predominantly homosexual (line 28) and to be involved in the gay lifestyle (line 25). And he was the person eager to explore everything that this lifestyle had to offer.

Importantly, the syntax of these comments supports and confirms the messages displayed through the speaker's word choices. Negative constructions, so common to the comments in lines 1–16, do not occur in these statements. Sentence subjects are first-person, singular references, and the indicated subject is always the agent, not the recipient, of verb action.

The shift from vague to concrete commentary, and from speaker-as-object to speaker-as-actor, occurs during the middle section of the interview (lines 17–25). It was at this point that the respondent moved away from discussing his 'illness' and focused instead on key events in his gender career. This shift did not result from the physician's prompting. The respondent volunteered the reflexive comment (line 17) which, when paraphrased (lines 20–21), formally stated the connection between AIDS and gay lifestyle implicit in his earlier remarks (another issue requiring listener inference), and which cued the physician to begin exploring the respondent's gender career.

The shifts in richness of speaker commentary and assertions of speaker agency[2] displayed within this text do more than coincide with speaker-controlled changes in text focus. They also show how AIDS-related references to the distant, anti-social other affect the overall form of a speaker's text and influence other areas of his text-based presentation of messages. In this case, someone who had nothing to say about his own erotic activity when the topic under discussion was HIV illness became quite willing to offer comment on that activity once the topic shifted to a more neutral, less disquieting domain. Initially, other parties — the roommate, his unidentified sex partners — were the significant actors in the discussion, with the respondent carefully positioning himself at distance from them, from his friends, and from anyone else he had to identify. Once the topic changed, so did the importance he assigns to his own actions, compared against the emphasis he placed on the actions of others in that regard. Not surprisingly, the respondent accounted for his illness by identifying his roommate as the risk-taker, while positioning himself as the victim of circumstances over which he had no control. Once the topic changed, innocent victim became active adventurer, eager to participate in new experiences — adventures and experiences which, by his narration, had no effects whatsoever on his subsequent illness.

AIDS AND THE SOCIAL CONSTRUCTION
OF PASSION

Health educators and policymakers continue to be perplexed by a contradictory condition widely reported by AIDS researchers and practitioners: gay men will report a high degree of 'correct' risk knowledge but still engage in high-risk erotic activities, all the same. Stall, Coates, and Hoff (1988) found this to be the only common theme in studies of effective AIDS education as of 1988; otherwise, studies to date disagreed quite openly as to factors actually promoting changes in AIDS-related risk behaviour. Reviews of the literature published since that time (see discussion in Bolton 1992) show that those disagreements have not been resolved.

Some researchers, hoping to bring greater clarity to these conditions, have carried out extensive interviews/discussions with gay men to elicit their rationales for participating in high-risk erotics. Bolton (1992, in this volume) cautions that comments offered in the objective environment of an interview setting may not coincide with the respondent's actual practice in real-life, erotic domains. Equally serious, I suggest, are instances where researchers elicit first-hand commentary about risky sex but use their own assumptions about erotic risk, rather than clues in the respondents' commentary, to interpret the respondents' explanations for their behaviour.

As an example of such an analysis, and its implications, consider the statements in Example II. The speakers here, two gay men, are discussing reasons for their participation in unprotected anal sex. Levine and Siegel (1992) use these examples to show how sexual passion, sexual desire, or lust become motivating factors for unsafe sex. The authors explain:

> Nearly all of the men offering this excuse felt their behaviour was uncharacteristic of them and attributable to uncontrollable urges, which overwhelmed their intent to use protection. These men typically described these urges as powerful biological needs and drives, which they dubbed passion or 'horniness.' (Levine and Siegel 1992:62)

Gay men who have been sexually active during their gender career will understand the issues (and the state of mind) which these respondents are describing. In that sense, explaining the appeal of high-risk sex in terms of 'horniness' seems a reasonable research conclusion. But that conclusion ignores other clues to their behaviour which the speakers built into their responses. Analyzing these statements as texts — that is, as products of choice-making, as intended constructions — will make those comments more accessible.

Important in that regard is the notion of text coherence, the central themes which underlie and give focus to each of these statements. I agree that 'overwhelming passion and lust' are important to text coherence in Respondent A's statement. He notes (lines 4, 6–7, 9–10): 'we had brought condoms ... (but) somewhere along the course of action, we forgot ... we both felt bad, stupid about it.... It just happened. It was passion.' But reading the comments as he constructed them shows that another issue — agency — needs to be taken into account here as well.

Respondent A described his first encounter with this partner by using a statement which is devoid of agency marking: 'There was unprotected oral sex and unprotected anal sex' (lines 1–2). Agency can be inferred from his comments (e.g., unprotected sex where he did not come suggests that the partner was the inserter in the activity), but agency is not formally marked as such in this description.

Example II

Respondent A

1 The first time we met there was unprotected oral sex. And he
2 is HIV positive.... There was unprotected oral sex and unpro-
3 tected anal sex where he did not cum.... And the second time —
4 we've only had sex twice — we had brought condoms, the whole
5 bit. You know what I mean, like we were all ready to go. And
6 you know, somewhere along the course of the action we for-
7 got to put, you know, to bring out the condoms ... and he did
8 cum inside of me. And you know we both felt bad, so stupid
9 about it. There hadn't even been drinking.... It just hap-
10 pened. It was passion.

Respondent B

1 Ah, I know there's one particularly hot guy. Well he, he
2 works in the movies, I guess. Just a stud, you know. Ah,
3 just completely rejecting the idea [of using a condom dur-
4 ing anal sex]. Ah, and so once, we did have a session and he
5 fucked the hell out of me. And I'm happy to say he just, he
6 couldn't cum at all. And even though I was so overwhelmed by
7 the passion of the moment that I would have permitted him
8 that pleasure, things sort of lucked out, as it were.

Source: Siegel and Levine 1992:62–63

Respondent A's description of their second encounter addresses questions of agency much more directly. Here, instead of using actor-less impersonal statements ('There was unprotected oral sex') as in the preceding lines, the respondent focused his sentences around first-person plural ('we') agency: 'we've only had sex twice ... we had brought condoms ... we were all ready to go ... we forgot to put, ... to bring out the condoms ... we both felt bad.' The passion to which he refers at the end of the statement (line 10) may have just happened (lines 9–10), but this was a shared happening: both parties jointly participated in its detail.

Respondent B presents a different picture of agency in his description of unsafe sex experience. Unlike Respondent A, he begins his comments with a description of his partner, using phrases ('particularly hot guy, ... just a stud,' lines 1–2), which suggest that the respondent was eager to have this erotic encounter. Apparently, as suggested by the statement in line 3, the partner was not willing to use condoms, though the absence of an identified actor in that statement leaves agency open to question. It is clear, however, that absence of condom use did not matter to the respondent. The text indicates that he allowed this hot stud to fuck the hell out of (him) (line 5, tense altered) and would have permitted him that pleasure (= cumming in his ass) given the passion of the moment (lines 7–8), had the partner been able to ejaculate.

As far as this text is concerned, agency in this encounter was an entirely one-sided affair. Even if the partner was the person who objected to condom use (ambiguous line 3), those objections did not create the conditions of risk within this encounter. Instead, the risk resulted from Respondent B's interest in having sex with the hot stud and willingness to do so regardless of stipulations. Notice how he uses the first-person singular ('I') pronoun to specify agency in the opening and closing lines of the text — the segments which establish his interest in the partner-to-be and make clear that he, not the partner, was in control during the erotic encounter. In contrast, he uses first-person plural reference only once: we did have a session (line 4), and indicates third-person agency only once: 'he fucked the hell out of me' (lines 4–5).

In other words, this text does not describe an encounter between two equally active parties — as was the case in Respondent A's narrative; instead, this text describes one event in the life of a single individual (Respondent B). The other character in that event is a necessary figure in the narrative, but is in no sense a focus for agency in its events.

These differences in text construction make it necessary to rethink the conclusions which Levine and Siegel (1992) drew from these statements. Lust and passion are issues in these discussion, and they do influence the respondents' decisions to participate in high-risk behaviour. However, lust and passion are secondary to the assertions of agency presented in these texts and to the effects which differences in agency had on risk-related decision-making in each case. Levine and Siegel are correct to note that their respondents use sexual passion as a means of accounting for the participation in unsafe sex. But a closer reading of the respondents' comments — as text — suggests the need to distinguish between different constructions of passion, particularly as each construction intertwines with, and is shaped by, different assertions of power within each erotic domain.

IMPLICATIONS

I suggested, in the opening of this chapter, that discussions of AIDS are rule-governed speech events. And the examples presented here have shown some of the ways in which assumptions about AIDS can produce regularities in language use within such domains.

Hence in Example I, we found a respondent constructing an explanation for his HIV illness which placed greater emphasis on unnamed persons and unspecified activities than it did on his own life experiences in this regard. The linguistic details in this portion of the text emphasize the other-as-actor and conceal direct references to his own risk-related activities even though, at a later point in the discussion, he seems quite willing to discuss those activities in some detail.

In Example II, we found speakers offering somewhat different interpretations of their participation in high-risk erotics. Once again, pronoun choices, verb forms, and other features of sentence and paragraph syntax parallel and reinforce the comments about lust and passion which each speaker conveys through choices in text meaning.

Such connections between language and experience are hardly surprising, though the significance is often overlooked in the search to identify barriers preventing people from making greater use of safe sex materials and other prevention-oriented resources. Levine and Siegel's reading of lust and passion, above, compared to that given by their respondents, is just one instance of this problem. Text-centred methods of linguistic research, of the sort illustrated in this chapter, offer powerful ways of identifying the forms of knowledge which underlie meaningful discussions of AIDS while making certain that the analysis of that discourse remains tightly focused around prevention needs.

238 William L. Leap

ACKNOWLEDGEMENTS

My thanks to Gilbert Herdt and to Ron Bueno (The American University) for helpful comments on earlier versions.

NOTES

1. The physician/anthropologist tape-recorded this conversation with the respondent's consent. He supplied me with a copy of the audiotape for transcription and linguistic analysis, and provided additional comments about the respondent's background once I had completed my review of the text and the information it displays.
2. Text-based references to agency identify the person or persons who initiated or controlled the action which is under discussion in a given text. Agency is a feature of text construction. Claims to agency may or may not coincide with the speaker's real-life experiences, though they certainly suggest the conclusion the speaker wants others to draw in that regard.

REFERENCES

Bolton, R. 1992. Mapping Terra Incognita: Sex Research for AIDS Prevention — an Urgent Agenda for the 1990s. In: *The Time of AIDS: Social Analysis, Theory and Method*, edited by G. Herdt and S. Lindenbaum. Newbury Park: Sage Publications.

Clatts, M.C., and K.M. Mutchler. 1989. AIDS and the Dangerous Other: Metaphors of Sex and Deviance in the Representation of Disease. In: *The AIDS Pandemic: A Global Emergency*, edited by R. Bolton. New York City: Gordon and Breach.

Leap, W. 1990. Language and AIDS. In: *Culture and AIDS*, edited by D. Feldman. New York City: Praeger Press.

Leap, W. 1991. AIDS, Linguistics, and the Study of Non-Neutral Discourse. *Journal of Sex Research* 28(2):275–288.

Levine, M., and C. Siegel. 1992. Unprotected Sex: Understanding Gay Men's Participation. In: *The Social Context of AIDS*, edited by J. Huber and B.E. Schneider. San Francisco: Sage Press.

Murray, S.O., and K. Payne. 1989. The Social Classification of AIDS in American Epidemiology. In: *The AIDS Pandemic: A Global Emergency*, edited by R. Bolton. New York City: Gordon and Breach.

Shilts, R. 1987. *And the Band Played On*. New York City: St. Martin's Press.

Stall, R., T. Coates, and C. Hoff. 1988. Behavioral Risk Reduction for HIV Infection Among Gay and Bisexual Men: A Review of Results from the United States. *American Psychologist* 43(11):878–885.

Part IV

The Study of Culture
and Sexual Risk

Chapter
TWELVE

Disembodied Acts: On the Perverse Use of Sexual Categories in the Study of High-Risk Behaviour

Michael C. Clatts

Research must be held accountable for the choice of its rationality; its basis — which we know is not the established objectivity of science — must be questioned.

Michel Foucault

Since the human immunodeficiency virus (HIV) was first identified in 1981, its spread has been largely associated with unprotected sexual intercourse. Early in the pandemic, the spread of the disease was believed to be confined to homosexual men, and indeed was represented as being somehow peculiar to so-called 'gay sex,' as if heterosexuals never have more than one sexual partner and never engage in anal intercourse.[1] The early association between the incidence of this disease and certain kinds of sexual behaviour, notably 'deviant' sexual behaviour, resulted in an enormous expansion in the study of sexual behaviour. Indeed, it is probably fair to say that a substantial part of virtually every dollar that is spent in AIDS prevention research, even in areas in which drug injection is prevalent, includes an examination of some aspect of sexual behaviour. One would think that nearly ten years later, after the expenditure of tens of millions of dollars, that we would have acquired a clearer understanding of the nature of the sexual behaviours that are associated with the spread of this disease. Minimally, one would expect that we would at least have a better understanding of what the questions ought to be, and how to best go about trying to resolve them. It is the thesis of this chapter, however, that we are not much closer now to understanding how to foster sexual risk reduction than we were ten years ago. Indeed, the discussion which follows is aimed at showing how we have been asking the wrong questions about sexual risk behaviour, and often, asking them in a manner that is ill-suited to the complex nature of the behaviours themselves. In some sense, the latter methodological problem is antecedent to the former, which might be said to be more fundamentally conceptual in nature, and so that is where the discussion begins.

SEX AS A BEHAVIOURAL CATEGORY

Although a number of large survey data bases on high-risk sexual behaviour have been amassed over the last ten years, much of this information remains difficult to interpret, and much of it is of very limited utility in fostering sustained changes in sexual behaviour. Particularly problematic is the fact that much of this research has employed rather narrow theoretical paradigms in which sexual behaviour is often used as the independent variable. This often ignores any substantial consideration of the broad diversity in gender roles and meanings that exist, or of the way in which both behaviour and meaning are shaped by interacting cultural, social, economic, and political factors. As Carrier and Bolton have pointed out: 'The usefulness of most AIDS-related studies of human sexual behaviors conducted since the epidemic began is limited because of the narrow range of methods employed to gather data (mostly survey research methods)' (1991:49).

The scope of this chapter does not permit an exhaustive treatment of the various kinds of methodological problems that attend contemporary sex research, particularly those which are specific to the study of risk behaviours associated with the transmission of HIV infection. I would like, however, to give a couple of examples from my own ethnographic work, which illustrate the lack of utility of the kinds of conceptual categories that underpin most survey research on risk behaviour and AIDS. They also highlight the dire results stemming from the use of these categories, for both our understanding of the spread of this disease and our capacity to develop appropriate education and prevention messages.

Take, for example, the story of Tina, an Asian-American who is approximately twenty years of age. Born a biological male, at the age of nineteen Tina initiated a process of making herself into a 'female' — including breast implants and regular female hormone injection. For several years prior to this, and reportedly since puberty, Tina had dressed as a female and used what she and others around her commonly identified as 'effeminate' speech patterns. Indeed, Tina divided her life history into two major parts, her childhood — a time that she described as 'before I became a woman' — and her early adolescence — 'when I knew I wanted a man,' a desire that she identified as consistent with her female gender identity. Her life story narrative is filled with descriptions of her body, including what she imagines herself to have looked like at various times in her life. Indeed, the way she imagined her body was as if it contained a 'woman inside.'

It is noteworthy that this also referred to her 'social skin' (cf. Turner 1980), since she did not identify as homosexual. 'It's not a gay thing,' explained Tina, 'I'm all woman.' This concept of self was consistent with her social behaviour. At the time of her interview in 1989, she was partnered with Roberto, a white, biological male of about the same age. Roberto was, by his own description, a heterosexual male who strenuously denied being involved in any same-sex activity. Over the course of more than a years' ethnographic observation, including a prolonged period of time in which Tina was away in prison, Roberto was involved in several relationships, all of them with biological females. Thus, neither Tina nor Roberto viewed Tina as male, and despite the facts of Tina's birth, both represented their relationship as heterosexual. Both anticipated that they would get married, and they talked of someday 'having' children, via adoption, as a fulfilment of their heterosexual marriage. Thus, although Tina was typically viewed as a 'homosexual' or a 'transvestite,' it must be noted that Tina did not view herself as such. Nor was she accepted as one by most of the individuals in the community who identified as 'butch fags.' This was so even though, in outward appearances, she resembled many of them, 'worked' a similar area in the prostitution stroll on the Lower West Side of Manhattan, was involved in similar sexual behaviours, and in fact had many of the same 'johns' as other cross-dressing, trans-gender individuals in this street scene. Finally, and again consistent with her concept of self, it is noteworthy that most of her close social relationships were with heterosexual females.

Despite the fact that she openly identified the kind of sex work in which others around her were involved as risky for AIDS, Tina did not believe that she was at risk. She associated risk with 'being gay,' and concluded that since she was not gay, she was not at risk. The early misrepresentation of AIDS by the medical community as a 'gay disease' (Clatts and Mutchler 1989), and a continuing predilection to employ stigmatizing gender categories that fail to distinguish between issues of sexual identity and issues of sexual behaviour, promote such concepts of risk. At the very least, they fail to correct them, often with dire results. About a year later, Tina tested positive for HIV infection.

Another example is illustrated in the case of Toni, a Hispanic female, now in her late thirties. Toni came to New York City from Puerto Rico when she was about ten years of age, and lived with an aunt in East Harlem. She found English difficult and had considerable trouble in school. This, coupled with the fact that the household in which she was living could not really support her, eventually led her, around the age of 13, to get involved in street prostitution. She explained that a male friend took her to midtown Manhattan where he hustled, suggesting that Toni, who at the time had very 'boy-like' body features, could probably 'pass.' Recalls Toni, 'He told me, most of them just want blow jobs; it's easy.'

Toni was able to pass and, for several years, worked on weekends as a 'male prostitute' in the Times Square area of Manhattan, while continuing in a heterosexual relationship with her boyfriend in Harlem. She was popular on the streets, and in fact was able to don the role of 'chicken' far longer than many of her male counterparts, some of whom she says did not know that she was female and heterosexual. The money she earned made a substantial contribution to her aunt's household. Like many of her male counterparts on the streets, Toni was engaged in oral sex and occasionally receptive anal intercourse. Nevertheless, she did not see herself as being at high risk for HIV infection, principally because she regarded herself as female and heterosexual.

As Toni became older, however, she found it increasingly difficult to pass as a male. In addition to her high voice and lack of facial hair, she had also developed breasts. Moreover, around this time she became pregnant, reportedly by a boyfriend. After the birth of her baby she once again found herself in need of money. Now several years older, and still without the education and training necessary to obtain a job, she returned to prostitution, this time as a 'woman.' Initially she supplemented her income from Public Assistance by working on the Lexington Avenue 'stroll' (an area in East Harlem in which street prostitution occurs).

With strikingly attractive physical features, she was again very popular among the 'johns,' and for a time was able to establish a regular clientele that she 'serviced' on a scheduled basis in her own home. She believed that she was at higher risk for AIDS at this time than in earlier stages in her life. However, her reasons for believing this stemmed largely from the identity of her clients, whom she described as 'junkies,' rather than from a concern about risk from sexual behaviour, per se. Indeed, she told a story about a very well-paying customer who was often unable to achieve an erection, a fact that made her wonder if he was 'half gay,' and whether or not he might give her AIDS.

Note that sex in this case is viewed as a commodity of exchange, much like any other kind of behaviour whose primary purpose is economic, a subject to which I will return in later discussions in this chapter. The sexual orientation of the person with whom Toni was engaged in sexual intercourse, either men who have sex with men or men who have sex with women, was irrelevant to her concept of self. As she described it, 'It's just like the guy at the newsstand.... He sells all these male porno magazines.... That doesn't make him gay.... It's just business.'

Note also the difficulty and misconceptions that arise when information about risk behaviour is forged in gender categories that focus attention on *who* is risky, rather than on *what* is risky. As an adolescent, and in the context of low-risk oral sex, Toni believed that she was safe because she was not 'gay.' Later, and in the context of high-risk vaginal sex, she acknowledged that she was at greater risk but for the wrong reasons. Her perception of greater risk stemmed not from the nature of the specific sexual behaviours involved but rather was a consequence of the social identity of her partners (i.e., 'junkies').[2] Indeed, she later described how she was eventually able to move out of street prostitution by setting up a 'private house' out of her own apartment. Here she sold sex and drugs to 'regulars' who came to her apartment, explaining that this allowed her to be 'safer' because she could pick and choose who she let in, and by extension, who she had sex with. It is noteworthy that the criteria she described were largely social and economic in character (e.g., 'he looked dirty,' 'he smelled bad so I sent him away,' 'that one don't have no money until the end of the month'). Condoms were used only when she thought she was at risk of becoming pregnant, and often not even then 'if the money was right.'

These examples illustrate some of the issues and obstacles that the existing approaches to AIDS prevention research are inadequate to address, particularly as they relate to sexual minorities and individuals involved in survival sex. They also demonstrate the way that a failure to distinguish between sex and gender may serve as a substantial barrier to acquiring the kind of understanding of risk behaviour that is critical to the development of effective prevention messages and strategies. Clearly, if we are to reach sexual minority groups with meaningful and effective HIV/AIDS prevention efforts, we must challenge the use of categories that serve to obfuscate the nature of risk. As Shedlin, Clatts, and Carrier (1992) have pointed out in reference to sexual categories in AIDS prevention research:

> None of the labels provides any real insight or understanding into the complex gender identity issues or range of sexual and drug behaviors which place these individuals and their clients/partners at risk for HIV infection. In terms of the development of prevention education materials for example, it can be seen that most have little relevance or appropriate advice or backup for biological males who identify as females, and who survive in an environment which seeks unsuccessfully to classify them by a whole range of mutually exclusive labels and terms.

These examples also underscore the inadequacy of the rigid and often static clinical and behavioural categories that implicitly superimpose some set of biological properties onto sexual behaviour and experience, independent of the processual factors in which these acts occur or the larger socio-cultural contexts in and by which they are signified. Rigid categories, such as 'heterosexual,' 'homosexual,' and even 'bisexual' take sexual activity and sexual identity out of time and place. The use of these categories makes it impossible to identify and map changes in concepts of self over the course of an individual's life span, or to locate an ever-emergent self within social, cultural, and economic institutions that are themselves dynamic in character.

Far from serving to clarify the import of social, economic, and political institutions on risk behaviour, this kind of approach to the study of sexual risk results in the production of enormous bodies of behavioural data, which, because it is devoid of any substantive attention to issues of time and place, is of very limited utility in the development of AIDS prevention strategies. Of particular concern here are the economic forces that underpin risk behaviour and that may represent acute barriers to risk reduction.

Even those studies that acknowledge the systemic economic in-equities that persist in these communities utilize this information for little more than descriptive purposes. Typically these conditions are held as constants, and dubious academic constructions, such as 'self-efficacy' and 'locus of control,' are used to explain variance in be-haviour. These same dubious entities then become the target for intervention, again with little or no attention to the structural condi-tions which give rise to perceptions of self, or to those that recreate these systems of power.

SEX AS A TRANSACTION

The identification of those specific sexual acts that most efficiently facilitate the transmission of HIV was certainly an important break-through in the early formulation of AIDS prevention information. The problem in terms of the application of this information is that we have never really got beyond a focus on who puts what part of their anatomy into what part of a partner's anatomy, with or without a condom, and on how many occasions, information that has proven to be largely irrelevant to understanding either the nature of sexual relations or how to foster sexual risk reduction.[3] As noted in the previous section, one of the reasons that rigid sex categories have proven to be so inadequate is that this kind of approach to the study of sexual behaviour has the result of removing behaviour from the socio-cultural institutions in which it is embedded and to which it gives rise (Geertz 1973). This is admittedly a complex issue, but at the risk of oversimplifying the discussion of sexual behaviour, I would like to comment on one aspect of high-risk sexual behaviour that is not likely to be ameliorated in any way by prevention strategies and policies that focus on such dubious behavioural goals as that of advising individuals to reduce their number of sexual partners.[4]

Take, for example, the case of Jake, a 23-year-old white male who has been homeless for the past nine years. Born in Massachusetts, and adopted from an orphanage at the age of three, he lived with his adopted parents and sister in a small town in Maine until he ran away for the very last time at the age of fourteen. He describes his early childhood as one filled with material comforts, but plagued with physical and sexual abuse. His father began raping him when he was only five years old, and his mother, while aware of the situation, did nothing to stop it: 'They didn't know how to treat a child.... My father's excuse was that he never had a father to know how to have a kid or be a father.... My mother's was that she wanted to believe that things like that couldn't really happen.'

Jake first began running away from home for short periods of time at the age of 10. He used to go over to a friend's house to hide but knowing he couldn't hide forever, he would call up his parents and ask to go home: 'He'd come pick me up, and I'd go back. He'd get me into the bedroom and that's it. Finally, I got sick of him beating me and using me. I got sick of him hurting me all the time.'

Jake made his way to Portland, Maine and was forced to fend for himself. He recalls learning quickly that he had something other people wanted, that he was a commodity. Since that time he has travelled across the United States, from Maine to California; has been in and out of jail for robbery, possession of drugs, prostitution, breaking and entering, and assault; and has been in and out of hospitals, rehabilitation programmes, and temporary adolescent and adult residences. He takes pride in his ability to survive against the odds but he recalls that 'hustling became serious work' when he became 'a drug addict.' Says Jake:

> As an addict, nothing else seemed to matter besides securing the next hit. When you first start, you set your limits. When I wasn't getting high, forty to fifty dollars just to blow me. When I started getting high, twenty bucks to blow me. Then, when I became an addict, my life changed. Five dollars for anything. Anything. Fucking me — anything! You do it just for the next hit. That's when you don't love yourself anymore.

Looking back, Jake recalled a time in which he thought that hustling was fun, but then it became a job.

> It's like a job. I stand out there from eight at night until four in the morning, selling my ass! That's not fun. It's not fun. It's work!... And the people, they treat you like shit. They don't care about you. All they care about is getting their nuts off. And sometimes, after they grab you and touch you, they don't want to give you nothing for it. That's not fair, if they touch you they got to pay for it. It's not a job to have. It destroys you. You get old fast.

In 1988, when he was admitted to a New York City hospital with tuberculosis, Jake tested positive for HIV infection. In the last three years he has had many of the opportunistic infections associated with AIDS, and his life is a daily struggle to manage intermittent episodes of diarrhoea, oral candiditis, upper respiratory ailments, and seizures. His last severe bout of pneumonia cost him a lung and doctors warn him that the next attack might be his very last. Despite it all, Jake continues to hustle around Times Square and West Village areas of Manhattan. He says that 'business' has been slow lately, and he attributes this to the fact that he's started to look sick, and word has got out that he has AIDS. Sometimes, he admits, he's able to use this 'AIDS-thing' to his advantage. Some tricks, upon taking him home and learning from Jake that he has AIDS, give him money just to go away. On most nights of the week, and in all kinds of weather, he can be found on the same corner of a Greenwich Village street, hustling for his next hit. Bitter and withdrawn, he stands on the corner watching the traffic, trying to make eye contact with drivers stopping at the traffic light, eye contact that will signal potential interest. He works all night, earning a few dollars a time for sex in a doorway, in a parked car, or in the apartment of a man whose name he does not know. By four o'clock in the morning he will have earned enough money to stay high on crack, and perhaps even enough to keep from getting dope-sick the next morning.

Over and over again, Jake has been told by health care providers that in order to get help 'he has to do his share' — a poignant phrase for the kind of supply-side economics that engenders poverty and homelessness. Poignant also for what it says about some of the fundamental assumptions that underpin much of AIDS prevention practice. For clearly, and quite apart from what he might like to do, the share that Jake is able to do is quite limited. Limited not by his intelligence, his creativity, or his dreams, but rather by his ability, any child's ability, to grow and mature in a world in which his value is subject to the vagaries of the street meat market (Clatts and Atillasoy 1993).

As this brief case study reveals, it is of paramount importance that we begin looking more carefully at the way in which high-risk sexual behaviour is embedded in systems of economic exchange, particularly those systems of exchange that typify many poor communities in both the industrial and nonindustrial world. For quite apart from the information an individual possesses about risk for HIV transmission, or what actions an individual may perceive as necessary in order to avoid it — or indeed what an individual might *wish* to do in order to avoid it — a number of complex structural constraints may serve as overwhelming barriers to an individuals' capacity to engage in consistent risk reduction. Most of the people in the world who will be at risk for AIDS in the coming decade, are at risk not because of a lack of knowledge, belief, or intention, but rather because of the larger social and economic circumstances that govern their lives.[5] Most will be subject to economic inequalities that have disparities of power and wealth at their core — inequalities exacerbated by factors of race, gender, sexual identity. Hence — and this is evident from the study of many other disease outcomes as well — economic constraints are a fundamental barrier to arresting the spread of this disease.[6]

Unfortunately, very little of the current research that is being done on sexual risk behaviour acknowledges the import of systemic poverty on sexual risk behaviour. Moreover, research paradigms that continue to place a premium on the study of behavioural frequencies and dubious notions of motive are unsuited to the task of identifying ways in which to foster 'actionable' changes in high-risk sexual behaviour. Certainly this fact reflects a failure of political will, but it should also call into question the kinds of priorities that have been established in the AIDS prevention research industry. To continue to pretend that a two-hour session with an AIDS educator, for example, can measurably increase 'self-esteem' in a person who has lived an entire lifetime in a context of violence, discrimination, and abject poverty, or that the problem of 'empowerment' lies solely in convincing the subject that he or she has power, regardless of whether this is the case, is to completely miss the mark about why people engage in risk behaviour.

At the very least, the assumption that these kinds of models are adequate research tools in the context of AIDS is based upon a particular kind of intellectual fiction. Such models hold the conditions in which the subject lives, as well as the factors that have brought him or her to these circumstances, as an analytic 'constant' (or minimally, as at a 'constant variance'). And yet we know that in everyday life this is simply not the case. It is precisely the force of the social and economic conditions in which an individual lives and works, what Schoepf (1988) has referred to as the 'political ecology of disease,' that will in large measure determine why some individuals, rather than others, have a substantially greater likelihood of becoming infected.[7]

It is noteworthy, moreover, that these same circumstances govern not only who will be exposed to HIV infection, but also who is more likely to become ill with AIDS-spectrum diseases. Clearly, an individual living in conditions characterized by poor nutrition, inadequate shelter, and ineffectual health care, all of which contribute to poor immune response, will be more vulnerable to developing opportunistic infections than someone who is not confronted by these kinds of circumstances. This is, of course, over and above the fact that someone living in these circumstances is also likely to have a very different experience of illness itself (Clatts 1992a).

CONCLUSION

We live in an age when we feel confident that we can see everything that we need to see through scientific lenses — that anything can be accomplished if we just assemble enough of the right technology to work on it. There is, I believe, a similar assumption driving much of what we, as social scientists, do in the name of AIDS prevention research: that if we could just muster enough resources for research — all the king's horses and all the king's men — we would be well on our way to finding the magic bullet for behavioural change (Clatts 1992b). At least with regard to prevention research, I have lost all confidence in this prospect. Moreover, I increasingly find myself wondering about the propriety of the endeavour itself.

It is probably true that the present emphasis in AIDS prevention research on identifying behavioural change models began with the best of intentions, notably the development of community-based, culturally sensitive prevention messages. I submit, however, that the process has gone terribly awry, that the undaunted search for quick-fix models forces us to crawl into very narrow boxes, that it jeopardizes our ability to see the world as it is, as well as our ability to offer constructive ideas about how to foster change within it. In my experience, such models inevitably end up trying to fit the subject to the technology, rather than the other way around. As such, and reminiscent of the colonialism of an earlier age, these models become tools of abuse and neglect, rather than reservoirs of comfort and relief. They lead us down conceptual paths that have little or no relevance to the way people actually live, and hence inevitably to strategies and policies that have no relevance to prevention. Still worse, they serve to fuel the metaphors of failure and blame that already characterize the representation of those who have contracted this disease, a fact that can only exacerbate the suffering they experience from it.

In an earlier paper on the topic of AIDS and the social representation of its sufferers, Kevin Mutchler and I pointed out the way in which cultural metaphors of sex and deviance have tended to control our attention by crystallizing specific constellations of ideas about disease, and orienting our thoughts in particular directions

(Clatts and Mutchler 1989). We were especially concerned that these metaphoric images and predications of AIDS, and of those afflicted by it, simultaneously obscure and block our orientation to other possible ways of seeing and knowing. We also pointed out that the experience of AIDS is a potent metaphor for the social and cultural predication of the self. For here we see, poignantly and tragically, the force that ideas can have in bending and shaping our experience to fit received categories of being and knowing.

Unfortunately, this is as true today as it has ever been, perhaps even more so given the rapidly growing magnitude of this disease. Thus, it is more critical than ever that anthropologists work to chronicle the experience of this disease, and the experience of risk for acquiring it, in ways that challenge received categories of being, including the boundaries that are said to pertain between facile notions of 'he' and 'she,' 'us,' and 'them.' It is imperative that we resist the tide of scientific opinion that wants to wrap experience up into tight little bundles of efficient commodities, and that we challenge ourselves and each other regarding the adequacy of the way in which we represent our ethnographic experience. In particular, we must remain alert to the manner in which the marketplace influences the assumptions that we bring to the task of ethnography. For to the extent that our assumptions are limited, so is our vision of the world. In the world of AIDS, when assumptions are limited, suffering grows.

ACKNOWLEDGEMENTS

I would like to thank Ralph Bolton, Deborah Hillman, Steve Koester, and Kevin M. Mutchler for the thoughtful comments that they have provided in the development of these ideas. Aspects of this chapter were originally presented at the conference 'Culture, Sexual Behavior, and AIDS,' Department of Anthropology, University of Amsterdam, July 24–26, 1992.

NOTES

1. Subsequently, however, it became clear that while differing in relative risk, a number of sexual behaviours are efficient mechanisms for transmission, irrespective of the sex or gender of the individuals involved. In addition, other behaviours implicated in the spread of HIV infection include the sharing of drug injection equipment. It is noteworthy, how-

ever, that even in communities in which drug injection is prevalent, sexual transmission accounts for an increasing number of new cases, a fact that serves to highlight the urgency of sexual risk reduction (cf. Clatts et al. 1990; Kronliczak 1990; Tortu et al. 1992).

2. Early in the AIDS pandemic, there was a common perception among drug injectors in New York City that AIDS was caused by the substance heroin itself, rather than by the exchange of fluids during the sharing of injection equipment (cf. Clatts 1989). Indeed, what might be called a lack of precision in much of the AIDS prevention literature may have inadvertently fostered this belief, focusing as it did on drug use and the drug user rather than on the specific behaviours implicated in HIV transmission.

3. As a number of others have pointed out, this social control approach to public health cannot be fully understood apart from the kind of political forces that marked the 1980s, particularly the Reagan administration's neglect of this disease, even as they exploited it in political rhetoric (cf. Patton 1985).

4. Such an approach to prevention is particularly irrelevant for fostering risk reduction among individuals who are involved in, and dependent upon, the sex economy for their very survival. Quite apart from this specific application, however, I should like to add that a focus on numbers of sexual partners is problematic for other reasons as well. First, no causal relationship between number of sexual partners and transmission of HIV has been established epidemiologically. Indeed, the focus on sexual partners repeats the classic mistake of inferring a cause from a correlation. Second, strategies that stigmatize individuals who engage in sex with multiple partners, and that attempt to eliminate some of the kinds of contexts in which this behaviour may occur, only serve to confuse the prevention message (see also Bolton 1992). Moreover, as Bolton et al. (1994) have shown in the context of gay saunas, for example, such strategies not only send the wrong message but may also have the effect of squandering important opportunities for AIDS education (see also Leap 1993).

5. For important discussions of this in the context of the spread of HIV infection in Africa, see Schoepf (1988).

6. For an examination of the role of homelessness, for example, in the frequency and persistence of risk behaviour in a national sample of drug injectors, see Clatts et al. (1993).

7. As noted, these circumstances are certainly very prominent in the spread of HIV disease in the so-called Third World. However, the examination of a wide variety of disease indicators demonstrates that these circumstances are not limited to these areas. Many urban communities in comparatively affluent industrialized nations are confronted with startlingly similar patterns of mortality and morbidity,

including widespread suffering and death associated with HIV disease (cf. McCord and Freeman 1990).

REFERENCES

Bolton, R. 1992. AIDS and Promiscuity: Muddles in the Models of HIV Prevention. In: *Rethinking AIDS Prevention: Cultural Approaches*, edited by R. Bolton and M. Singer. Philadelphia: Gordon and Breach Science Publishers.

Bolton, R., J. Vincke, and R. Mak. 1994. Gay Baths Revisited. An Empirical Analysis. *GLQ* 1:255-273.

Carrier, J., and R. Bolton. 1991. Anthropological Perspectives on Sexuality and HIV Prevention. *Annual Review of Sex Research* 2:49–75.

Clatts, M.C. 1989. Ethnography and AIDS Intervention in New York City: Life History as an Ethnographic Strategy. In: *Community Based AIDS Prevention. Studies of Intravenous Drug Users and Their Sexual Partners*. Rockville, MD: National Institute on Drug Abuse.

Clatts, M.C. 1992a. At the End of the Rainbow: The Meaning and Experience of AIDS. Paper presented at the Annual Meetings of the American Anthropological Association, Chicago, Illinois, November 23.

Clatts, M.C. 1992b. All the King's Horses and All the King's Men: Some Personal Reflections on Ten Years of AIDS Ethnography. Paper presented at a conference on 'Culture, Sexual Behavior, and AIDS,' Department of Anthropology, University of Amsterdam, July 24–26, 1992. Forthcoming in *Human Organization*.

Clatts, M.C., and A. Atillasoy. 1993. Where the Day Takes You: Homeless Youth and the Structure of the Street Economy. Paper presented at the Annual Meetings of the Society for Applied Anthropology, San Antonio, Texas, March 10.

Clatts, M.C., and K.M. Mutchler. 1989. AIDS and the Dangerous Other: Metaphors of Sex and Deviance in the Representation of a Disease. *Medical Anthropology* 11(2–3):105–114.

Clatts, M.C., R. Davis, S. Deren, and S. Tortu. 1990. Sex for Crack: The Many Faces of Risk Within the Street Economy of Harlem. In: *Community Based AIDS Prevention Among Intravenous Drug Users And Their Sexual Partners: The Many Faces of HIV Disease*. Proceedings of the Second Annual NADR National Meeting. Bethesda, MD: National Institute on Drug Abuse.

Clatts, M.C., M. Beardsley, S. Deren, S. Tortu, and R. Davis. 1993. Homelessness and Changes in HIV Risk Behavior in a National Sample of Drug Injectors: Implications for Public Health Policy. Forthcoming.

Geertz, C. 1973. *The Interpretation of Cultures*. New York: Basic Books.

Kronliczak, A. 1990. Update on High-Risk Behaviors Among Female Sexual Partners of Injection Drug Users. *NADR Network* (Special Issue). Bethesda, MD: National Institute on Drug Abuse.

Leap, W. 1993. Condom Avoidance in a Health Club Locker Room: Elites, Erotics and the Ethnography of AIDS. Paper presented at the Annual Meetings of the Society for Applied Anthropology, San Antonio, Texas, March 10.

McCord, C., and H. Freeman. 1990. Excess Mortality in Harlem. *The New England Journal of Medicine* 22(3):173–177.

Patton, C. 1985. *Sex and Germs*. Boston: South End Press.

Schoepf, B. 1988. Women, AIDS, and Economic Crisis in Central Africa. *Canadian Journal of African Studies* 22:625–644.

Shedlin, M., M.C. Clatts, and J. Carrier. 1992. Rethinking Our Paradigms: The Challenges of HIV/AIDS Research on Sexual Minorities. Paper presented at the Annual Meeting of the Society for Cross-Cultural Research, Santa Fe, April 5.

Tortu, S., M. Beardsley, and S. Deren. 1992. AIDS Risk Among Female Sexual Partners of Injection Drug Users: Implications for Prevention. Paper presented at a conference of the College for Problems of Drug Dependence, Boulder, Colorado.

Turner, T.A. 1980. The Social Skin. *Not Work Alone*, edited by J. Cherfas and R. Lewin. London: Temple Smith.

Chapter
THIRTEEN

The Social and Cultural Construction of Sexual Risk, or How to Have (Sex) Research in an Epidemic

Richard G. Parker

For more than a decade now, the unchecked spread of HIV/AIDS around the world has made our profound ignorance concerning human sexuality painfully evident. The long-standing neglect of research on sexual behaviour, and, consequently, an almost complete lack of understanding concerning the complexity and diversity of sexual expression, has made it almost impossible to respond to AIDS by drawing on a pre-existing data base or body of knowledge. The absence of a more fully developed tradition of theory and method for conducting sex research has restricted the development of new studies, offering AIDS researchers little foundation for the assessment of sexual practices relevant to the spread of HIV, and has limited their ability to contribute significantly to the design of more effective strategies for AIDS prevention (see, for example, the discussions in Abramson 1988, 1990, 1992; Abramson and Herdt 1990; Chouinard and Albert 1990; Gagnon 1988; Herdt and Lindenbaum 1992; Parker 1992; Parker and Carballo 1990; Parker, Herdt, and Carballo 1991; Turner, Miller, and Moses 1989, 1990).

These points are of course hardly novel. On the contrary, many similar concerns have already been raised elsewhere (see, for example, Bolton 1992; Herdt 1992; Parker 1992). As the HIV/AIDS epidemic (or, better, epidemics [Gagnon 1992]) continues to gain force, however, apparently escaping the vast majority of our efforts to contain it (as well as the conceptual models that we have constructed in order to understand it), the limitations in our understanding of sexuality and sexual risk in the face of HIV/AIDS nonetheless pose a series of theoretical, methodological, and procedural questions which cannot be ignored. Perhaps more than anything else, we are confronted with the urgent need to rethink the models that have guided the dominant response to AIDS thus far. In this paper, then, I try to sketch out what I see as some of the major tendencies that have characterized sex research in relation to HIV/AIDS over the course of the past decade. My goal will be to critically examine the development of sexual behaviour research during this period in order to identify some of the basic problems that may have limited the kinds of insights that it has offered — problems that will continue to limit our understanding in the future if we are unable to respond to them.

In seeking to review the development of sex research in relation to HIV/AIDS over the course of the past decade, at least two major problems are worth careful consideration: (1) the fundamental limitations in the dominant theoretical and methodological paradigms that have been used in carrying out research; and (2) the equally fundamental limitations in the research agenda that has guided the study of sexual behaviour in relation to HIV/AIDS. Clearly, these issues are closely interrelated, since the lack of theoretical and methodological development is almost surely linked to the failure to define a more meaningful research agenda, and vice versa. Nonetheless, I would like to briefly examine each of these issues in turn, in order to identify some of the problems that they have raised for research on sexual behaviour in relation to AIDS thus far, as well as to use them as a point of departure for thinking about more effective research activities in the future.

THEORY, SEXUAL NATURALISM, AND THE CONSTRUCTION OF MEANING

The lack of pre-existing baseline data on human sexuality, and, consequently, the urgent need for data collection on behaviours that may be linked to HIV transmission, have of course been widely discussed (see, for example, Chouinard and Albert 1990; Turner, Miller, and Moses 1989, 1990). Somewhat less attention has been given, however, to the serious limitations of dominant theoretical and methodological paradigms that have been employed in carrying out such research (see Abramson 1992; Abramson and Herdt 1990; Bolton 1992; Parker and Carballo 1990; Parker, Herdt, and Carballo 1991). The limitations of such paradigms are perhaps most glaring at a theoretical level, as sexual behaviour research within the context of AIDS has almost never been driven by a theory of sexual behaviour. Indeed, in most instances, it has not been driven by any theory at all — the emphasis has been on the urgent need for descriptive data (such as knowledge, attitude, and practice (KAP) studies), apparently based upon the hope that theoretical insights will emerge from such data if we only have enough of it. When, occasionally, a theoretical framework for conceptualizing sexual behaviour has been invoked, it has been at best a minimal one — most commonly the conceptualization of sexual desire as a basic human drive, but a drive that is shaped somewhat differently in different social and cultural settings, and that must therefore be described as it manifests itself within these settings (see, for example, WHO/GPA/SBR 1989; Carballo et al. 1989).

This lack of theoretical development is not, of course, new to AIDS research. On the contrary, it is very much a product or result of the particular tradition of sex research that has been incorporated within the field of public health more generally (and hence, the study of sexual behaviour in relation to HIV/AIDS in particular) — what has been described as a kind of 'sex modernism' running from early writers such as Havelock Ellis through Kinsey and his colleagues on up to more current sexologists such as Masters and Johnson (see Robinson 1976). Emerging, in many ways, as a response to the moral strictures of Victorian society and science, the primary focus of this tradition has been an attempt to 'demystify' and, in particular, to 'naturalize' human sexual behaviour — an attempt to describe, as exhaustively as possible, the forms of sexual expression that exist 'in nature' (Robinson 1976; see also Weeks 1981, 1985, 1986).

The importance of such a perspective should not be underestimated, as it is principally responsible, particularly following the work of Kinsey and his colleagues, for opening up the field of sexual behaviour as an object of scientific investigation rather than as the domain of religion or morality (see Robinson 1976; Turner, Miller, and Moses 1989). At the same time, its legacy, particularly as it has been incorporated into the field of public health (and by extension, the vast majority of AIDS research), has clearly been problematic — a kind of extreme empiricism, which, in the absence of a more convincing theory for the explanation of human sexuality and sexual diversity, has focused almost exclusively on documenting behavioural frequencies within a relatively limited range of population groups (especially in perceived 'high risk' populations such as gay men or female prostitutes, though increasingly in the more nebulous 'general' population as well).

Increasingly, over the course of a number of decades now, work carried out in a variety of (principally social scientific) disciplines has tended to challenge this naturalist view, focusing instead on what has been described as the 'social and cultural construction' of sexual conduct (see, for example, Gagnon 1977; Rubin 1984; Weeks 1985). In fields such as cultural anthropology, sociology, social psychology, and history, attention has increasingly focused on the social, cultural, economic, and political forces shaping sexual behaviour in different settings, together with the complicated meanings associated with sexual experience on the part of both individuals and social groups (see, for example, Gagnon and Simon 1973; Herdt and Stoller 1990; Parker 1991; Weeks 1981, 1985, 1986). For the most part, however, the impact of such developments has been extremely limited, particularly within the context of public health and the health sciences (still largely the domain of the medical profession rather than of social scientists), and a more naturalist approach, in spite of its theoretical limitations, has largely continued to dominate the discussion of sexual behaviour and sexual health.

The result of this general lack of theoretical development (again, particularly within the health sciences) has been a relative poverty in the conceptual frameworks of much sexual behaviour research in relation to HIV/AIDS. Sexual desire has been treated, in many ways, as a kind of given, and the social and cultural factors shaping sexual experience in different settings have largely been ignored, even when lip service has been paid to their potential importance. In keeping with the dominant tendencies in much health behaviour research, emphasis has been placed largely on the individual determinants of sexual behaviour and behaviour change, and the diverse social, cultural, economic, and political factors potentially influencing or even shaping sexual experience have more often than not been ignored. A range of theoretical perspectives based on quite distinct premises (and therefore suggesting a very different reading of the factors shaping sexual conduct) have been largely absent from the field of AIDS research, and the various insights that such perspectives might potentially offer have rarely been incorporated in AIDS research findings (see Abramson and Herdt 1990; Bolton 1992; Parker, Herdt, and Carballo 1991).

A series of methodological limitations can be associated, in large part, with the theoretical limitations described above — again seriously inhibiting the quality of the sexual behaviour research that has been carried out in response to AIDS. Throughout this period, the dominant focus has been on the use of survey research methods (once again, an inheritance from Kinsey and his colleagues), and the key question addressed in the design of research has almost inevitably been how to make these methods more effective in the different contexts in which AIDS research must be carried out — in developing countries, for example, or among problematically defined target populations such as homosexual men or intravenous drug users and so on (see Turner, Miller, and Moses 1989, 1990).

Such an approach has fit reasonably well within the framework of a research agenda defined in terms of epidemiological questions, for example, or of psychological models of behavioural change. Counting the frequency of sexual acts, if carried out effectively, can clearly offer important insights concerning the course of the HIV/AIDS epidemic in specific settings. In much the same way, depending upon one's assumptions, measuring psychosocial indicators may offer insight into the propensity for risk reduction. These frameworks, and the methodological approach stemming from them, have been much weaker, however, as a way of providing a multi-dimensional, and hence fuller, understanding of sexual behaviour more generally — and this, in turn, has had serious consequences, especially in seeking to move from primary epidemiological questions to the questions that must be confronted in intervening through health promotion and education (see, in particular, Bolton 1992; Parker 1992; Parker and Carballo 1990; Parker, Herdt, and Carballo 1991; de Zalduondo 1991).

Here, in thinking about the complicated questions involved in AIDS prevention, it is clear that not just the frequency of a given behaviour is important. The subjective (psychological) and inter-subjective (social and cultural) meanings associated with it may be far more important (see Parker 1992; Parker and Carballo 1990; Parker, Herdt, and Carballo 1991; de Zalduondo 1991). The social construction of sexual excitement and desire, ways in which sexual identities are formed and transformed, the relations of power and domination that may shape and structure sexual interactions, and the social/ sexual networks that channel and condition the selection of potential sexual partners may all be salient issues that must be taken into account in developing more effective strategies for AIDS prevention. Yet, to the extent that sexual behaviour research in relation to AIDS has largely closed itself off from a wider range of theoretical frameworks, it has also closed itself off, at least in part, from any number of potentially important methodological approaches that might well lead to new, and perhaps quite different, insights about such issues — approaches such as ethnographic description, linguistic analysis, and so on (see, for example, Bolton 1992; Carrier and Magaña 1991; Herdt 1992; Herdt, Leap, and Sovine 1991; Herdt and Boxer 1991; Parker 1992; Parker and Carballo 1990; Parker, Herdt, and Carballo 1991; de Zalduondo 1991).

RESEARCH PRIORITIES, MONEY, AND POWER

The lack of theoretical and methodological development characterizing much of the sexual behaviour research carried out during the course of the first decade of the AIDS epidemic has also clearly been exaggerated or aggravated by the absence of more systematic planning and the failure to articulate a coherent research agenda capable of directing or guiding long-term research activities within an international or global framework (see Mann, Tarantola, and Netter 1992). We (the AIDS research community in general, and [social science] sex researchers in particular) have been unable to define and implement a more comprehensive research agenda on the full range of sexual behaviour and sexual diversity that might truly be capable of guiding epidemiological insights rather than simply following upon their heels. In the absence of such an agenda, changing demands (and fashions) on the part of policy makers, and often funding agencies as well, have tended to shift more rapidly than behavioural research on sexuality (or any other topic) can accompany. An early emphasis on descriptive research has thus given way, increasingly, to a focus on intervention research (in my opinion at least, a generally positive development). Research attention to certain behavioural groups (such as gay men) has given way to a focus on others (such as heterosexual women) — again, sometimes for good reason. And so on. Yet such changes have taken place without the benefit of any kind of wider framework or vision concerning the long-term research issues that must be addressed in the study of sexual behaviour.

Changes of direction are of course expected in the development of behavioural research in any area. In the case of research on sexual behaviour within the context of the international AIDS pandemic, however, the lack of a wider research agenda developed on a global level has all too often led to the lack of sustained research development — to the abandonment of work that has only just begun, or the inability to implement studies that fail to fit the model of this year's fashions. Only a few years ago, it was virtually impossible to find funding for studies of (obviously important questions such as) women's sexual behaviour in relation to HIV/AIDS. Today, it is equally or more difficult to find funds for studies of homosexuality (apparently already considered out of date). The limitations implicit in such shortsighted visions are all too evident, and pose a serious threat to our ability to develop a longer-term understanding of the international AIDS pandemic. Globally, in a world in which research priorities are often established far from the sites where research must actually be carried out, the results of such disparities can be a fundamental distortion of reality. Just one example here might be the way in which reported changes in gay and bisexual behaviour in San Francisco or Amsterdam have sometimes been used to suggest that it is unnecessary to investigate (or invest in) questions of same-sex behaviour change in Rio de Janeiro, Bangkok, Mexico City, Lagos, and so on. And this is the case in spite of the fact that preliminary studies of same-sex interactions in every one of these non-Western sites have made it clear that homosexuality is structured, organized, and experienced in profoundly different ways than in the gay communities of Western Europe or the United States — and that the course of the HIV/AIDS epidemic in each has thus demonstrated any number of important differences when compared with the industrialized West (see Daniel and Parker 1993; Werasit, Brown, and Siraphone 1991; García et al. 1991; Aina 1991).

Ultimately then, together with the limitations of existing theoretical and methodological models for the study of sexual behaviour in relation to HIV/AIDS, the lack of a meaningful research agenda (developed within a global framework) has made it almost impossible to elaborate a set of coherent and consistent research priorities. Throughout the course of the past decade, sexual behaviour research in response to AIDS has thus been faced with the peculiarly intense pressure of rapidly changing priorities — an almost constant sense of 'putting out fires' in which sexual behaviour research activities have consistently lagged behind the identification of epidemiological 'hot spots.' In seeking to respond to key issues being raised by the epidemiology of AIDS, early studies of gay and bisexual behaviour (such as the Multicenter AIDS Cohort Studies carried out in the United States, or, later, the Homosexual Response Studies supported by WHO/GPA in a range of different developed and developing countries) were initiated very quickly. Later, as our understanding of the potential shape and size of the epidemic began to change, so too did our understanding of the topical areas that must be addressed — studies of heterosexual behaviour in the (so-called) general population, of women's sexual practices, and so on, have gradually followed (see Chouinard and Albert 1990; Turner, Miller, and Moses 1989). In general, however, AIDS case reporting and, to a lesser extent, seroprevalence rates, combined with our own sometimes distorted perceptions of these issues (rather than a clearly thought out, theoretically and methodologically grounded research agenda), have tended to define priorities — and sexual behaviour research, with few exceptions, has tended to offer little guidance in pointing the direction for epidemiological inquiry.

FROM EPIDEMIOLOGICAL MODELS
TO AIDS PREVENTION

Given these facts, it is perhaps especially worth noting that one of the very few (possible) exceptions to the general rule would seem to be the record of ethnographic work carried out over the course of the past decade in response to AIDS. It is symptomatic that ethnographic studies of sexual meanings have been fundamental in calling into question the hegemony of epidemiological categories — the relevance, not only for prevention but even for epidemiological purposes, of groups such as men who have sex with men, female commercial sex workers, or the female partners of male injecting drug users (see, for example, Carrier and Magaña 1991; Kane 1990, 1991; Kane and Mason 1992; Parker 1987; de Zalduondo 1991). Ethnographic research, preoccupied with the nuances of local knowledge, the social and cultural particularities of sexual experience and the complex networks of power that condition not only the spread of

HIV but the ways in which social systems respond to AIDS (see for example, Misztal and Moss 1990), has in fact developed one of the few bodies of knowledge that would appear to offer insights that might meaningfully guide epidemiological inquiry in different settings rather than simply being carried in its wake (see also, Herdt 1992; Herdt, Leap, and Sovine 1991).

Yet, ironically, even if ethnographic studies and cross-cultural analysis have shown promise in opening up new understandings, particularly in relation to sexuality and HIV/AIDS, such approaches have received relatively little attention or support as part of a broader, institutionalized research response to the international AIDS pandemic. The international research agenda, even in the social sciences, has continued to be largely overdetermined by epidemiological concerns, and the potential insights of other approaches, based on different theoretical foundations, have been largely ignored. And, in much the same way that the biomedical establishment has continued to define the kinds of approaches that will dominate the research agenda in relation to sexuality, the complex relationship between knowledge and power in the field of AIDS has been all the more problematic within an international framework.

It is by now abundantly clear that available resources for research on HIV and AIDS generally in the developing world add up to but a fraction of the resources available for such work in the industrialized West (see Mann, Tarantola, and Netter 1992), and this is clearly all the more true in relation to social and behavioural research in particular. The constantly changing, sometimes contradictory, priorities concerning what are considered to be relevant research topics would seem to be especially pronounced in the definition of an international research agenda in relation to sexuality and sexual behaviour. In spite of the obvious epidemiological (not to mention preventive) importance of increased understanding concerning sexual behaviour in some regions of the developing world (again, this time in geographical terms, epidemiological 'hot spots' such as Central Africa, for example), a variety of factors (which, depending on the setting, have ranged from a lack of local research capacity to moral and political reservations on the part of local authorities or to a lack of donor support) have combined to limit significant sexual behaviour research primarily to developed countries. While a number of initiatives have been planned to respond to this situation (such as the sexual behaviour research supported by IDRC, some of the work initiated by WHO/GPA/SBR, by AIDSCOM, AIDSTECH, AIDSCAP, and so on), diverse circumstances and rapid changes in policy and personnel have meant that relatively little has actually been done. And even where work has been initiated, the tendency has often been to simply apply the dominant research methodologies developed for the study of sexual behaviour in the quite different research settings found in many developed nations. Even though the application of survey research methods has often proven problematic, as well as expensive and slow to implement, for example, there has been very little attempt to respond to these limitations through methodological innovation — to develop research methodologies and research agendas that will be better suited to the actual research conditions and priorities that in fact exist at a global level.

CONCLUSION

Remarkably, then, more than ten years into a rapidly expanding epidemic transmitted above all else through sexual contact, we have still failed to develop the theoretical and methodological tools that might offer a fuller understanding of sexuality in relation to AIDS as well as to other aspects of health. Indeed we have been unable to formulate and articulate a coherent vision of the sexual behaviour research needs that must be confronted at a global level, and to create concrete mechanisms for more effective interaction between sex researchers, policy makers, and funding agencies in order to define the most important research priorities that currently confront us. As a result, in spite of the fact that a good deal of sexual behaviour research has been carried out in recent years, the production of concrete results capable of contributing to a more effective response in the face of HIV/AIDS and other related health concerns has in fact been relatively limited.

Ultimately, I would like to suggest that it is only by changing, however slightly, the frame of reference — by focusing not simply on sexual behaviour, but on the complicated nuances of sexual meanings, that we might hope to begin to move beyond the limitations of so much of the work that has been carried out thus far. We must begin to realize that the most fundamental questions that we need to answer are in fact related to both subjective and intersubjective meanings, and emerge not from a naturalist framework but from a focus on the social construction of human reality. Within such a perspective, research on sexuality (independent of, or in relation to, HIV/AIDS) must necessarily be understood as more than a simple exercise in the counting of sexual acts. On the contrary, it is only by focusing on the fuller social, cultural, economic, and political dimensions of sexual experience that we may begin to build up understandings capable of providing a foundation for the kinds of policies and practices that may ultimately enable us to respond to the spread of the HIV epidemic.

As we take stock of where we have come over the course of the past decade, and begin to think about where we hope to go in the future, there can be little doubt about the importance of addressing such issues as concretely and as rapidly as we possibly can. It is unfortunately all too clear that after more than a decade of AIDS (and AIDS research), the epidemic is winning. There is much to do if we hope to confront it.

REFERENCES

Abramson, P.R. 1988. Sexual Assessment and the Epidemiology of AIDS. *The Journal of Sex Research* 25:323–346.

Abramson, P.R. 1990. Sexual Science: Emerging Discipline or Oxymoron? *The Journal of Sex Research* 27:147–165.

Abramson, P.R. 1992. Sex, Lies, and Ethnography. In: *The Time of AIDS: Social Analysis, Theory, and Method*, edited by G. Herdt and S. Lindenbaum. Newbury Park, CA: Sage Publications.

Abramson, P.R., and G. Herdt. 1990. The Assessment of Sexual Practices Relevant to the Transmission of AIDS: A Global Perspective. *Journal of Sex Research* 27:215–232.

Aina, T.A. 1991. Patterns of Bisexuality in Sub-Saharan Africa. In: *Bisexuality and HIV/AIDS: A Global Perspective*, edited by R. Tielman, M. Carballo, and A. Hendriks. Buffalo, NY: Prometheus Books.

Bolton, R. 1992. Mapping Terra Incognita: Sex Research for AIDS Prevention — An Urgent Agenda for the 1990s. In: *The Time of AIDS: Social Analysis, Theory, and Method*, edited by G. Herdt and S. Lindenbaum. Newbury Park, CA: Sage Publications.

Carballo, M., J. Cleland, M. Caraël, and G. Albrecht. 1989. A Cross-National Study of Patterns of Sexual Behaviour. *Journal of Sex Research* 26:287–299.

Carrier, J.M., and R. Magaña. 1991. Use of Ethnosexual Data on Men of Mexican Origin for HIV/AIDS Prevention Programs. *Journal of Sex Research* 28:189–202.

Chouinard, A., and J. Albert, eds. 1990. *Human Sexuality: Research Perspectives in a World Facing AIDS*. Ottawa: International Development Research Centre.

Daniel, H., and R. Parker. 1993. *Sexuality, Politics and AIDS in Brazil*. London: The Falmer Press.

Gagnon, J.H. 1977. *Human Sexualities*. Glenview, IL: Scott Foresman.

Gagnon, J.H. 1988. Sex Research and Sexual Conduct in the Era of AIDS. *Journal of Acquired Immune Deficiency Syndromes* 1:593–601.

Gagnon, J.H. 1992. Epidemics and Researchers: AIDS and the Practice of Social Studies. In: *The Time of AIDS: Social Analysis, Theory, and Method,* edited by G. Herdt and S. Lindenbaum. Newbury Park, CA: Sage Publications.

Gagnon, J.H., and W. Simon. 1973. *Sexual Conduct: The Social Sources of Human Sexuality.* Chicago: Aldine.

García, L., J. Valdespino, J. Izazola, M. Palacios, and J. Sepú. 1991. Bisexuality in Mexico: Current Perspectives. In: *Bisexuality and HIV/AIDS: A Global Perspective,* edited by R. Tielman, M. Carballo, and A. Hendriks. Buffalo, NY: Prometheus Books.

Herdt, G. 1992. Introduction. In: *The Time of AIDS: Social Analysis, Theory, and Method,* edited by G. Herdt, and S. Lindenbaum. Newbury Park, CA: Sage Publications.

Herdt, G., and A. Boxer. 1991. Ethnographic Issues in the Study of AIDS. *Journal of Sex Research* 28:171–187.

Herdt, G., W.L. Leap, and M. Sovine. 1991. Introduction: Anthropology, Sexuality, and AIDS. *Journal of Sex Research* 28:167–169.

Herdt, G., and S. Lindenbaum, eds. 1992. *The Time of AIDS: Social Analysis, Theory, and Method.* Newbury Park, CA: Sage Publications.

Herdt, G., and R. Stoller. 1990. *Intimate Communications: Erotics and the Study of Culture.* New York: Columbia University Press.

Kane, S. 1990. AIDS, Addiction, and Condom Use: Sources of Sexual Risk for Heterosexual Women. *Journal of Sex Research* 27(3):427–444.

Kane, S. 1991. Heterosexuals, AIDS, and the Heroin Subculture. *Social Science and Medicine* 32(9):1037–1050.

Kane, S., and T. Mason. 1992. 'IV Drug Users' and 'Sex Partners': The Limits of Epidemiological Categories and the Ethnography of Risk. In: *The Time of AIDS: Social Analysis, Theory, and Method,* edited by G. Herdt and S. Lindenbaum. Newbury Park, CA: Sage Publications.

Mann, J.M., D.J.M. Tarantola, and T.W. Netter, eds. 1992. *AIDS in the World.* Cambridge: Harvard University Press.

Misztal, B.A., and D. Moss, eds. 1990. *Action on AIDS: National Policies in Comparative Perspective.* New York: Greenwood Press.

Parker, R.G. 1987. Aquired Immunodeficiency Syndrome in Urban Brazil. *Medical Anthropology Quarterly* 1(2):155–175.

Parker, R.G. 1991. *Bodies, Pleasures, and Passions: Sexual Culture in Contemporary Brazil.* Boston: Beacon Press.

Parker, R.G. 1992. Sexual Diversity, Cultural Analysis, and AIDS Education in Brazil. In: *The Time of AIDS: Social Analysis, Theory, and Method,* edited by G. Herdt and S. Lindenbaum. Newbury Park, CA: Sage Publications.

Parker, R.G., and M. Carballo. 1990. Qualitative Research on Gay and Bisexual Behaviour Relevant to HIV/AIDS. *Journal of Sex Research* 27:497–525.

Parker, R.G., G. Herdt, and M. Carballo. 1991. Sexual Culture, HIV Transmission, and AIDS Research. *Journal of Sex Research* 28:77–98.

Robinson, P. 1976. *The Modernization of Sex*. New York: Harper.

Rubin, G. 1984. Thinking Sex: Notes for a Radical Theory of the Politics of Sexuality. In: *Pleasure and Danger*, edited by C. Vance. Boston: Routledge and Kegan Paul.

Turner, C.F., H.G. Miller, and L.E. Moses. 1989. *AIDS, Sexual Behaviour, and Intravenous Drug Use*. Washington, DC: National Academy Press.

Turner, C.F., H.G. Miller, and L.E. Moses. 1990. *AIDS: The Second Decade*. Washington, DC: National Academy Press.

Weeks, J. 1981. *Sex, Politics, and Society: The Regulation of Sexuality Since 1800*. New York: Longman.

Weeks, J. 1985. *Sexuality and Its Discontents: Meanings, Myths, and Modern Sexualities*. London: Routledge and Kegan Paul.

Weeks, J. 1986. *Sexuality*. London: Tavistock.

Werasit Sittitrai, T. Brown, and Surapone Virulak. 1991. Patterns of Bisexuality in Thailand. In: *Bisexuality and HIV/AIDS*, edited by R. Tielman, M. Carballo, and A. Hendriks. Buffalo, NY: Prometheus Books.

WHO/GPA/SBR. 1989. *Survey of Partner Relations: Research Package*. Geneva, Switzerland: World Health Organization.

de Zalduondo, B.O. 1991. Prostitution Viewed Cross-Culturally: Toward Re-Contextualizing Sex Work in AIDS Intervention Research. *Journal of Sex Research* 28:223–248.

Chapter FOURTEEN

Theory and Method in HIV Prevention: The Philippine Experience

Michael Lim Tan

It was in 1984 that the Philippine government first confirmed a clinical case of AIDS in the country. As in many developing countries, the initial public response was one of indifference, with the problem perceived as a 'foreign disease' and, later, as a 'sex worker disease.' Such perceptions were reinforced by the demographic pattern of initial reports, with most of the identified HIV positive cases involving women sex workers servicing US military bases in the country.

Starting in 1988, the Philippine government, mainly through foreign grants, began to intensify its HIV prevention activities through information, education and communication (IEC) campaigns. The result has been a number of research projects conducted mainly in order to support the IEC campaigns. This chapter will concentrate on some of the operational research activities. Specifically, I will be referring to projects in Metro Manila with which I have been involved, either as a consultant or as a project director: (1) a knowledge, attitudes, and practices (KAP) survey conducted by a private market research firm in 1989 in Metro Manila among 'sentinel groups' (young adults; overseas workers; sex workers and men who have sex with men) with a total of 900 respondents, the results of which I was contracted to analyse and synthesize in 1990–1991 (Tan 1990, 1991); (2) an IEC project for medical and nursing students that included a survey of 960 students in Metro Manila universities, implemented by the Health Action Information Network (HAIN) (Tan et al. 1992b, 1992c); (3) an IEC project for male sex workers, implemented by HAIN (Tan et al. 1992a); and (4) an ongoing IEC project for men who have sex with men, implemented by The Library Foundation.

My involvement with these projects grew out of an interest in the opportunity to gather more information on sexuality and gender issues in the Philippines. This interest is, in turn, based on my teaching courses on Sex and Culture and on Medical Anthropology at the University of the Philippines and on my work with HAIN, a non-governmental organization servicing community-based health programmes. As with other social scientists in developing countries, I felt that the problem of AIDS had raised the challenge of bringing back into public discourse frank and open discussion of sexuality and gender issues. As I reflect on the HIV prevention projects that have supported research over the past two years, I feel that much has been accomplished. At the same time, I am disturbed by numerous questions that arose in the course of my work: questions that I will discuss in this chapter.

These concerns can be broadly categorized into three divisions that I will use as a framework for my discussion: (a) theory, (b) method, and (c) application of research.

THE PHILIPPINE SOCIO-CULTURAL CONTEXT

Before tackling specific issues, I will briefly discuss facets of Philippine society and culture that affect HIV/AIDS and the work being done in this area. The Philippines went through periods of colonization under Spain (1571–1898) and the United States (1898–1946), often described in the media as '300 years of the convent followed by 50 years of Hollywood.' The description can be misleading, implying two different and discrete socio-cultural 'waves' crashing on precolonial culture and eventually creating a homogenous 'Filipino culture.'

The Spaniards did introduce their strongly patriarchal and erotophobic brand of Roman Catholicism, but this found continuity with the fire-and-brimstone moralism of American Protestant evangelicals. The US colonial period also introduced secular — often medical — explanatory models that could co-exist with or even reinforce religious paradigms, e.g., the labelling of homosexuality as a disease or the use of Freudian explanations ('weak' father/'dominant' mother models that represent an inversion of *machismo* roles) to explain sexual orientation.

A positivist tradition in social research, established during the US colonial period, tends to limit analysis to superficial expressions of sexual and political cultures without adequately addressing the dynamics of these cultures, including the interaction between religious and secular sexual ideologies, or between dominant and popular cultures. There is, for instance, the frequently cited work of the Jesuit psychologist Bulatao (1966), who described 'split-level Christianity' — sharp differences between expressed norms and actual behaviour — and attributed this to the coexistence of 'Christian' and 'pagan' theological systems in the Philippines. Bulatao's work includes examples of sexual behaviour. His article calls for an individual change of values (presumably in the direction of 'Christianity') as the solution.

It is not surprising that with the spread of HIV and AIDS, such forms of moralistic analysis have once again emerged, often creating common ground for conservatives and progressives who target 'moral decadence' as the cause of HIV.

The lack of a critical tradition in research into sexuality can be serious. When we began the HIV prevention programmes, one of our major problems was the lack of published studies on sexuality in the Philippines. In fact, the only noteworthy publications on general issues surrounding sexuality in the Philippines have been produced only in the last two years, consisting of three books by a Filipino clinical psychologist and sex therapist, Margarita Go-Singco Holmes (1990, 1991, 1992). Another reflection of the lack of scholarly research is the fact that there are only two publications, now both quite dated, that are worth citing for Filipino 'men who have sex with men,' one by the late anthropologist Donn Hart (1968) and the other a four-country study by sociologists Frederick Whitam and Robin Mathy (1986), both articles concentrating on transvestite cultures.[1]

As the HIV/AIDS problem grows in the Philippines, the urgency for action-oriented research has become even more pressing, but HIV prevention and control programmes will remain off-course as social scientists and programme implementors fail to recognize their own cultural blind spots. These contradictions are found even among people involved in HIV/AIDS work and are best exemplified by *Poisoned Blood*, a film documentary produced by a Filipino AIDS activist in which AIDS is depicted as a product of the moralism of Roman Catholicism; the US colonizers' 'sexual permissiveness'; the US military bases in the Philippines; the non-illegal status of homosexuality; and the Marcos dictatorship's promotion of sexual tourism.

THEORETICAL ISSUES

Much of the literature on sex and culture has focused on debates between social constructivists and essentialists. A provocative article by Vance (1991), dealing with anthropology and the study of sexuality, suggests that the debate has little impact on many anthropologists (as well as social and behavioural scientists). Vance argues that the research has in fact been dominated by what she calls the 'cultural influence model' (878–880), one that recognizes the role of society and culture in shaping sexual behaviour and attitudes but which continues to accept, as a given, a universal and biologically determined 'bedrock of sexuality' (878).

I share Vance's concern over the lack of theoretical discussion, particularly for a developing country such as the Philippines where the need for such debates has been pushed aside because of the dominance of biomedical researchers, who use social scientists simply to gather 'baseline data.' The absence of debates on theories and models raises serious questions about the validity of the social and behavioural research being conducted, since such research, in the absence of theoretical grounding, is more vulnerable to reducing sexuality to 'quantifiable' behaviour — number of times for particular forms of sexual activity (receptor/insertor; anal, vaginal, oral; same sex, opposite sex; frequency of condom use) — divorced from its socio-cultural context.

Even attempts to recognize the socio-cultural context of sexuality, and to adopt some form of cultural relativism, are inadequate when it comes to dealing with realities, and I use this term in the sense of what is 'real' subjectively for the individual, as well as what is 'real' objectively, for an outside observer.

Let us take the phrase 'men who have sex with men,' abbreviated as 'MSM,' now widely used in HIV/AIDS programmes. The phrase was introduced, apparently by Western researchers, in an attempt to introduce neutral language as opposed to what was construed to be Western constructs: 'gay' or even 'homosexual.' I realize that it is difficult to produce a more appropriate phrase than 'men who have sex with men,' but the label is very much behaviourally fixated, precluding identity and, more importantly, gender. I must emphasize, and I will elaborate on this later in the paper, that usage of the term MSM has produced some rather positive and intriguing results. My point here is that 'men who have sex with men' is also a 'Western' term that emerged, consciously or not, out of an essentialist perspective (i.e., limiting sexuality to object choice) and that IEC campaigns integrating this term into a plan of action could restrict the potentials of such projects to reach this population, mainly because it shunts off cultural contexts that are important in understanding behaviour.

I am not suggesting a universalist interpretation of 'gay' or 'homosexual.' What I am suggesting is that these terms evolve in the context both of local cultures, as well as of the 'global village.' In the Philippines, for instance, the term 'gay' has been incorporated into daily discourse and although it has different uses in different settings (e.g., it is more often used as a noun rather than as an adjective), the term does carry meaning, including a sense of sexual and social identity for many Filipinos.

To be even more specific, I will cite the case of The Library Foundation's HIV prevention workshops for 'men who have sex with men.' Organizers faced a minor crisis when they had an applicant who self-identified as being 'a gay' but had no sexual experience, either with other men or with women. He was allowed to join the workshop. One organizer explained, 'He's a gay. He's an MSM.' It was an extraordinary instance of an academic, behaviourally oriented term — men who have sex with men — being appropriated, and transformed, into a social marker.

The issue here goes beyond semantics. The danger lies in the use of behaviour as a starting point, and ending there. If social science research dissociates itself from the study of dynamic socio-cultural contexts, explanations for behaviour will be greatly weakened. Already, we find many examples of HIV social science research reduced to inputs that reflect behaviourist psychology (although, again because of the poverty of discussions on theory, there may be an eclectic mixture of different schools of thought from psychology). Thus, many research projects concentrate on health psychologists' behavioural change models, resulting in an often futile search for 'psycho-graphic' (i.e., personality) traits that facilitate or hinder the initiation and maintenance of behavioural change. I refer specifically to the classic work on 'locus of control' (internal versus external) by Rotter (1966) which has since been widely adapted by health psychologists for health belief models (Wallston and Wallston 1978). Unfortunately, the cross-cultural validity of 'locus of control' — as a construct and as a variable (or variables) — remains dubious (see Rogers 1991). Yet, so much of the research in HIV/AIDS projects in the Philippines — following US models — attempts to measure this locus of control and its correlations with behavioural change for HIV risk reduction.

Not surprisingly, this correlation could not be established in the Philippine studies, since Rotter's model, as applied, fails to consider many significant macrovariables that shape, as well as determine, this locus of control. In retrospect, this should have been anticipated, since the concept of internal locus of control, presumed to be one of, if not the most important determinants of behavioural change, fails to consider the possibility that there may in fact be a collective locus of control that is neither externally nor internally oriented. To further explain this point, in my review of the 1989 survey of sentinel groups, I found a significant correlation between 'group affiliation' (another form of locus of control revolving around small peer groups) and the possibilities for behavioural change.[2]

METHODOLOGICAL CONCERNS

Support for HIV/AIDS research, specifically into the social and be-havioural aspects, has often been in the form of one-year grants where the research component is meant to support IEC activities. By necessity, the research has to be much like orthodox sex: short, quick, almost mechanical.

For researchers in developing countries, this often means the use of instruments drawn up in the United States or Europe (more often the former). Surveys that can be easily quantified for data processing and analysis are therefore the norm. I am not anti-empiricist, having conducted several surveys with the usual dose of means and stand-ard deviations and analysis of variance. What does alarm me is how the instruments are formulated: usually through what I call a 'pick-up sticks' approach, combining questions and scales from a range of US surveys. In one questionnaire I reviewed I found a psychogra-phics section that lifted seven statements from Rotter's I–E Scale for locus of control (out of the original version with 29 *paired* statements involving forced-choice responses). Moreover, there was a hodge-podge array of statements from the Eysenck Personality Questionnaire and the California Psychological Inventory. Together, these were supposed to measure locus of control, group orientation, rationality, conformity, assertiveness and moralism in an attempt to draw up a psychographic profile of sentinel groups and to relate these to behavioural change.

More disturbing was the fact that the statements had been translated with a lack of linguistic equivalence and, more importantly, conceptual equivalence and cultural appropriateness. The problems in translation lead us back to problems in the theoretical (or atheoretical) framework, i.e., an assumption that behaviour, and its 'determinants,' can be easily transformed into measurable variables without due consideration for the subtle texture of culture. I will cite two examples here. First, a statement lifted from Rotter's I–E Scale for locus of control — 'I have often found that what is going to happen will happen' — was totally distorted in its translation into Filipino, being transformed into the statement that: 'Usually, what one expects to happen will happen.' Second, a statement — 'I am aggressive' — was used as a measure for 'individualism,' which was in turn presumed to be in direct opposition to 'conformity.' The underlying assumption was that 'individualism' presented a better prognosis for the chances of behavioural change, an assumption that is, of course, controversial. The problem here is complex because the statement is itself culturally inappropriate. 'I am aggressive' was rated as a positive trait (as one measure of individualism — another questionable assumption), failing to consider that aggressiveness is unacceptable in the Philippines, especially because *agresibo* has pejorative sexual connotations.

Cross-cultural differences can create other problems, not just in translation. In the survey I reviewed, and in many other surveys conducted in conjunction with planning for IEC materials, Likert scales are almost always used. Yet my experience with surveys in the Philippines is that 'strongly agree' and 'somewhat agree' is a distinction of minimal value. In the words of a peasant health worker, the distinction is *burgis* (bourgeois): 'You either agree or you don't. There is no 'somewhat.' Yet survey after survey in HIV projects insist on using such scales. Because of this, HAIN's surveys now use 'agree,' 'disagree,' or 'don't know/not sure,' which, incidentally, does make data processing simpler and more rapid, if this is the objective.

I must reiterate that, while I am not against surveys and questionnaires, I do have serious questions about the validity and reliability of surveys that are not triangulated with qualitative methods, not just in data collection but also in data interpretation. For instance, among medical and nursing students, we encountered what seemed to be a contradiction in attitudes toward homosexuality. In our self-administered questionnaires used by the students, 27.4 per cent agreed with the statement 'Homosexuality is a disease' and 86.4 per cent agreed with the statement 'It is a sin to have sex with another person of the same sex.' At the same time, 47.6 per cent of the respondents felt that 'Homosexuality is merely a different kind of lifestyle.' The inclusion of three different questions in the survey itself, supplemented by focus group discussions, showed that the figures were not necessarily contradictory; in fact, it showed how the medical and nursing students compartmentalize their attitudes toward homosexuals and homosexuality. Moral statements elicited more rigid responses while a secular label, 'disease,' tended to be used less often. Straddling religious and medical stigmatization was the statement on 'different kind of lifestyle,' a neutral area where some degree of tolerance could be expressed. Whether these views reflect homophobia, and how they may affect the medical and nursing students' willingness to work with homosexuals, would of course be separate issues that need other research methodologies to complement the survey findings.

There are rapid qualitative methods that can be used, but they do tend to take more time, and this seems to discourage social and behavioural scientists from utilizing them, despite the fact that such methods, including focus group discussions, can generate vital information. Another example comes from our work with medical and nursing students, where we persistently found agreement with the statement that: 'People with AIDS should be isolated.' We found this important enough to feed back to the students in a final consultative workshop. The explanation was simple: one student said that among medical and nursing students, the concept of 'isolation' does not mean discrimination against people with AIDS (PWAs), since 'isolation' here could have meant protecting PWAs from opportunistic infections, rather than protecting society from the PWAs. The logic is clear, and it certainly is not limited to Filipino medical and nursing students. For anthropologists, it is important that we recognize the 'cultures' from which people come, including the 'biomedical' culture that plays such a dominant role today.

To summarize, the rich texture of culture is all too often sacrificed in surveys. Often, it is not the survey itself that may be flawed, but research design that reflects disembodied empiricism and non-critical adoption of Western research 'instruments.' For an area as amorphous as sexual behaviour, such methodologies are clearly inadequate and may even be counterproductive.

APPLIED PERSPECTIVES

If social scientists are to contribute anything substantial to HIV prevention, it will have to come from the way our research contributes to the actual implementation of 'interventions.' In the Philippines we have found that social science research is most useful when it is integrated into all phases of an IEC campaign. As an example, I will paraphrase two of the exchanges we had in a session (predominantly in English) with 'men who have sex with men' where we attempted to synthesize 'values (read culture), sexual behaviour, and AIDS':

Segment 1

Workshop participant:
  You can't generalize about situations: it's different if it's a lover, or a casual pick-up, or a call boy [male sex worker]....
Facilitator:
  Good point. What if Mr. X (a popular male actor) offered sex but refuses to use a condom?
(Brief silence, then laughter)
Several participants:
  Why not?
Facilitator
  So, never mind all this talk we've had about safe sex?
Workshop participant
  Of course, who cares about safe sex if it's Mr. X.
Facilitator:
  In other words, he is *so* good looking that the experience would be worth it, to die for, right?
(Laughter)

Segment 2

Workshop participant:
  I've wondered if there's a difference between how Westerners and Filipinos look at condoms. Is it easier to talk about safer sex with Westerners?

Facilitator:
Certainly, there's no problem with talking about condoms if
you're out on a date in the States. You can even compare
brands ... but this does not necessarily correspond to
actual behaviour when you get to bed.
Workshop participant:
I'd like to share my views on that, being an *Afamista* (a person
who prefers Caucasians). When I do it with a foreigner, I think
of myself as representing the Philippines, and that I have to
project our country, meaning, I have to show him the 'full
beauty and splendour of the Philippines' (lifted from an
advertisement of Philippine Airlines) ... so ...
(Laughter, applause)

The session from which the two excerpts were derived was introduced only after we had conducted eight workshops, realizing that
all the talk on safer sex was so divorced from the 'real' world outside
of the workshop site. So much of the processing could have been
relegated to post-workshop follow-up sessions but we decided to
formulate a 'bridging session,' using focus group discussions, to
synthesize the discussions half-way through the two-day workshops, after participants had gone through intensive sessions on the
basics about HIV/AIDS and on sexual issues. The bridging session
allowed an integration of 'culture' and 'sexuality,' helping participants to identify, on their own, the parameters of their sexuality
and to relate these to their sexual behaviour.

Earlier I referred to the problems with the use of the phrase 'men
who have sex with men' because of its behaviourist origins and its
ambiguity. Yet the ambiguity can be viewed positively precisely because it generates cognitive tension (not necessarily dissonance) that
can, if properly handled, become a channel for challenging socially
generated stereotypes that the participants have internalized. To elaborate, the use of the label 'men who have sex with men' did allow
workshop participants and facilitators to explore the range of sexualities that exists within this particular population. Perceptions of
gender status and roles were easily evoked, allowing participants to
be more introspective about the processes of socialization and encul-
turation that shape sexual behaviour and stimulating a critical
awareness of 'self,' in whatever ways the participants wanted to
interpret 'men who have sex with men' in relation to macrosocial
variables. Then, and only then, could HIV prevention be properly
contextualized and made meaningful. An example was a session
where the 'girl role' among gay men (which in an extended discus-

sion translates into an imperative to take on the role of a receptor in anal intercourse) was discussed. One participant actually expressed his concern that he was 'abnormal' because he had never felt this 'girl role.'

Such comments show the complexity of popular perceptions. It is therefore important that they are evoked and 'processed' in the workshops, allowing participants to map out these perceptions and to understand factors that may inhibit behavioural change, either at the level of motivation or, later, of sustaining the change as they reintegrate into the 'real world' outside of the workshops.

In the case of medical and nursing students, we found it important to go beyond lectures on epidemiology and to process their perceptions of so-called high-risk groups. Their concepts of 'the other,' versus 'myself,' are vital in understanding the powerful role of sex and sexuality in the creation and maintenance of social boundaries and how these boundaries will affect the provision of health care — whether through preventive educational programmes or actual care for people with HIV and AIDS. It is encouraging that several Philippine non-governmental organizations (NGOs) working with HIV/ AIDS programmes have now created an informal coalition that allows dialogue among the different groups, precisely to help each other in becoming more conscious of the processes of moral exclusion. These have taken place through forums involving so-called target groups (e.g., male sex workers with 'men who have sex with men') as well as through dialogues between policy-makers and programme implementors (e.g., between overseas recruitment agencies and groups conducting HIV prevention workshops with the overseas contract workers). Such dialogues have become all the more important when set against a broader socio-political background, such as the rapid expansion of feminist organizations and the emergence of gay and lesbian organizations that challenge existing norms.

All these developments would not have been possible without a conscious effort to take up the entire IEC project as a process involving research as ethnography and ethnology. Despite the many problems we have faced (and the problems we anticipate), these processes of documentation and dialogue give grounds for optimism about the future of social and behavioural research in HIV/AIDS prevention projects. More importantly, the projects have proven to be exciting as we develop new perspectives, and methodologies, for the study of sexuality and society.

NOTES

1. Not surprisingly, proposed solutions to the HIV problem can border on the ridiculous, such as a recently proposed bill in Congress that would establish red light districts in every province and city, to be managed by the Health Department with monthly testing of the sex workers. Defending the bill on television, the sponsor insisted this was the only way AIDS could be controlled and that he had his bishop's endorsement for the bill. Ludicrous as the bill may be, it is only one of many examples of the broader social and political context that has to be documented and analysed, including the instances of cultural contradictions and cultural accommodation.

2. I would like to mention, in passing, other debates that I have found important in our work: materialism versus idealism; positivism versus interpretivism; universalism versus relativism; and romanticism versus rationalism. It is beyond the scope of this chapter to go into detail on all of these debates, but in terms of the realities of responding to the problems of HIV and AIDS in developing countries, I must assert the view that it is *not* a luxury to enter into debates on theories, paradigms or models. Any claim to a scientific approach to HIV and AIDS must be based on a serious attempt to identify the social matrix in which 'knowledge, attitudes, practices and behaviour' are grounded. Even ethnographic research, if conducted in an environment that disregards theoretical reflection, will prove to be sterile.

REFERENCES

Bulatao, J.C. 1966. *Split-Level Christianity*. Quezon City: Ateneo de Manila University Press.

Hart, D. 1968. Homosexuality and Transvestism in the Philippines. *Behaviour Science Notes* 3:211–248.

Holmes, M.G. 1990. *Life, Love, Lust*. Quezon City: Anvil.

Holmes, M.G. 1991. *Passion, Power, Pleasure*. Quezon City: Anvil.

Holmes, M.G. 1992. *Roles We Play in Family Life*. Quezon City: Anvil.

Rogers, W.S. 1991. *Explaining Health and Illness*. New York: Harvester Wheatsheaf.

Rotter, J.B. 1966. Some Problems and Misconceptions Related to the Construct of Internal and External Locus of Control of Reinforcement. *Journal of Consulting and Clinical Psychology* 45:489–493.

Tan, M.L. 1990. Synthesis of an AIDS KAP Survey Among Sentinel Groups in Metro Manila. Unpublished document submitted to the Department of Health and the Academy for Educational Development.

Tan, M.L. 1991. Comments on Methodologies in the 1989 AIDS KAP Metro Manila Survey. Unpublished document submitted to the Department of Health and the Academy for Educational Development.

Tan, M.L., et al. 1992a. *Final Report: HIV/AIDS Prevention Project for Male Sex Workers in Metro Manila.* Quezon City: Health Action Information Network.

Tan, M.L. et al. 1992b. *Final Report: HIV/AIDS Prevention Project for Medical and Nursing Students in Metro Manila.* Quezon City: Health Action Information Network.

Tan, M.L. et al. 1992c. Responding to HIV and AIDS: Medical and Nursing Students in Metro Manila. *Health Alert* 8:5–19.

Vance, C.S. 1991. Anthropology Rediscovers Sexuality: A Theoretical Comment. *Social Science and Medicine* 33:875–884.

Wallston, B.S., and K.A. Wallston. 1978. Locus of Control and Health: A Review of the Literature. *Health Education Monographs* 6:107–116.

Whitam, F.L., and R.M. Mathy. 1986. *Male Homosexuality in Four Societies (Brazil, Guatemala, the Philippines and the United States).* New York: Praeger.

Chapter

FIFTEEN

Rethinking Anthropology: The Study of AIDS

Ralph Bolton

Before I begin this intellectual exercise, I would like to ask you to stand for one minute and to reflect silently on the people whom you know who are living with HIV or AIDS. I suspect that, like me, most of you are here today because of your concern for loved ones for whom this epidemic is a personal ordeal [moment of silence].

In recent years it has been my custom to dedicate my writings to friends who are living with HIV, as a tribute to their courage and as an expression of my gratitude for the part they have played in my life. Extending that practice, I would like to dedicate this talk to my first lover, to the man who transformed my life, giving me the gift of

---

This chapter is the text of a keynote address as delivered at the opening of the Amsterdam Conference 'Culture, Sexual Behavior, and AIDS' on which this volume is based.

wholeness and helping me to attain a higher level of personal integrity and happiness. I owe him a debt I can never repay, but I hope
he will accept this dedication as a token of my esteem. I am honoured
by his presence in the audience today. Little could we have imagined
when we met each other on a snowy winter's night on a pier in
Trondheim that ten years later we would find ourselves together in
Amsterdam under these trying circumstances. [Bjørn Olav Berg died
in Oslo, Norway, on February 15, 1993.]

I wish the organizers of this conference had settled on someone
else to present this discussion — for reasons which have nothing to
do with modesty, or false modesty for that matter. The first reason is
quite personal. I'm tired. I am in shock and almost immobilized by
the daily intrusion of this epidemic into my personal life. While HIV
has not ravaged my body, it has seared my soul, and at times I fear
that it threatens my sanity as I witness the impact of the epidemic on
the lives of people I love. AIDS forces us constantly to rethink our
lives and our knowledge in the most profound ways, to rethink
everything, all at the same time. Sometimes I become paralysed by
the process for fear of making mistakes with disastrous consequences. I recall how a not-so-innocent question in a letter to an HIV-positive friend lead him to come out to a boyfriend about being seropositive, which resulted in a serious rupture in their relationship and
tremendous psychological stress on my friend. Was I right to suggest
this course of action? We must constantly face the question of how to
act responsibly when there is so much uncertainty and so much at
stake.

Furthermore, I seethe with barely controllable rage. I am not
apologetic about that rage since rage is a sane and reasonable response to the irrationality so often manifested in dealing with this
epidemic; it is a rage fuelled by an unwillingness to see friends and
lovers go quietly into the night. It is a rage that does not lead to a loss
of objectivity but one that is produced by objectivity, and by seeing
all too clearly the horror we are experiencing. We need *more* rage,
more outrage, in the face of the truly outrageous. If there are three
things that have been in short supply in this epidemic, in my
opinion, they are rage, reason, and compassion. I do fear, however,
that the expression of my rage in this forum may be inappropriate
and misdirected, and for that I am sorry.

The second reason is that I am not certain I have anything profound to say to you; most definitely I am not in a state of mind to give
you a nice upbeat, inspirational message. It's not that I'm insuffi-
ciently familiar with anthropological research on AIDS to be able to

present a cool, dispassionate analysis of anthropology's role in this epidemic; quite the contrary in a sense. But as I read the literature I tend to have the feeling that I'm not really learning anything new anymore. Yes, of course, there are additional facts I come across: the seroprevalence rate here, the percentage of prostitutes who use condoms there, etc. Really useful and valuable findings or observations, however, are rare. So much of what I encounter is mere repetition. Whenever I read something on AIDS, I ask myself, 'What have I learned from this piece?' and that I learn so little now has nothing to do with knowing a lot, but with the fact that so few new and important facts are being generated. Even worse, though, is that the more I think about AIDS, the more I fear that I no longer have a sense that I know much that counts. I certainly don't have the answers to the important questions, and I may not even have the right questions. Yet, my task is to raise questions for your consideration. I'm afraid of having no wisdom to offer you, only my personal prejudices, for whatever they are worth.[1]

The third reason for my reticence in giving this talk is that I am frankly not enthusiastic about adding still another piece to the programmatic literature. Many of the publications to date consist of programmatic statements about what anthropology can contribute, and few are serious substantive contributions. There seems to have been too much effort devoted to convincing ourselves and others (most likely funding agencies) that we have something to offer and too little actual demonstration of the usefulness of anthropological approaches to AIDS.

And finally, what I am going to say may be as painful to hear as it is painful to say, because I intend to be ruthlessly critical of anthropology as applied to AIDS during the first decade of the epidemic, and quite possibly my assessment of the situation may be wrong — if so, I know you will correct me in the two days of our discussions here, but I assure you that I am not merely playing devil's advocate on these issues; I do believe that my interpretation is reasoned and accurate. Still, I retain some slight hope that the contents of this conference will invalidate, or at least mitigate, my views; certainly from reading the titles of your presentations, it seems possible that you will prove my pessimism to be unfounded and that you will instill a faith that I don't currently have. Perhaps by the end of this conference you will have generated a set of questions which we need to address; if so this conference will be a success, especially if some of you then go out and find the answers quickly.

WHAT'S IMPORTANT?

From time to time I reread *The Plague* by Camus, a book I assign in my AIDS courses. The last time I did so, I was struck by a passage which can stand as the theme of my remarks, and, indeed, if you remember nothing else from this talk, I would urge you to recall this passage:

> The essential thing was to save the greatest number of people from dying and being doomed to unending separation. And to do this there was only one resource: to fight the plague. There was nothing admirable about this attitude; it was merely logical. (Camus 1972:126)

This text suggests some questions that each of us should ask ourselves: How does my work contribute to what is essential? Has my work, has our work, saved any lives? Can we in fact, when being honest with ourselves, make a link between what we are doing and keeping people from dying?

In the various programmatic statements you will find lists of suggestions (cf. Bolton 1989; Frankenberg 1988; Herdt 1987; Herdt and Boxer 1991; Parker and Carballo 1990). Paul Farmer (1992), for example, has indicated five tasks or roles for anthropologists, which we share with others concerned about the epidemic: (1) explaining why AIDS is fast becoming an illness of the disadvantaged; (2) using ethnology as cultural critique; (3) countering false information; (4) documenting the effects of misinformation and joining forces with community groups in using such information to develop cultural activist responses to the epidemic; and (5) witnessing, honouring the memory of persons who have died from AIDS.

Ronald Bayer has asked

> What is the duty of researchers, physicians, and intellectuals? It is to hold up a mirror that can reflect an uncompromising picture of the suffering caused by the HIV epidemic in the hope, faint as it is, that a collective conscience can be moved. At this moment in the world history of the AIDS epidemic silence would be an unforgivable dereliction of professional moral responsibility. (1992:531)

While statements such as those by Farmer and Bayer are laudable, this is not enough, I submit, if only because the hope is too faint, as Bayer puts it, that the collective conscience will be moved. If this is all we can do, it would be better to be out on the streets with ACT UP or engaged in personal campaigns to save lives.

I reject the notion that we should merely bear witness, that our only role should be to record this catastrophic event in human history, although I am not inherently opposed to interpreting and witnessing the epidemic, to efforts to create meaning in the face of meaninglessness: this we do by our very involvement in AIDS issues. But I would prefer to leave those tasks to humanists, to artists who have shown themselves much more competent at this than we have been, perhaps because they understand that emotions are central to understanding this phenomenon, whereas we have utilized rational and linear models which are intrinsically inadequate to the effective representation of a world turned upside down. As anthropologists, if we are to go beyond merely interpreting to stopping AIDS, I would contend that there are only three important general arenas of research where anthropological expertise is crucial and where we should be concentrating our efforts. These are: (a) preventing new cases of AIDS through the generation of knowledge that improves the effectiveness of efforts to reduce the incidence of high-risk behaviours which facilitate the transmission of HIV; (b) promoting knowledge about how to enhance the quality of life of people living with HIV or AIDS; and (c) learning how to overcome obstacles to the implementation of the knowledge we have gained or can obtain on issues related to prevention and to improving the lives of men, women, and children who are already infected.

I think we have largely failed in all three of these arenas. Prevention efforts have enjoyed limited success — behaviours have changed to some degree in some places, but no thanks to our research nor to that of other social scientists. Instead, credit must go to situational factors over which we have had no control and to the insights and work of people living in afflicted communities. Improvements in the quality of life of the infected have come about mostly through the struggles of the infected themselves to learn how to live with HIV, from their lived experiences. As for the third, the record is so dismal, it leaves everything to be done. We have not even managed to figure out how to get the United States government to remove its unenlightened policy of immigration restrictions on HIV-positive individuals.

I would ask you: What do we need to know that we do not already know? What *are* the significant unanswered questions? I can think of only one absolutely fundamental one and that is one on which we are not doing much research, perhaps because we know intuitively that we cannot answer it. That question is, 'How can we produce the political action necessary to implement radical prevention programmes?' A second question of great importance is, 'What is the best way to live with HIV, to improve the quality of life for people living with

HIV/AIDS, and hence for all of us?' On most other matters we have known the critical information now for at least five or six years; the point is to apply it.

Self-congratulatory attitudes of AIDS researchers are unjustified. How often have we heard the mantra, 'We have learned more in a shorter time about this disease than about any other disease in history'? But has what we have learned yielded a cure or even truly effective therapies? Has it reduced high-risk behaviour and hence the number of infections? Has it saved lives? No. At best it has lengthened some lives by a year or two, and at a cost that is hard to measure, in the suffering caused by the highly toxic therapies themselves. We have antibody tests that cause people to commit suicide, and that have not been shown to have an overall positive effect on behaviour change, and yet they are the main armament in the prevention strategy of the US government, despite a recognition by CDC authorities that they do not work — when all of us should just assume that we are seropositive and live accordingly.

AIDS RESEARCH AND RETHINKING ANTHROPOLOGICAL THEORY

When I read publications by anthropologists on AIDS, I am forced to ask myself, 'Is it anthropology?' And my conclusion is, in most cases, no, not in theory nor in methods. And, consequently, I would assert that there is no such thing as the anthropology of AIDS. Perhaps I'm hopelessly old-fashioned and prepostmodern, but I thought anthropology had something to do with holism and in-depth understandings of human behaviour and culture usually based on thorough field research in a community. There's damned little evidence of that in the so-called anthropological literature on AIDS. So let's turn to theory in anthropological AIDS research.[2]

My reading of the current state of anthropology, in general, and the literature on AIDS to which anthropologists have contributed, in particular, suggests to me the following basic propositions, which I will illustrate primarily in the area of research on sexuality:

1. Anthropology was not prepared to cope with AIDS.
2. Most anthropological work on the epidemic has been atheoretical.
3. We have employed inappropriate theoretical paradigms.
4. We have abandoned our uniquely anthropological perspectives and knowledge.

Anthropological Unpreparedness

An emphasis on cultural relativism has been a strength of anthropology for decades, but it may also be a source of tremendous weakness. Cultural relativism may have been invented to constrain the rapaciousness of colonialist societies, but it is now used to justify tolerance for the perpetuation of injustice and the failure to take responsibility for human misery. I had an argument recently with a colleague who could not understand why I would say that I condemn and would actively work to eliminate anywhere in the world discrimination against gays and lesbians, that it was necessary to speak out against societies in which homosexuality is punished by imprisonment or death, and that I cannot tolerate, in the name of cultural relativism, the right of any society to discriminate against my people. We, as anthropologists, have failed to contribute to the cause of fundamental human rights. In part this is because we have exoticised 'the other,' thereby contributing to differentiating ourselves from others. Instead of fostering the oneness of humanity we have stressed its divisions, thereby making it possible to consider AIDS a disease of 'the other.' An emphasis on cultural relativity and human differences, instead of building on human similarities and oneness, has permitted us to relinquish responsibility for human welfare.

The anthropology of sexuality is a notoriously barren wasteland. In this domain especially, anthropology, and other disciplines as well, have been mired in the sterile debate imported from history, sociology and literary criticism between essentialists and social constructionists, which is merely a modern version of the ancient nature/nurture controversy. We reinvent anthropology alright, like reinventing the wheel. But then it's understandable — if you don't have new ideas then at least invent new terms and by all means make your writing obscure and capable of multiple interpretations (keep them guessing) to keep the game going, to promote your career, to get a piece of the action. It's a silly game that might be tolerable if there weren't more important tasks to get on with. The theory game as it is played in anthropology is actually a deterrent to producing resolution. If we were really serious we could solve problems. I have the suspicion that we don't really want to because then the game would be over.

Perhaps the one branch of the discipline of which this is less true is indeed medical anthropology, which has not been as totally seduced by anti-scientific fads, perhaps precisely because when we deal with sickness and death we are less inclined to accept the illusion that everything is illusion. This may explain why medical anthropology is one of the most vibrant areas of the discipline. Perhaps your work is informed by postmodern theory, structuralism, evolutionism, or other theoretical paradigms, but I'm sceptical that it is, and if it is, I wonder what these theories really tell us about how to answer the major questions I posed.

The Absence of Theory in AIDS Research

In reality, much of the anthropological work on AIDS is atheoretical. In some ways this does not disturb me because it has the virtue of being unpretentious, and further, if it generates basic information that is actually useful for answering the questions noted above, then it has merit. Unfortunately, I'm not sure that it does provide the critical data. More on that below. You might object that no research is theoretically uninformed inasmuch as implicit assumptions guide the kinds of data we collect.

The Adoption of Inappropriate Paradigms

When theory has informed our work explicitly, it has not worked out well. The Health Belief Model, for example, has been utilized in one form or another by many of us, with extremely disappointing results. Moreover, when one looks at this model its components are rather pedestrian and not particularly helpful in telling us how to design effective prevention programmes. I used to argue for higher levels of funding for social science research, but when I see large amounts of money being spent to prove that those who like condoms are more likely to use them, I'm not impressed and would rather those limited funds be spent in other ways. Or, take still another profound finding: those who report that they intend to use condoms are more likely to use them than those who say they do not intend to use them.

Other theories incorporate variables which are not possible to manipulate in the short run, and I would suggest that to work on theories that involve variables about which nothing can be done is a waste of time and resources. So we learn that individuals with low self-esteem (the root cause of all evils in the world, along with greed) are more likely to engage in unsafe sex than are those with high self-esteem; will this knowledge help us to construct prevention programmes? Are we really naïve enough to think that we can reme-dy self-esteem problems while trying to promote safe sex?

The problem with many of the approaches that have been tried is that they are based on inappropriate, naïve, and rational models of human behaviour. Yet, AIDS and sex both involve irrationality. AIDS is fundamentally a problem of rationality; to give but a few examples: (1) Do you understand my uninfected friends who say they wish they were infected? (2) Do you understand the loss of the will to live — a problem commonly found among the elderly who are 'left behind' when all their peers are dying? Suicide in the face of tremendous pain is not irrational, nor is risk behaviour when there is a loss of the will to live — which should be easily understood when everything meaningful in one's life has disappeared, friends, loved ones. (3) Irrationality is at the base of religious systems which refuse to permit measures that would save lives because they place more emphasis on saving the 'soul.'

In addition, our approaches have tended to be individualistic, a searching for individual 'deficiencies' to explain seemingly irrational behaviour. The concept of 'relapse' comes to mind here as a good example of blaming the victim. Instead of focusing on cultural and social conditions which provide the context for behaviour, we have reduced the problem to one of the individual actor. For anthropologists to be doing this is odd indeed.

Instead of seeking guidance from rationalistic theories, I suggest it might be better to draw on some other bodies of literature for insights: the literature on the holocaust, on war and post-traumatic stress syndrome or general theories of risk-taking (hardly ever mentioned). The literature of the health sciences was probably the last place we should have expected to find answers to this crisis. This could only be done by those who view AIDS as just another problem rather than the apocalyptic occurrence that it has become in some of our communities.

Finally, our theories have tended to be unremittingly negative, fear-inducing, and anti-pleasure. Little wonder, then, that they have not produced results.

Abandoning Anthropology

For the most part one finds in the anthropological literature on AIDS almost no references to theoretical insights we have gained from work on other problems. It seems at best that 'an anthropological approach' consists of calling for 'cultural sensitivity.' Have we nothing else to offer? Calls for cultural sensitivity are problematic, too. Whose culture? I recall sitting in on a discussion, as an observer, of

AIDS experts assembled from around the world and having to listen to one Third World delegate express his satisfaction that the epidemic would eliminate such social evils as prostitution and homosexuality. As an observer I had no right to speak out, but the closeted gay men who were present and who were full participants did not respond, for fear of offending this delegate's 'cultural sensibilities.' All of us could think about bodies of anthropological literature which might give us useful insights. Sexuality is about the search for the ecstatic; indeed most forms of HIV transmission involve pleasure in some form — drugs, sex. Is the literature on altered states of consciousness relevant here? Transmission occurs in many societies, particularly among people who are marginal in occupation, in prestige, outlaws. Can theoretical work on stigma and prejudice provide us with guidance? What about the applicability of Victor Turner's work on ritual and on the significance of such body fluids as blood, milk, and semen, or the applicability of John M. Roberts' work on expressive culture?

RETHINKING SEX: WHAT IS IT?

When you read the research on sexuality that has emerged during this epidemic, you get an extremely impoverished and naïve view of what sex is. If you didn't know better, you would think that sex is about cocks, cunts and assholes. The discourse on sex by AIDS researchers sounds like the product of parochial school education, and has about as much relevance to the lived experiences of sexually active men and women as the notion that sex is 'about' reproduction. Only the sexually innocent could think this is what sex is about. *Pleasure and Danger* was the title of one book on sexuality. We have focused almost exclusively on the dangers of sex, thereby contributing to the right-wing, erotophobic agenda. So we hear a great deal about sex as murder and now as suicide. To be sure, sexual risk-taking as suicide is a real phenomenon, but part of the ongoing negative assessment of sexuality and a further stigmatization of those who choose to die rather than continue to live in a world in which all meaning has been lost with the deaths of friends and lovers. Where's the joy of sex? We have become part of the machinery for turning sex into a dangerous and despicable activity. Where in the literature do you find discussions of:

1. sex as play
2. sex as stress-seeking

3. sex as adventure
4. sex as transcendence
5. sex as fun
6. sex as fantasy
7. sex as interaction and connectedness
8. sex as pleasure
9. sex as time-out, as a break from everyday reality, which for many people, especially in the hardest hit communities, is grim
10. sex as liminality
11. sex as self-testing of one's limits
12. sex as growth
13. sex as a source of community, as communitas
14. sex as giving
15. sex as sharing
16. sex as ecstatic experience
17. sex as theatre
18. sex as an endorphin-induced high
19. sex as spirituality
20. sex as an expression of emotions
21. sex as a source of meaning
22. sex as power — those doing research on women and AIDS have begun to elucidate this point
23. sex as aesthetics
24. sex as sacrifice
25. sex as beauty
26. sex as ritual?

The list could continue; it is far from exhaustive of the richness and complexity of sexuality, not only in the forms it takes but in its meanings. Oh, yes, and then what about *love*. Where does this fit in? We hear about people engaging in unsafe sex because of power relations; we see a focus on specific high-risk behaviours, and on self-esteem and other personality variables, but probably the biggest reason for unsafe sex is love; love involves risk-taking, giving, trusting ... and yet where is the research on this topic? We have done lots of work on prostitutes, as if the exchange of money was a determinant risk, when my reading of the literature is that prostitutes are more likely to become infected in their relations with lovers than with clients. But then I ask myself, how much of the research on prostitutes is being done because of a concern for sex workers and how much because of a concern primarily for their clients and a worry about the possible spread of HIV among mainstream, middle-class heterosexuals? Sex and positive relationships are closely linked. We have countless studies in which 'promiscuity' is a variable and which never mention love in this context as if love could not be involved in 'casual' encounters. Sex is about love as well as lust — but this seems to have been overlooked, probably because of absurd stereotypes of promiscuous sex, of the sexuality of gay men, of sex workers, of drug users, and of people in other cultures. Only normal, monogamous, heterosexual, bourgeois, middle-class white folks truly know love, and they are not at risk; that seems to be the assumption (Bolton 1992a).

I think there are fairly obvious reasons why not much worthwhile research on sex has been done during this epidemic, among them, the following:

1.   We don't have a tradition of such work in anthropology; I discussed this above.

2.   One cannot do sex research if one is not comfortable with one's own sexuality or sex in all of its manifestations. I suspect that most of us have never completely gotten over our own sexual hangups. To investigate sexuality one must be open to exploring the full range of sexualities. In anthropology we are always asked to shed our cultural preconceptions, but in the domain of sexuality, given the cultural backgrounds of most anthropologists in the US at least, this may be more difficult to accomplish than in other domains. And yet it must be done if we are to understand other people's sexuality. Then, too, sex researchers may themselves be relatively inexperienced sexually, and this will be reflected in the quality of their work; or they feel compelled to maintain a presentation of self as a model of probity, as conforming to the sexual morality of their own culture, regardless of whether they do or do not, in fact, conform. Must they pretend to know less than they know?

3.   There is still a strong stigma attached to sex research, a stigma that is even more pervasive than the one associated with AIDS research, which by now at least has a certain chic value

attached to it. If we are not willing to be stigmatized, we don't study it, or we do so in the most sterile and clinical ways; if we are unwilling to say that bourgeois social norms on sex are not important, we don't do it.

4. Good sex research, just like good sex, requires body and soul in addition to mind, and academics tend to be people for whom the wisdom of the mind substitutes for, rather than complements, the wisdom of the body. Perhaps it is impossible for those with an Apollonian approach to life to really comprehend sexuality, which is essentially Dionysian, especially for people we need to reach with effective prevention messages, i.e., those whose sexuality perhaps places them at higher risk. Sex is about ecstasy and the release of conscious control over the mind — just the opposite of intellectual activity; the contrast could hardly be sharper.

We need to keep in mind that what makes this epidemic so difficult to deal with is the fact that HIV transmission occurs, or the risk of such transmission exists, precisely in the context of some of the most meaningful and emotionally charged experiences of human life, indeed in the very experiences that are life-giving: (a) from mother to child, whether in utero, perinatally, or in breastfeeding, that intimate act which is the ultimate symbol of love; (b) from donor to recipient in the life-sustaining context of the gift of blood in transfusions; (c) between individuals in the shared ecstasy of sexual encounters; (d) in the bonds between those who share in chemically induced ecstasy; (e) in the rituals of manhood or womanhood, such as scarification, which create bonds of solidarity and identification between generations or within them; and (f) even potentially, albeit extremely rarely, in the bond of caring represented by the physician/patient relationship. It is in these contexts of the most fundamental relationships of human caring and love that HIV intervenes.

RETHINKING METHODS

Toward the end of his life, George Peter Murdock, an anthropological theorist, remarked that the crowning glory of the anthropological enterprise, its unique and lasting contribution to humanity, was to be found not in its theories but in the ethnographic record it had created. If anthropological theory related to AIDS has been deficient, the ethnographic record is even worse. Full-scale ethnographic work on

AIDS is almost non-existent, Paul Farmer's (1992) work on AIDS in Haiti being the exception that proves the rule.

Instead, anthropologists doing AIDS research have tended to adopt wholesale the piecemeal, quick-and-dirty methods which we generally associate with other disciplines, or with marketing research. Instead of doing participant observation we have seen study after study based on such methods as surveys, rapid assessment procedures, and focus groups, and when what passes for ethnography is done, it is usually work that has been delegated to underlings, to hired assistants rather than carried out by a fully trained, professional ethnographer. These methods all have as a critical feature the effect of keeping distance between us as anthropologists and the people we are studying.

If I may use a gastronomic analogy: In my view survey research is comparable to eating at an automat or cafeteria, Rapid Assessment Procedures are the McDonald's equivalent, and focus groups are perhaps a step up — Burger King. They are fast foods and just about as satisfying. Quick-and-dirty instead of down-and-dirty seems to be the motto of AIDS researchers. I don't have the time here to detail my objections to the use of these methods as substitutes for ethnography, which they have become. But I can assure you that when they are used in the domain of sexuality, they represent an incredible naïvety.

In adopting these methods we have privileged etic over emic, data quantity over data quality, reliability over validity, and statistical significance over real significance. How can I attack these things when the intentions of the researchers are surely good? But if you'll permit a cliché, the road to hell is paved with good intentions. We may not pay for our sins, but many of the people we pretend to serve with our research will pay for our mistakes, and they will pay dearly, with their lives.

Of course you can get reliability on surveys when you are measuring cultural concepts rather than behaviour. And by now most people with any smarts at all know what to say on surveys, which may be why we have reported findings that the less educated and minorities are said to be doing riskier sex — they have not yet been quite as indoctrinated in what to say or to be as sophisticated in giving the interviewers what they think the interviewers want to hear. What we have, as a result of a concern for large sample sizes and massive surveys, are reliable data with low validity. Frankly, I would prefer to have accurate information on a small number of cases than such garbage. Ah, but we find reliability, we are told. Of course, you are likely to get high reliability but not for the reasons you think, not because people are reporting their behaviour accurately but because it is even easier to report ideology consistently.

Ethnography as it has been practised in this epidemic is a sick joke, not entirely absent but done in a slipshod manner. How many people do you know who are involved in full-time field research in the traditional anthropological sense? How many of you are involved in serious ethnography? We have become part of teams, we are forced to do fieldwork in short shifts. Have we prostituted ourselves?

Of course, institutional support and rewards are forthcoming for this abandonment of our traditional methods. If you examine the list of anthropologists on the Program Committee of the VIII International Conference on AIDS, for example, only one can make a credible claim to be doing serious ethnography. The others are doing epidemiology or rapid assessments or, in one or two cases, no AIDS research at all.

Adding another call for qualitative research seems to be such a futile exercise; how many have made this call before, yet how little is such research being funded? Do you honestly believe that anyone will fund me to do research on gay sex clubs or on gay culture? If you know of a source of funding, let me know. Almost no ethnography has been done in ten years on gay culture in relation to AIDS. Those doing work on intravenous drug users and sex workers have fared somewhat better, but even for them, ethnography tends to be done as an afterthought, as an add-on to 'real' research; ethnographers are called in after the quantitative data are collected and the number crunchers cannot make sense of them. We have become public opinion pollsters, we have delegated the collection of data to subordinates, we have become the servants of others with more power over funds. We have served the masters much as anthropology in the first half of this century served the interests of colonial powers. We have been bought out and I dare say not at a high price.

Give me the lone ethnographer any day over multimillion-dollar team projects. I have come to the conclusion that there is an inverse correlation between the number of authors on a study and the likelihood of finding anything of value in it, and that the amount one learns is inversely proportional to the amount invested (within certain parameters). We have research by committee, and therefore it is not surprising that what we read in the literature is so useless. Give me one thoughtful ethnographer who is totally immersed in the problem. Thinking is an individual process; it takes only one person to be insightful, whereas it takes many to crunch numbers, to compress the garbage being produced.

As I read the publications coming from big multicentre projects, funded by megabuck grants, I am appalled when I think how much we could be learning if only a fraction of that amount were to go for serious ethnographic work. The cost of one WHO conference alone would fund dozens of ethnographers for a year or two — and their work would save lives, whereas most of these conferences, AIDS research centres, and big projects do nothing for anybody except the researchers themselves.

RETHINKING PREVENTION

We have known the essential facts about HIV transmission since at least the mid-eighties, eight or nine years. And we witnessed dramatic behaviour changes in the early years of the epidemic, at least in major gay communities in the US. But this change was not the product of research. Indeed, I would claim with confidence that behaviour change slowed down or stopped the moment social scientists and health educators stepped into the picture and started applying inappropriate models in their attempts to manipulate sexuality, when professionals replaced the people whose lives were at stake in the running of prevention programmes, and when sex-negativity, as mandated by the Centres for Disease Control, replaced sex-positivity as the basic approach to prevention. Recommendations emanating from the prevention research industry in the US have not only not helped, they have been counterproductive and dangerous. We need to sweep aside most of the work done on prevention and start afresh. It is time for us to do some bolder thinking about prevention, and to come up with new and radical prevention proposals. For example, why not have programmes of prevention in gay communities in which one hires attractive men to go out and have sex and in the process to educate their partners about the joys of safer sex, a kind of safe sex sexual surrogate programme? Why not develop more extensively programmes which teach people how to have good sex that is safe sex? We already have some programmes like this but their reach is quite limited despite the fact that they seem to be the most effective means of reducing risky behaviour. In essence, we need to develop approaches that are pleasure-enhancing rather than pleasure-reducing; it doesn't take a Ph.D. to tell which will work better.

I would like to make two proposals on prevention, one theoretical and the other pragmatic. First, I wish to propose that, contrary to prevailing dogma on sexual transmission prevention, the way to halt transmission is to liberate sexuality, not to return to a conservative sexual ethos. Promoting pleasure will do what the opposite will not. We need to focus on the pleasures, not the dangers, of sexuality. We need to increase the sum of sexual gratification, not reduce it. I am reminded of an anti-STD campaign I saw in Norway ten years ago in which there were billboards that said something to the effect that 'last night so many people had sex and so many got an STD.' It is not our duty to reduce the amount of sex that people have, only to reduce the number of those who become infected with HIV as a result of sex. Ironically, perhaps, we may reduce HIV transmission by increasing the amount and the quality of sex people have.

I would argue that we, as anthropologists, have a responsibility to create culture, not merely to interpret it. We are not merely people who study culture, we participate in it and we must help to shape the future. In this connection we need to do our part to create a new sexual culture. We need to carry forward the sexual revolution, creating a truly liberated sexuality rather than leading the forces of counterrevolution; we need to have a new sexuality which will continue after the problem of AIDS has been solved because there will be other diseases down the road. Our goal should be the elaboration of healthy sexualities, which may be a prime ingredient in being able to reduce problems in other domains of culture as well, such as violence. A repressive sexual counterrevolution will not solve the problem of AIDS, but it will definitely contribute to other problems as a manifestation of increased unhappiness and frustration. This calls for imaginative work, just the opposite of the tedious accountancy to which we have been subjected in the sexual epidemiological literature. It requires listening to and learning from people on the sexual fringe who are exploring these questions. I have been reading the literature of intelligent and articulate practitioners of sadomasochism recently; their writings are much more insightful and knowledgeable about sex and about AIDS prevention than those of the health promotion specialists working on these issues.[3]

A second proposal would be to establish an AIDS Corps similar to the Peace Corps to take charge of prevention programmes. That is to say, we should pay persons with HIV who are interested to become active in prevention on a full- or part-time basis. It is clear that the most effective prevention agents are persons with HIV/AIDS; we've exploited them as volunteers in our efforts when prevention is not their most pressing problem — their problem is how to live with a life-threatening condition. Many gain much from helping others. Why should we not promote a programme that employs those who are interested and able to participate? These people may be the most creative agents for the development of effective prevention, at least in part because of their often superior knowledge of risky behaviour and its contexts. It will bring seropositivity out of the closet and reduce its stigma. This is the kind of programme that the Global Program on AIDS could promote instead of spending more money on expensive international consultants and conferences and still more on meaningless surveys.

In all of our prevention activities, we need to ask the questions, 'Are we doing more harm than good? Are we part of the problem or part of the solution?' Our noble intentions are no guarantee that we are either blameless or effective in reducing HIV transmission.

RETHINKING ETHICS

Ethical issues arise wherever we turn in AIDS work. Thus we are faced repeatedly not only with the question of what can we do that will help to stop the dying, but also what can or must we do that will be morally justifiable in pursuit of this objective. Like all of you, I must confront ethical issues every day in this epidemic, in my personal life as well as in my professional decision-making. It is my view that while these issues are important, we cannot afford to spend much time agonizing over them; we need to consider them seriously, resolve them quickly, and then get on with the job as best we can. I will comment briefly on several examples from my own work.

Participant observation on sex. Several years ago I was presented with a conclusion by the government agency with which I was affiliated that gay men in Belgium were already well informed about AIDS and that they had changed their behaviour to such a degree that it was not necessary to emphasize prevention in that population, thereby freeing resources to work on prevention in the 'general population' (where HIV transmission was much less of a problem). To check this assertion, I drew on information gained through sexual activity with informants in which I discovered that safe sex was definitely not the norm, and that the official position on this issue was based on invalid data. This sexual participant observation in the community in which I was working has been challenged by some as unethical because I did not inform my sexual partners that their behaviour might be used by me to draw conclusions about the sexual behaviour patterns of Belgian gay men. This is not the place to analyse this case in detail (see Bolton 1992b). The question I wish to raise is, quite simply, 'When is it ethical to utilize information gained in daily interaction with members of the communities we study?' In this instance, I used such information to correct the false conclusion that resources need not be devoted to the community I was studying because risky behaviour was no longer practised.

In studying AIDS, we cannot avoid studying sexual issues. Unfortunately, Western attitudes and preconceptions on sexuality impede work in this area. At best anthropologists have kept silent on the topic of sex in the field; at worst they have perpetuated hypocritical pretences and ethnocentric injunctions about sex with people in the societies they study. It is considered acceptable to share meals with informants, it is okay to invade the privacy of their funerals or the intimacy of their sickrooms, but God forbid we should share in their sexuality, i.e., in one of the most meaningful aspects of their lives. For many anthropologists, it may be too threatening to become so intimately involved, but in my view sexual aloofness serves not only to maintain the distinction between the self and the 'other,' but also to prevent us from the fuller identification with the people we study that is provided by sharing in non-trivial domains of life.

Impossible research? For some time I considered the possibility of doing research on so-called adult bookstores, i.e., stores that sell and rent various forms of erotica. In many places in the US and Europe, these establishments provide opportunities for on-site anonymous sexual encounters in video booths. I was interested in them particularly because they might be suitable locations in which to conduct prevention activities, especially those directed toward hard-to-reach men who have sex with men but who do not self-identify as gay and who therefore are not exposed to prevention messages found within gay communities. These venues are frequented by many closeted married and bisexual men who tend to regard themselves as not at risk for HIV because they are not gay.

But is it ethically possible to do such research? I have refrained from applying for support to conduct such research because of the possible negative consequences that could result. In particular, I have agonized over the possibility that such research could call attention to these venues of public sex and thereby lead to restrictive legislation aimed at closing these businesses, which are already under siege in many places by anti-pornography forces. Such an outcome, analogous to the closing of baths, would do more harm than good. Some research, which would be useful under other circumstances, simply cannot be done because of the possible hazardous consequences given the current political conditions.

Prison research. Recently I served on a human subjects review committee which considered a colleague's proposal to study stress among HIV-positive prisoners. Prison research is always fraught with ethical dilemmas because of the difficulty of insuring that participation is truly voluntary. In this instance, the case was made more difficult due to the fact that the facility in which the research was conducted segregated HIV-positive prisoners from others. Should one collaborate with a system that violates prisoners' rights? Would the research increase the stress to which the prisoners were already subjected, thereby perhaps being detrimental to their health? Would the possible findings of this study of the effects of stress warrant the risks inherent in carrying it out?

Research on persons with HIV/AIDS. Doing research among persons with HIV or AIDS is fraught with difficulties. Because of a personal friendship with a man who has chosen to use a stress-reduction strategy, exclusive of medical intervention, to cope with his seropositive status, I have become interested in the effects of this type of coping strategy and have considered doing research with those who have chosen this approach to living with HIV (my proposal to do this research was rejected, I might add). However, one common component of this strategy is to reject participation in all forms of discussion of AIDS issues as a means of keeping AIDS both out of sight and out of mind. Doing research with these individuals would violate a major element in the strategy and, if carried out, except under the tightest of constraints, would be ethically impossible.

There are many difficult ethical issues in this epidemic, but only too rarely are the real ethical issues the ones being addressed by the ethics establishment. Below are some of the things I find highly unethical:

1. doing research that stigmatizes individuals or groups

2. doing shoddy research and making recommendations, on the basis of such work, that cannot be supported

3. supporting any anthropological use of scarce resources for research on issues that do not have serious potential to contribute toward a reduction in human misery (whatever the cause)

4. fighting by scientists over glory and power and interpersonal feuding which prevents common aims from being achieved, and I am not referring here only to the notorious and destructive competitiveness between Gallo and Montagnier — even in anthropology we have seen interpersonal squabbling among AIDS researchers

5. physicians refusing to attend to the sick, whether because of their fears of contracting HIV or of their disdain toward members of populations with large numbers of AIDS cases

6. insurance companies ridding themselves of subscribers with HIV/AIDS or who are perceived to be at high risk for AIDS

7. the failure of our institutions to find ways to assure that the best quality of medical care is available to everyone in the world afflicted by this disease

8. price gouging by pharmaceutical companies, a common phenomenon

9. bureaucratic obstacles of all kinds, those which slow access to promising drugs, those which impede urgent research, and those that prevent the implementation of adequate prevention programmes

10. failing to have an all-out war on AIDS

11. merely documenting the epidemic

Unfortunately, debates over lesser issues serve to distract our attention from the truly immoral actions that are so pervasive in this epidemic. Research-related ethical issues need to be dealt with swiftly because they are inhibiting work that needs to be done; fear of violating traditional ethical standards alone may be preventing needed research and preventing funding agencies from supporting such work.[4]

RETHINKING OUR WORK: GUIDELINES FOR AIDS RESEARCHERS

Based on the preceding discussion, in this section I would like to offer some points which I think we all need to consider as we reflect on what we are doing as anthropologists and as men and women concerned about doing what we can to help end the AIDS pandemic. The list, I hope, may serve as a basis for discussions on how we should proceed with our work.

1. *Be honest.* Be scrupulously honest, especially with the people your work is intended to serve. We have seen too many lies and too much deception during this epidemic. For example, we have told people that using condoms won't reduce their pleasure, a lie that is obvious to any man who has ever used one. Such dishonesty is counterproductive. Yes, be scrupulously honest, but lie through your teeth if you must when dealing with government authorities in order

to get resources to do what must be done. AIDS challenges us to eliminate hypocrisy from our lives, from our science, but AIDS must also embolden us to go to the heart of the matter and to act now; there is no time for anything else. AIDS is a great teacher of the lesson that today counts more than any other: the past cannot be changed, and the future cannot be lived until it arrives, so savour the moment. AIDS should help us to re-order our priorities.

2. *Be courageous.* Cowardice has been rampant during this epidemic, yet we so often see that when courageous people take the lead, the opposition falls like so many paper tigers. I do not wish to underestimate the power of the enemy, of people whose own agendas do not include the goal of ending this disaster; such power is sometimes real, but more often it is imaginary and it feeds on cowardice. I am reminded of such simple projects as having condom machines installed in university bathrooms, where fears of reactions from trustees and parents lead many administrators to oppose the action; in such cases, when concerned members of the communities insisted on having machines installed, they usually won. As the tee-shirt says, 'Just Do It!'

3. *Think carefully about what you do, about your priorities.* Don't waste your precious time. We are too few and there is too much to be done. If we, as anthropologists, are to have much impact, we must choose our work carefully. We are too few in number to waste our energies; perhaps several hundred anthropologists worldwide dealing with AIDS? Unless research informs policy, is it worth doing? Should we do research because there is funding for it even when we know it is not high priority for saving lives?

4. *Protect yourself.* Go out and party! Unless you are a hopelessly Apollonian case, be sure to get your share of ecstatic experience to revitalize your spirit and restore your own well-being. Burnout is a clear danger for all of us who are committed to this battle; protect yourself against it.

5. *Take risks.* We ask people with AIDS (PWAs) to take risks when we give them experimental drugs which may be harmful, and we feel justified in doing so because of the greater good to be derived from finding a cure; we ask health care workers to take some risk in treating patients (however slight that risk may be); we can do no less in taking risks that may involve financial, reputational, and career losses. An important lesson that has been learned during the first decade of AIDS is that without taking risks nothing gets done. By failing to take professional risks we incur an even greater risk, that of losing more of the people we love to this disease.

6. *Be intolerant of irrelevant work.* We need to refuse our support for anthropological research that does not address important practical issues. I recall being on a grants committee for the Social Science Research Council some years ago and being often the lone voice in asking what would be the impact of the study on human lives, on the prospects for improving the quality of life. Anthropology is under attack — a recent issue of the newsletter of the American Anthropological Association discusses this; we have not sold the value of our discipline to the public, and we are reaping the consequences. In hard times we get cut as a result and others who control funding for research do not take us seriously. We are hampered by our decades of focus on the exotic and esoteric, by our reputation for being specialists on trivial and irrelevant subjects. Changing this situation will require that we systematically discourage research on topics with no practical implications.

7. *Refrain from doing any work that further stigmatizes or revictimizes persons with HIV or groups perceived as being at high risk for AIDS.* In all of our work, we should be doing whatever we can to eliminate the stigma that attaches to people with HIV/AIDS and to many of the populations which have suffered the most to date from this epidemic or who are blamed for the spread of AIDS, e.g., intravenous drug users, gay men, people of colour, and sex workers.

8. *Do work that emancipates and empowers, work that builds community.* Anything that isolates the individual and reduces human interaction is to be discouraged. Do not lend your support to such actions. Instead, we should be working to strengthen the communities of the people with whom we work. The Norwegian government, for example, provided broad support to gay organizations for activities in addition to those directly related to AIDS prevention on the wise proposition that strong communities would be more successful in doing prevention work than would communities in disarray. It is such enlightened policies that our work should bolster.

9. *Keep uppermost in mind the audience you intend to reach.* Think carefully about the intended audience for your work. In this connection, I think we would be wise to work as closely as possible with individuals and organizations (NGOs) on the front lines in the battle against AIDS, either in designing and implementing prevention programmes or in developing programmes of assistance to people with HIV/AIDS. We should be producing work that is useful to them. For some of our work, the primary audience should be policymakers and those who influence them, even though I'm sceptical about the prospects that they will actually listen to us. Do NOT write primarily

for professional anthropologists. Of course, we need to share our results with each other, but if that is all we do, we will have no impact on this epidemic.

10. *Work where you can be most effective.* The job we face is enormous and the options on where to concentrate our work are varied. I strongly suggest that we should devote our energies to working as much as possible in our own communities, in those situations where we have the greatest impact. If you are gay, then work among gay men, for example. If you are a specialist on Thailand, then work on AIDS in that country. In view of the urgency to implement solutions, time is too short for you to build up expertise on a population with which you are not already thoroughly familiar. And the last thing we need is to have instant specialists trying out their ideas on cultures on which they are fundamentally ignorant.

11. *Work in partnership with your intended beneficiaries.* As a corollary to point 8, we all should be working as closely as possible with agencies and communities who will be using the results of our research. It is their agendas and needs which should drive ours, not vice versa.

12. *Always remember that lives are at stake.* In contrast with 99 per cent of anthropological work, your work may save lives or it may kill. It is important to keep in mind that your work may have a significant impact. This is not an academic game aimed purely at entertaining and enlightening yourself and a few colleagues. It's the real world.

13. *Get it right the first time!* And as a corollary to point 12, do only first-class work. AIDS is a case where what we say may matter; it may mean the difference between life and death. Wrong messages based on bad research should constitute scientific malpractice. Perhaps we need to propose that social scientists be subject to threats of class-action malpractice suits to keep them from doing harm, to force them to behave responsibly, and to stop creating hazardous wastes in the form of research that is poorly designed and executed or in the form of recommendations not backed by evidence that meets rigorous quality standards.

14. *Radicalize your thinking, break free from constraints, be creative.* AIDS research has been exceedingly cautious and conservative. 'Normal science' may lead to incremental advances in knowledge and understanding, but truly revolutionary solutions are more likely to emerge from creative departures from orthodoxy. Serendipitous discoveries cannot be forced, but we can encourage them by being

sceptical of received wisdom and by being open to radical alternatives to conventional approaches.

15. *Cast a wider theoretical net.* Too much research on AIDS has been derived from a limited range of theoretical possibilities. This is true in both the biomedical and the behavioural spheres. There is grave danger inherent in too quickly restricting research efforts to a few dominant paradigms which may prove to lead to dead ends. It is crucial that we entertain a wide array of theoretical options on many of the issues that confront us.

16. *Contribute your services to those engaged in political action.* It should be obvious to everyone that political pressure and political pressure alone produces significant progress in this epidemic. Think of such issues as access to experimental drugs, funding for AIDS research and prevention programmes, and reductions in pharmaceutical prices. We should be offering our talents as researchers to activist organizations in an effort to assist them in being effective.

17. *Don't tolerate shoddy work.* I recall reading an article produced by a project in which I was a subject; an elaborate discussion of the causes of risky behaviour was offered in which the only measure of risk was number of partners. I called one of the authors to complain and was told she didn't really approve of the report; I talked to another man at the project who disclaimed responsibility even though he was a co-author and who said he too had objected; he volunteered that the primary authors were erotophobic and homophobic, and this explained their emphasis on the concept of number of partners. But why hadn't these people stopped the publication? One of them even told me that her name was listed as a co-author despite her reservations simply because the contribution of her agency to the project had to be acknowledged through co-authorship. We must do everything possible to protest the production and publication of work that fails to meet acceptable scientific standards, especially when that work has the potential to have a disastrous impact on public policies related to AIDS.

18. *Question everything.*

CONCLUSION

By now, I assume that I have angered almost everyone by something I have said. If I haven't then this talk is a loss. What we need is a lot more anger and passion. If your anger induces you to reflect about what you are doing, then I will have done my job. To attenuate your anger just a bit, however, so that you will attend to the message and not kill the messenger, let me assure you that these criticisms are directed as much at myself as they are at my colleagues (Bolton n.d.). I would also note that there are important exceptions to my criticisms of anthropological praxis during this epidemic; the exceptions give hope that we might anticipate more worthy research by anthropologists in the near future.

Let me say that I am grateful to this epidemic for very little; but one thing I am grateful for, and that is the opportunity it has given me to meet some truly special people among colleagues who are working on AIDS, many of whom are in this audience. Their commitment has been a source of inspiration and their friendship extremely meaningful. It is because of that friendship and our mutual dedication to this cause that I can risk offending you, and because you are the only hope we have. I do continue to have faith in the potential of this group of scholars to have an impact on the course of this tragedy. Moreover, let me acknowledge that most of what I have learned during this epidemic, other than what I have learned from seropositive friends and informants, I have learned from you.

In closing, I must apologize for the overwhelmingly critical and pessimistic tone. Perhaps this stems from an approaching burnout, or from an anxiety born of knowledge that I may not have the strength and will to persist as this epidemic comes closer and closer to my loved ones; others of you have been affected even more brutally, you have had loved ones die in your arms, you have ministered to the sick, and your courage is inspirational. For others, though, this may still be a disease of 'the other,' of drug users when you are not one, of people in Third World countries or in poverty-stricken enclaves in urban America when you are not from there. But for gay men, regardless of serostatus, we witness this from the inside as we watch our communities struggle valiantly against this threat, communities whose unity and very existence have been forged in the fires of sexual ecstasy, societal oppression, and now the spectre of death.

NOTES

1. Since this article is based on an oral presentation and to save space, I have dispensed, for the most part, with standard scholarly practice of including citations to publications which illustrate or elaborate on the points I am making. The reader, I hope, will forgive this omission in view of the primary goal of this presentation, i.e., to stimulate discus-

sion rather than to 'prove' the correctness of my arguments. Further, since my work on AIDS has been carried out in the United States and Western Europe, the issues I raise in this talk necessarily reflect my assessment of the situation in these countries, with special emphasis on the US. My conclusions may or may not apply to the work of anthropologists in the Third World. I hope they do not.

2. For the past five or six years, one of the roles I have played is that of bibliographer of the anthropological literature on AIDS, publishing in 1991 a bibliography which has been updated quarterly in the *AIDS & Anthropology Bulletin* of the AIDS & Anthropology Research Group. The original publication runs to 35 pages, but this may suggest an exaggerated productivity since my co-authors and I included in that publication anthropologically relevant publications by other social scientists and also unpublished papers (Bolton, with Lewis and Orozco 1991). Recently we had occasion to prepare a more realistic version of the bibliography restricted to published anthropological writings; it is much more modest (Bolton 1992c). What this suggests is that after a slow start (Bolton 1989) there is now a lot of professional activity on AIDS, but the research is not getting into print very fast. I am puzzled by the reasons for this. Perhaps we will see an explosion of articles shortly, but I doubt it. Perhaps there are few outlets for this work. Certainly most of the major, specialized AIDS journals, with their emphasis on biomedical and epidemiological research, are not suitable for or sympathetic to the publication of ethnographic analyses. Is it that we don't go on to complete our writings and our analyses once they are presented as conference papers? Norris Lang and I issued a call for papers for a special issue of a journal to be devoted to AIDS in the Third World; yet we received only three submissions and had to cancel the effort.

3. The best anthropological paper on prevention through safe sex promotion is one by Clark Taylor and his associate, David Lourea (1992). Taylor's work is not funded, of course, although he has received some support from companies that produce lubricants and condoms. Pharmaceutical companies are not likely to be interested in prevention, nor it would appear are governments if prevention means being sex-positive; they would seem to prefer seropositivity to sex-positivity. We might hire sex experts to do sex research and education. We should fire the health educators; nay, I'd go further to suggest that we round most of them up and put them on a Nuremburg-style trial for their complicity in promoting genocidal prevention messages such as reduce your number of partners, get tested, and know your partner. Those who have promoted sex-negative, fear-mongering approaches to prevention have blood on their hands.

4. I recently watched a documentary about the Tuskegee experiment in which one of the doctors involved still could not see that there was

anything wrong with the work he did as part of that project, which in retrospect seems to us totally reprehensible. May it serve as a warning, that a generation from now, what we are doing in this epidemic may also be viewed as having been morally indefensible. To document this epidemic, to serve as the body counters, or, even worse, the sexual accountants, instead of doing what needs to be done to stop this epidemic may be the moral equivalent of letting people with syphilis progress to advanced stages rather than intervene to cure them, all in the name of science. We have known what needs to be done since very early on in this epidemic, and we have sat back and watched it grow. It may be that when the full horror of this tragedy is over, the ethical standards by which we will be judged will not be those which currently prevail, at least not as narrowly construed by so many professional ethicists.

REFERENCES

Bayer, R. 1992. As the Second Decade of AIDS Begins: An International Perspective on the Ethics of the Epidemic. *AIDS* 6:527–532.

Bolton, R. 1989. Introduction: The AIDS Pandemic: A Global Emergency. In: *The AIDS Pandemic: A Global Emergency*, edited by R. Bolton. New York: Gordon and Breach.

Bolton, R. 1992a. AIDS and Promiscuity: Muddles in the Models of HIV Prevention. In: *Rethinking AIDS Prevention: Cultural Approaches*, edited by R. Bolton and M. Singer. Philadelphia: Gordon and Breach Science Publishers.

Bolton, R. 1992b. Mapping Terra Incognita: Sex Research for AIDS Prevention — An Urgent Agenda for the 1990s. In: *The Time of AIDS: Social Analysis, Theory, and Method*, edited by G. Herdt and S. Lindenbaum. Newbury Park, CA: Sage Publications.

Bolton, R. 1992c. Selected Publications on AIDS by Anthropologists. In: *The Anthropology of AIDS: Syllabi and Other Teaching Materials*, edited by R. Bolton and E. Kempler. Washington, DC: American Anthropological Association, AIDS and Anthropology Task Force.

Bolton, R. 1995. Coming Home: The Journey of a Gay Ethnographer in the Years of the Plague. In: *Doing Lesbian and Gay Ethnography: Anthropologists Reflect on Fieldwork, Writing, and Representation*, edited by E. Lewin and W. Leap. Champagne: University of Illinois Press. Forthcoming.

Bolton, R., M. Lewis, and G. Orozco. 1991. AIDS Literature for Anthropologists: A Working Bibliography. Anthropology, Sexuality, and AIDS, edited by G. Herdt, W. Leap, and M. Sovine. *Journal of Sex Research* 28(2): 307–346. Special Issue.

Camus, A. 1972. *The Plague*. New York: Vintage Books.

Farmer, P. 1992. New Disorder, Old Dilemmas: AIDS and Anthropology in Haiti. In: *The Time of AIDS: Social Analysis, Theory, and Method*, edited by G. Herdt and S. Lindenbaum. Newbury Park, CA: Sage Publications.

Frankenberg, R. 1988. AIDS and Anthropologists. *Anthropology Today* 4(2):13–15.

Herdt, G. 1987. AIDS and Anthropology. *Anthropology Today* 3(2):3–5.

Herdt, G., and A. Boxer. 1991. Ethnographic Issues in the Study of AIDS. Anthropology, Sexuality, and AIDS, edited by G. Herdt, W. Leap, and M. Sovine. *Journal of Sex Research* 28(2):171–187. Special Issue.

Parker, R., and M. Carballo. 1990. Qualitative Research on Homosexual and Bisexual Behavior Relevant to HIV/AIDS. *Journal of Sex Research* 27(4): 497–525.

Taylor, C.L., and D. Lourea. 1992. HIV Prevention: A Dramaturgical Analysis and Practical Guide to Creating Safer Sex Interventions. In: *Rethinking AIDS Prevention: Cultural Approaches*, edited by R. Bolton and M. Singer. Philadelphia: Gordon and Breach Science Publishers.

Chapter SIXTEEN

Half-Way There: Anthropology and Intervention-Oriented AIDS Research in KwaZulu/Natal, South Africa

E.M. Preston-Whyte

This chapter deals with a number of the concerns which emerged from the papers and ensuing discussions at the Amsterdam Conference on 'Culture, Sexual Behavior, and AIDS' upon which this volume is based. Many of those present expressed a commitment not only to study, but to become involved in ameliorating the ravages of a disease which they had experienced both as researchers and as the friends and lovers of people who were suffering from, and had died from the disease. The anguish and anger of the opening addresses set the tone for the conference, and in his concluding remarks, Richard Parker positioned the anthropological response to AIDS in the long, chequered, and controversial history of anthropology as an applied discipline. There was no doubt as to his chosen course of action: intervention and a total commitment of skill and professional insight to the struggle against HIV and AIDS. That he found the current state of theory and method in the study of human sexuality in relation to the task of AIDS intervention wanting, epitomizes the challenge which he argued faces the discipline of anthropology in the decade to come.

Parker's sentiments were echoed by other speakers and a start was made to meet his challenge by a number of papers which reported on what may be conveniently labelled 'action anthropology' in the field of AIDS intervention. Most were using forms of participatory research aimed both at behavioural change in high-risk sexual behaviour — into which category this chapter falls — and in the exploration of community responses to death and dying as a result of AIDS in different cultural and structural settings.

The context of the research reported here is Southern Africa, and my comments arise from the experience of AIDS research in the African community of KwaZulu/Natal. The discussion has two major objectives. First to suggest why and how 'traditional' anthropological methods of qualitative research can be developed as a basis for AIDS intervention, and, second, to indicate some of the problems which such a course of action will surely entail. While the discussion is committed to intervention, it raises a number of caveats about the uncritical acceptance of intervention as a legitimate and necessary aim of anthropology and questions, in particular, some of the solutions which characterize much interventionist anthropology of the metropole.

The last point surfaced on a number of occasions at the conference in the guise of calls that 'local voices' — that is perspectives representative of places other than Europe and the United States of America — be heard in the AIDS debate. One way for this to be achieved is for anthropologists to work not so much with (for we have always done this) as *in partnership* with local people to develop appropriate strategies for intervention. The argument is advanced here that the traditional research methodology of anthropology, based on the qualitative techniques of participant observation and in-depth ethnographic interviewing, is already 'half-way' to achieving this goal. Although the specific locale, and to a large extent, the cultural context of my remarks are unique, the claims for anthropology and particularly action anthropology in the field of AIDS echo other intervention studies, and specifically the work of the CONNAIS-SIDA Project in Zaïre (Schoepf et al. 1992, and in this volume). More significant, much the same research experience and success with adapted qualitative techniques has been reported from very different cultural contexts; witness the work of Worth (1989) among poor inner city American women drug users and partners of drug-dependent men.

Yet another theme to dominate the conference was that 'living with' HIV and AIDS is a more appropriate form of discourse than 'dying' from AIDS. This sentiment was poignantly expressed in the personal tributes offered to friends and colleagues struck down by the HIV virus. It was here that anger and anguish surfaced and the introspection of 'insiders' studying their own condition provided the key to understanding and, perhaps, expiation. Expressed most clearly in relation to the community of men who have sex with men and epitomized by the opening address given by Ralph Bolton, and in the already large European and American anthropological literature (Patton 1990; Illingworth 1990; Herdt and Lindenbaum 1992) on the topic, it seems inevitable that similar anger and introspection will characterize both the experience and research of anthropologists as the heterosexual spread of HIV and AIDS takes the centre stage of the pandemic. The lesson of the Western response to AIDS is that the impetus for change and coping is precipitated by this anger. In the case of women as lovers and mothers, as well as the sufferers and transmitters of the disease, anger will have to be tempered with the strength to cope not only personally and within relationships with lovers and friends, but within the family and community context.

'LOCAL VOICES' OR THE CULTURAL CONTEXT

In most poor Third World situations, living with HIV and AIDS will be done without the benefit of the medical and health infrastructure taken for granted in the West (Barnett and Blaikie 1992). The challenge of the next decade in Third World countries is not one to medical and interventionist behavioural science alone, but to community response on the part of one and all — men, women, children, the old and the young, leaders and followers, rich and poor, educated and uneducated. In Africa, for instance, AIDS is 'everyone's' problem but, as Elizabeth Ngugi (1992) and others have pointed out, in Africa this usually means in practice that women bear the brunt of day-to-day risk and coping (Ankrah 1991; Bassett and Mhloyi 1991). It is here that intervention research in the field of AIDS will overlap with applied anthropology in the field of socio-economic development and the empowerment of minorities. It will also, as this chapter shows, face issues of gender and development which are in turn the counter of local-level and village politics in many developing countries.

Coping with the epidemic outside Europe and America and particularly the nature of appropriate preventative strategies was an important theme introduced at the conference by anthropologists representing what might once have been 'the other' — people of cultures very different of the West. The call, initiated by Christine Obbo, but echoed by Michael Tan, was for 'local voices' to be heard: the answers which the West advocates — and the use of condoms as the primary protective mechanism was mentioned specifically — may not suit other cultures, and the imperialism of the West echoes hollowly in the villages of rural Africa and Asia.

How are these 'local voices' to be heard and, more important, how are they to make themselves felt in their own countries and, often more to the point, in the consciousness of international donor and health aid agencies? It is clear that the intervention of foreign anthropologists is not needed to bring to light items of culture which are relevant for AIDS intervention — these are no mystery and exist in popular consciousness as 'local knowledge' in the sense used by Geertz (1983). It is a matter rather of persuading the West and, in particular, those in decision-making positions in the international health arena that local cultures have something to offer in the fight against AIDS. It is here that local anthropologists have a role to play: that of scribe and interpreter, the go-between or culture broker (Wolf 1956; Geertz 1959), whose task it is to translate local cultures not only to overseas donor agencies, but to the medical profession whose own culture is not sympathetic to what is regarded as the irrationalities of a non-scientific world view.

But the path of the anthropologist as culture broker is fraught with danger: even when it is local anthropologists who are involved, it is but a small step from being the handmaiden of colonialism (Asad 1973) to being the tool of aid agencies and governments. Both Frankenberg (1992) and Clatts (1992, and in this volume) offered timely warnings in this direction, albeit from Western experience. The burden of their argument is that 'culture' usually means something very different to anthropologists and non-anthropologists: to the latter and particularly those in positions of power 'culture' is a convenient catch-all, a universal explanation for the apparent irrationality demonstrated by the failure of people to comply with what is regarded as 'best' for them; anthropologists are often employed to get around just such 'cultural problems.' When they take the side of the apparently irrational local culture they are replaced by more amenable social scientists — such as sociologists and psychologists — who share the world view of those holding the purse strings. Frankenberg (1992:8) made an elegant appeal to his colleagues to attempt the almost impossible:

> Culture has come out. It is too late to drive it back into the closet....
> Like other comings-out ... there is no guarantee of subsequent materialization of desired outcomes. Anthropologists need to educate themselves and others about the use of so power laden a concept.

The first step in this direction is to resist not only the oversimplification but the reification of culture. Culture is not an immutable fact and it is certainly not a simple (or even a complex) variable which can be programmed into a universal (or even a local) model. It is mutable and it can be changed — witness the events of this century — but changes have consequences, and in the fight against AIDS in Third World situations, it is with a world already beset by change and transformation that anthropologists are dealing. It is also a world of dependency and powerlessness. Culture in Africa inheres not only in local custom but in the realities of political economy: the presence of international aid agencies continues the colonial encounter.[1]

Instead of reifying particular items of culture, the holistic anthropological perspective conceptualizes local cultures and cultural items as part of a dynamic and often complex set of historically determined structural features which constrain action and interaction. At one level local knowledge may claim to explain the acceptance of many sexual partners as 'part of our culture' or as a 'legacy of polygyny,' but at another level the need for more than one lover is part of the political economy of contemporary survival in both emotional and financial terms. The complexity of these intertwined levels of cultural explanation are well illustrated by an examination of AIDS and HIV in the local situation of KwaZulu/Natal.

THE RESEARCH CONTEXT OF THE ARGUMENT

Prior to 1987 HIV infection in the heterosexual population of South Africa was absent or rare. It is now spreading in all race groups although the epidemic is at a more advanced stage among African South Africans with a generally higher prevalence appearing among African women in comparison with African men. Teenagers are at high risk; those most affected fall into the 15 to 44 age category with infection from mother to baby giving increasing cause for concern

(S.S. Abdool Karim et al. 1992). Although infection in Kwa-Zulu/Natal falls into this general pattern, there are indications that the epidemic is advancing particularly rapidly in this region with the incidence of HIV-1 infection being highest in the 15 to 25 age group.[2]

A detailed breakdown of the KwaZulu/Natal survey results to mid-1991 shows differential infection in terms of both age and sex. Within six months the prevalence of infection rose from 1.6 per cent to 3.6 per cent in the 15 to 19 age group, suggesting that 2 per cent of all the people surveyed between these ages became infected with HIV in the six months between November/December 1990 and June/July 1991. An analysis of the 1990 figures showed the male infection rate to be 0.6 per and the female rate 1.6 per cent. Even given the fact that the absence of male migrants from the area surveyed resulted in an under-representation of men in the sample, these are startling figures and indicate the risk to which women are subject. Read in combination with the statistics on age, it is clear that the vertical transmission of HIV from mother to unborn child is likely to grow. It is in interpreting and explaining individual risk that an appreciation of the major features of the cultural context become important.

Although intravenous drug use is minimal and gay relationships are not characteristic of the African community, multi-partner sex between men and women is the norm. While people wish their partners (and this includes spouses and long-term lovers) did not have sex relations with other people, few are confident on this score. Women accept that men have other partners and although they may react violently to evidence of this, they seldom end the relationship on this score — or even consider that they have the grounds for doing so. Men aver that women should not have other partners, but, on the evidence of their own experience, admit that many do. It is not that there is an acceptance of permissiveness — merely that sex is a common counter in the interaction of men and women and is accepted pragmatically. Pre- and extramarital sex are censured by the Christian churches, and parents try to insist that daughters remain chaste until marriage. Since there is less emphasis on socializing boys in this ideal, and male sexuality is generally valued and openly encouraged by peers and older men, their success is limited and sexual intercourse is initiated from twelve or thirteen years of age (Preston-Whyte and Zondi 1991, 1992).

It requires but little specific anthropological insight to point to the features of the macro environment which operate against sexual exclusivity — politics and poverty are the bottom line. Apartheid has separated spouses for decades, institutionalizing multi-sex partnerships in which migrants with wives in the country set up relationships with women in town, and poor women in both urban and rural areas depend on sex to earn money for survival. As the current violence and its accompanying lawlessness and social disruption has spread, sex has become the counter of female survival in a more immediate sense. Many women are forced to submit to male sexual demands in order to avoid violence and death; the kin and neighbourhood networks, which once provided a safety net against this type of exploitation, have been disrupted in many areas. Sexually transmitted diseases (STDs) abound and are not controlled by the limited health services available. Girls and boys follow their parents into multi-partner sexual lifestyles which inevitably result in high levels of STD infection among the youth which follow them into adult life. This trend is as evident from the study of STD clinic registers today as it was forty years ago when first reported in the medical literature on Southern Africa (Kark 1948).[3]

Of the relatively few men who have had experience of condoms, most have used them as part of the treatment for STDs rather than as part of normal sex. Those who, in response to the current AIDS scare, have begun to use condoms, do so with casual and non-marital partners rather than with wives. Very few women in town and fewer in the country have seen condoms, but most accept the negative stereotypes about them which abound — that they cut down sensation, are disliked by men, and, worst, get lodged in the vagina. As talk about condoms grows, misconceptions proliferate. One of the latest going the rounds blames contraceptives themselves for the spread of AIDS; another whispers that because the condom holds bodily fluids, its use plays into the hands of sorcerers. With such a bad press it is hardly surprising that condom use is not widespread, and this situation of neglect and suspicion is as characteristic of the youth as it is of older people (S.S. Abdool Karim et al. 1992). There is more to it than this, however. As in many Third World situations, poverty and insecurity ensure a high value being placed on fertility and children (Caldwell 1982; Caldwell, Caldwell, and Orubuloye 1990), while mistrust of the ruling white regime has made all forms of contraception suspect for years (Abdool Karim, Preston-Whyte, and Abdool Karim 1992a, 1992b).

Yet another level of understanding needs to be fed into the situation of macro deprivation and political mistrust: the personal motivation of individuals and the meaning they assign to sex. We are only now beginning to explore this complex and sensitive area, but previous anthropological work has suggested that sex cannot be understood in isolation from the paramount importance placed by most people on fertility and the birth of children. I have argued elsewhere (Preston-Whyte and Zondi 1992) that, whatever the circumstances, both women and men welcome the birth of a child and children are valued even when born outside marriage — as is the case in as high as 70 per cent of births in the African community. Fertility overrides sexual control and exclusivity, opening the way for birth and marriage to be effectively dissociated in much contemporary practice. Taken together with high bridewealth payments which accompany (de Haas 1987) and often serve to delay marriage, this leads to birth and sex outside marriage being accepted pragmatically.

The above means, in turn, that the pressure to prevent pregnancy is not strong; the major candidates for contraception are older women who have children and younger women for whom pregnancy may mean the loss of employment or the end of professional training. This is the situation, however, of only a very small minority of young women. For most the chances of post-school education and more than the least skilled of jobs is slim and the birth of a baby seems neither a problem nor 'the end of the world.' Indeed, it may be attractive, and this, in turn, makes contraception seem unattractive and unnecessary. For women who do choose contraception, the most usual methods are the pill and injection, both of which can be taken without the knowledge of men and which it has been the policy of state contraceptive services to promote. In the context of AIDS the role of the condom in preventing birth is highly problematic. While it may not inhibit the very young, it will certainly stay the hand of both men and women who believe that birth is part and parcel of sexual and social fulfilment and a sine qua non for the achievement of human maturity. This leads directly to issues of gender and differences in the perception, of men and women and of older and younger women, of the advantages and disadvantages of condom use. It is here that the importance of local cultural meanings is evident, as is the need for 'local voices' to be heard. It means also that no single strategy for promoting 'safe sex' will suffice; different strategies designed to suit the heterogeneous population will be necessary, and these, being highly specific, will need to be based on detailed and nuanced research. In the next section of this chapter I explore the potential of anthropological methods in producing this type of information and intervention.

ANTHROPOLOGY: LISTENING TRANSLATED
INTO ACTION?

It is anthropologists more than most social scientists who have developed and internalized the skill of listening to what people are saying, of sinking into the community and following the often tortuous web of cultural explanation and behaviour. The ethnographic method is based on intensive and long-term interaction between researcher and research participants, in-depth interviewing with individuals and small groups seeking to map nuances of cultural meaning, and, above all, an emphasis on building mutual trust between researchers and their research communities. 'Being there,' in the sense of living and participating in the community of study, has always been the distinguishing feature (and the essential rite of passage) of anthropology and it is this we believe that allows us to observe behaviour as well as discuss beliefs and attitudes. In facing the AIDS crisis these features of the normal anthropological approach to research can be profitably used to lay the foundation for the development of successful intervention programmes. The title of this chapter — half-way there — attempts to capture this point.

What is implied is that the in-depth knowledge and understanding which 'being there' brings, and the rapport which long-term involvement with people develops, puts researchers in an ideal position to pursue intervention work. 'Being there' also allows for the monitoring of the progress and success of particular intervention strategies for it allows a check to be kept on changes in attitudes and meaning, and on reactions to, in this case, the inevitable progress of illness, death and accommodations to the stark realities of life and living with AIDS.

HALF-WAY THERE?

Put simply, I suggest that the closeness of the relationship which anthropologists establish with their research participants, and which is necessary for the interactive exploration of cultural meaning and process, can be used and extended for the mutual exploration and creation of *new* meanings, some of which may be successful in changing behaviour to meet the AIDS crisis.

What traditional anthropology does well is allow researcher and research participant to visualize together, and so together understand, the mechanics of the present. On the basis of this, it is, I believe, possible for them to project what 'could be' in the future.

Together, researcher and research participant would engage in what might be termed the 'imaginative (re)creation' of the future and could, in doing this, be 'half way' to bringing about change. The trust and, I suspect, the intellectual satisfaction on both sides, without which cultural understanding is impossible, can thus be used as a springboard for discovering how best to proceed with intervention. This may, in its turn, prove to be, to use the discourse of action-research (Whyte 1991), empowering for both parties.

While my argument is that the traditional techniques of anthropology (and in particular what is often referred to as the 'ethnographic method') lay an ideal foundation for exploring possible interventions, I am also aware that they may need to be extended and broadened in some directions. If intervention is to be long lasting, new and innovative interactive strategies need to be pioneered, and in this we may look fruitfully at the techniques of related disciplines. Here I report specifically on collaboration between anthropology and drama — but I think that there are many other possibilities. What is important, I suggest, is that in seeking to intervene, anthropologists agree to move outside and extend their traditional methodology. With any such move, however, problems of a practical and, in the case of AIDS, an ethical nature, are inevitable. Before discussing some of these I will describe briefly three multidisciplinary research projects which have been undertaken in KwaZulu/Natal and which I believe illustrate the advantages of the research strategy outlined above.

AIDS RESEARCH IN KWAZULU/NATAL

A major focus of attention of all three projects has been the influence of gender issues in the spread of HIV infection and the risks to which women and adolescents, in particular, are open. The first study comprised a preliminary experiment in qualitative AIDS research designed to generate a questionnaire on condom use for administration in urban African schools. As a result of the problems encountered with translation and administration, it was decided to abandon the original idea of a large-scale survey in favour of smaller in-depth and group interviews. A number of the insights discussed below come from the research team's early experience of exploring both the ideational and behavioural aspects of adolescent sexuality (S.S. Abdool Karim et al. 1992). The second was a four-month pilot study for AIDS intervention in rural schools using drama lessons and performance as the point of entry and contact with the children (Dalrymple 1991;

Dalrymple and Preston-Whyte 1992). The third study aimed to assess the ability of African women to protect themselves from HIV infection and included the piloting of some preliminary intervention strategies.[4] The fieldwork was carried out by a number of researchers, some of whom are graduates in anthropology, under the direction of team leaders, of whom two out of six are anthropologists.[5] The others were medical doctors and an epidemiologist. Fieldwork was conducted in three areas, a rural community, an informal shack settlement, and in a black suburb of urban Durban. The major field techniques were individual and group interviews combined with an adapted form of participant observation on the part of those team members who were living in their study communities. In addition to the social scientists on the team, we recruited and trained a number of local people to assist both in the initial research and in the pilot interventions. The intention is that these community-based researchers will continue the work either formally (if they can be attached to health services) or informally after the research period is over and that the project will thus leave its intervention strategies well rooted in the communities concerned. Where appropriate, we worked through and with the structures of local community government, informing and gaining the backing of influential community leaders at all stages of the research. Since many of the latter were men, this strategy served to draw men as well as women into all phases of the study.

Talking about sex. Our first surprise was the willingness shown by young and old, men and women, uneducated and professional, to talk about sex. When introduced via the topic of AIDS, they opened up and discussed their own sexual experiences and their perceptions of those of their peers. This has occurred both in individual interviews and in group sessions. The reticence we anticipated has not fully materialized, and herein lies an important lesson for intervention. The fear and concern engendered by AIDS has to a large extent broken down barriers to discussing sex — if the discussion *is* within the AIDS arena. More important, this openness in discussing sex can be put to good use in intervention. Handled with care, discussions of sex may help to alter people's attitudes to, and assumptions about, sexual behaviour. Let me explore this possibility with a concrete example.

Young black girls, who invariably began by stating that they could not see their way clear to argue with their lovers about condom use, have come to realize through group interaction (involving both the group leaders and each other), that such a stance *is* possible. They may even, through sharing experiences, begin to get the courage to 'try' themselves and to suggest, on the basis of their experiences, how they and others might go about insisting on 'safe sex.' I believe that the very experience of being able to talk about sex, sometimes with other girls, but, more critically, in groups which combine girls and boys, helps to break down the cultural inhibitions which have made it impossible for them to discuss sex with their partners. They may also move towards being able to negotiate the use of condoms or reduction of partners. Eventually what is afoot is the development of new patterns of action. Here I believe we and our research participants work together in (re)creating the future and contributing to the invention of alternative patterns of sexual interaction and, possibly, the giving of new meanings to old ones.

The above may present an overly optimistic view — getting people to talk about sex may simply mean that they voice stereotypes or engage in discussions at a fairly superficial level, reserving to themselves their 'real' opinions and 'gut reactions.' Just as problematic is the fact that we do not ordinarily have adequate vocabularies for discussing much sexual activity. Intercourse (of all sorts) is something which is done rather than spoken about. In fact it is often what is *not* said which is important and it is the forms of nonverbal communication which need to be tracked. How, when we cannot expect to observe the relevant behaviour, are we to come up with the information? It is here that we have to be 'methodologically' inventive, as indeed the work of Coxon (1988, and in this volume) and of Henriksson and Månsson (in this volume) demonstrate.

'Talking about' sex has yet another inherent problem: sex is not a topic normally verbalized in precise terms. Both the sex act itself and its preliminaries are often shrouded in inexact 'cover words,' jokes, or vulgar or obscene language. The women in our studies reported that little discussion occurred between them and their sexual partners on the topic of intercourse itself. In order to talk about sex we may have to teach people a vocabulary which is largely new to them — and which so far has been often drawn from medical discourse. Does this 'new language' in fact distance people further from the reality of action? Alternatively it could, perhaps, be argued that this new language is in a sense 'liberating' in that it (hopefully) might supersede the constraints of the previously gender-based discourse which has moulded sexual interaction. In this way space might be opened up for a new kind of personal introspection and (as important) interpersonal negotiation.

Participation and demands for intervention. The second surprise which we encountered in our research was that the people we interviewed turned the tables on us and began to take over the interviews. *They* wanted answers about AIDS and HIV and were not willing to be passive informants. Our first intimation of this was in the work in schools when we were inundated with eager questions from the pupils we had come to 'interview.' They clamoured for information and would not let the fieldworkers leave the classroom without some response. In the case of the condom study in urban schools it was fortunate that the interviewers were trained medical personnel who could answer most of the pupils' questions. Although the research had not been designed as an intervention project, we decided that the seriousness of the AIDS threat presented an ethical obligation to provide our research participants with the correct medical facts. Almost without realizing it we were drawn into the beginnings of intervention when we ended each interview with an information session which often turned into an informed discussion. These sessions, in themselves, proved invaluable sources of information as those present assimilated and commented upon the information we brought them.

In contrast to the condom study, many of the researchers in the drama project were medically unprepared for the questions which the pupils fired at them and the first crisis we faced as a research team was to arrange hasty medical briefings. We decided to explain to people that we needed to know what they thought, even if it was incorrect, and that we would return with the answers to their questions. As in the condom study these information sessions turned into group discussions and we encouraged the teenagers to voice their fears and opinions, not only about AIDS and HIV, but about courting and sex in general. Later we used the same technique of open discussion to evaluate the impact of the drama programme which we were developing. In fact, the pupils became part of the research process itself as they contributed both their views and their reactions to the programme as it developed.

More than this: our informants, young and old, have begun to interact with us and from them came what we soon realized were often sensible suggestions as to how to deal with the threat of HIV infection. Our 'informants' soon became research participants in the fullest sense of the term. As they have become more and more willing to explore their understandings of both HIV and the ways in which it is spread, and might be contained, they have become participants in the research and initiators in the thrust taken by intervention.

Almost immediately people began also to ask if we could provide them with condoms. In the case of youngsters at school this presented us with a dilemma. What would be the reaction of parents and teachers to condoms being made readily available? Was it ethical for us to distribute condoms without the agreement of parents? We suggested that condoms be obtained from the local clinic — only to be told that they had run out — which we verified. Some of the youngsters also confided that they were embarrassed to go to the clinic for condoms, while others pointed out that they had to travel great distances from either work or home to visit a clinic. Could we refuse help when it was asked? What use was our programme if people who wanted condoms could not get them?

At this point we made a decision to make condoms available to all the people who contributed to our research. In the case of the early studies this was not always possible, as we had not negotiated such a controversial move with the principals of the schools before we began the research. In the drama project we gave a supply of condoms to the school principal for distribution by the teachers. This did not prove a success as we later found that the condoms had not reached the pupils. We then arranged for a supply to be given to the school nurse for distribution on request.

The provision of condoms has now become part of the research strategy of all our projects. We ask all people who receive them to report on how they fared with introducing them into sexual encounters. Just such a technique for collecting 'hard' data on the problems encountered in using condoms had been part of the research proposal for the third study, but we had been unsure how to get it underway. In fact, the initiative came from our research participants, many of whom are now enthusiastically 'trying' and reporting both successes and failures.

Action: trying to influence others to change. Some of our research participants have taken us yet further along the road to intervention, and it is here that both we and they have looked to interactive strategies not normally part of the anthropologists' tool kit. I was drawn into the school drama experiment as an adviser on qualitative research methodology when the project leader realised that little was known about the sexual practices and attitudes of the children who were to be the focus of study. In turn I learnt from the drama team how to go about participating with the children in learning the 'facts' about AIDS — but it was the children and their teachers who showed us how to make the message meaningful to them and their community.

It was planned that the children in the school, after having seen a play produced on AIDS by the drama team, should devise their own play. They were given drama lessons and time was set aside for rehearsals in class. Eventually the enthusiasm made it possible for the play to be produced at an open day to which parents, teachers, and community leaders were invited. This was suggested by the school principal and was an overwhelming success, not least because teachers and pupils translated the AIDS message into their own terms, devising new words to local songs (many used in the context of coming-of-age ceremonies) and combining the whole within the framework adopted in the community for celebrating important communal events and particularly those associated with education. In the process of reinterpreting the information on AIDS and HIV in their own terms the children and their teachers actively integrated the new knowledge we had given them into their existing 'cognitive maps' of sex and illness and, at the same time, created a set of new meanings which had resonance, both for themselves and for their audience. We believe that it can, indeed, be claimed that this process allowed 'local voices' not only to be heard, but that the teachers and pupils were full participants in developing intervention.

The theme of drama has come up spontaneously in the community-based AIDS project. In the urban leg of the research we are working with a number of self-initiated youth groups which meet in the vicinity of the home of one of the research team.[6] Hearing of our interest in AIDS, a member of one of the youth groups suggested that he write a play about AIDS and the use of condoms and that it be acted by the group of which he is the leader. This is now underway and, if successful, it is planned to bring the team and their play to perform on the campus of the university. We also have plans to video the play for use with other youth groups. The initiator of these ideas is an anthropology graduate. Although employed as a field researcher, she has found that far from confining herself to interviewing — and, as described above, distributing condoms and following up what happened when they were used — she is suddenly an actress into the bargain! It is fortunate that she is willing and able to follow this course. Looking back at the course of the research, she is aware of how she has responded to the lead of her research participants, first in giving them condoms and then in entering with them into play production. In a nutshell her 'methodology' has been as follows: first, simply to 'be there,' and so build trust through participating in the group life of local youth; second, to make herself available to them, both for discussions of sex and AIDS and in the distribution of condoms; and third, to give assistance in devising a play about AIDS. 'Being there' has, indeed, put her 'half-way' to intervention.

PROBLEMS: PRACTICAL, ETHICAL
AND EPISTEMOLOGICAL

In the course of the projects outlined above we have had to make many serious and quick research management decisions — to begin intervention in the form of providing medical information, to give out condoms, and, latterly, to encourage self-initiated play production. The time expended on the rehearsals for the play will cut into the time which might have been spent on more traditional research or other intervention strategies. The researcher discussed above will have to limit the number of youth groups she works with, and she may have to abandon a proposal to initiate work with voluntary associations attended by older women. In addition, the demands of the research are making it difficult for her to keep up with the routine writing of notes and reviewing of where the research is leading.

Indeed as the project is gaining momentum, we are finding on all fronts that the demands of our research participants are becoming heavy — they want to talk and talk and talk. They need advice and moral support as they try to introduce condoms — and not least when they fail or when their lovers prove difficult. As we encounter people who are HIV positive and are ailing we will need counselling skills. Already some of our research participants need help because they are afraid that they may be HIV positive. Should we send them for testing — or is it better not to advise this when it is both costly and there are no adequate counselling facilities available for black people?

Looking ahead, what will we do when we suspect — or know — that our research participants (or worse still, members of our research team) are HIV positive? Do we respect their confidentiality or do we tell their partners and so possibly save lives? Many of the people who have tested positive, and who we and other local researchers have interviewed, have not told their families or partners. And they admit to not using condoms or refraining from sex with either one or more partners. Women are afraid of being deserted by their partners, the more so if they are not married; many cannot survive without the economic support or the physical protection of men, and most do not want to run the short term risk of losing their lovers and the fathers of their children. In the face of such confrontations our commitment not to break the traditional rules of confidentiality observed by most anthropologists is strengthened. But this is not necessarily the opinion of all of the research team and particularly of those who are not anthropologists. Neither is it the opinion of some of our research participants who argue forcibly that 'infected people' should be 'locked up.'

Inevitably, also, we are being asked to do favours and become involved in issues which are not strictly connected with AIDS research or intervention. These calls come both from some of our research participants who see us as a resource to be used to their own benefit regardless of our research agenda, and also from lobbies both within and outside the academic arena for research to be 'relevant' and, furthermore, empowering. If decisions are made to widen our field activities to include these time-consuming demands, how do we account to our funders, and also to our peers, who look for the speedy publication of our results — results which are often held up by the need to become involved in action?

STRANGER, FRIEND — AND AGENT FOR TRANSFORMATION?

In theory the idea — and as suggested in much of the earlier part of this chapter, the practice — of AIDS intervention research sounds extremely appealing: it raises, however, a hornets' nest when the implications of such an approach are explored. Thus, on the one hand such a programme is well suited to a climate in which 'action anthropology' is highly rated and where the call is for research to be 'democratic' and participatory — as is certainly the case in South African research circles today. On the other hand it makes, as we are finding to our cost, demands on fieldworkers which are at variance with some of the traditional strengths of an anthropological perspective — the ability of the anthropologist to be both an observer and a participant, a part of the community and observer of it, both stranger and friend.

We have to consider seriously whether we are running the risk of being turned into practitioners rather than thinkers;[7] have we time for reflection and analysis, or are these the first attributes to be jettisoned as time becomes precious and we are overtaken by the swell of events and the demands of action? Above all, does intervention imply an emotional commitment to a programme which has its origins in our own cultural milieu and which may easily be merely another form of intellectual imperialism — this time spurred by our belief, not in progress or socio-economic 'development', but threats to human survival or to social formations as we know and value them, and which *we* construe as part of human survival?

Criticisms which echo these sentiments uncomfortably closely have come to us from groups of older women who form the focus of study in the shack area outside Durban. Although poverty and deprivation are widespread throughout black KwaZulu/Natal, in shack settlements these are the very counters of day-to-day experience. Many, if not the majority, of households in the area are headed by women (Dubb 1974; Preston-Whyte 1978, 1981) who find access to formal employment not only difficult, but extremely poorly paid (Preston-Whyte and Rogerson 1992). The informal sector is the resort and repository of survival for them and their children and sex is merely one of the strategies adopted to survive. Most of the women know about AIDS from the mass media, but because few deaths have as yet occurred, many do not believe in the reality of the threat. Some regard injunctions to safe sex and the use of condoms as a plot on the part of whites to cut black population numbers. When we begin to enquire about numbers of sex partners and call for changes in sex habits and the use of condoms, many respond with calls for more relevant assistance: water, job creation, better health services, the vote. Gender issues, such as the inability and, more critical, the hesitation of women to take the initiative in sex, soon surface in discussions of condom use. It is not only in our own perception that the answer lies in empowerment for women: the groups we are consulting make the same point. 'Bring us a female condom,' they insist, 'or give us jobs so we are not dependent on men.'

Some raise the issue of how the community benefits from research, and they demand that research be accompanied by concrete help — they have mentioned the purchase of a candle-making machine or sewing machines, which at the moment are the particular priority formulated by the groups we have been visiting. But each group is likely to have its own demands and priorities, and we have to ask to what extent we can meet these, or should feel the obligation to do so. Our research team has already accepted what we see as an ethical responsibility to provide adequate medical information, to distribute condoms, and to become engaged in community-driven intervention strategies such as play production. Were we to provide the candle-making machine who would supervise its use and market its products? We cannot become 'developers' as well as AIDS interveners, and if we try, we may well make all the mistakes already perpetrated by a long succession of 'do-gooders,' including some well-meaning and concerned anthropologists who have not had the skills to engage successfully in socio-economic development.

A more critical question than merely becoming involved in socio-economic development is the issue of the empowerment of research participants who, as individuals or groups, are subject to discrimination or oppression. Here the dominating ethical call is to become involved in political action on both the state and domestic fronts. Black South African women are oppressed both as citizens and in terms of gender relations in the community and home. Is it, however, the job of all researchers to empower their research participants on all fronts? I would resist such a call simply because it is not feasible — again such a course of action will lead to our spreading our energies too thin — and also because we cannot give the adequate back-up which empowerment projects need, not only to be successful but to avoid creating more problems than they solve. In any case I have suggested that the very process of making the open discussion of sex possible among women, and between women and men, is empowering in terms of action to resist infection. It may well lead to empowerment on other fronts also (PANOS 1992).

DOING AND THINKING

Finally, I turn to the most difficult problem of all. What does combining research and intervention mean for the analysis and understanding of the ongoing research process? The inroads which 'action' makes on reflection have been mentioned: even routine note taking tends to be squeezed out as pressing calls are made on the time of field workers. The reflexivity without which good anthropological interpretation is not possible is even more critical as we seek actively to change the situation we are studying. How, for instance, do we separate what people think — thought — before we arrived and started talking to them, from the changes which the research process itself sets in motion and, indeed, was designed to initiate? One way to do this has been suggested above: ask people to give their existing views, then provide them with information and, subsequently, in group discussions, record their responses to the added knowledge. This may sound fairly simple, but in practice it is extremely demanding and each item of change or what appears to be change has to be critically assessed.

Adopting an 'action' approach has other implications. If we seek to involve our subjects in the process of change, should we not recognize that we will also change and that, if our research is a truly participatory venture, we should change in response to the 'local voices' we have promoted? To accept and monitor the changes in our own perceptions is, perhaps, the greatest challenge of all, as it necessitates personal introspection as much as professional reflexivity. A significant start has, however, been made in this direction (Herdt and Lindenbaum 1992).

For anthropologists working in teams which include fieldworkers drawn from other disciplinary backgrounds and also community-based liaison personnel the role and process of reflection and re-flexivity raises a number of problems. Team members as well as leaders need to reflect and consciously monitor their impact on re-search participants. Some of our fieldworkers find this not only difficult, but personally challenging: they ask if this is a way of checking on whether they are they doing their job or not, and they perceive the requests for regular self-examination as an indirect way for their work to be judged by the research leaders. They ask if the continual debriefings and requests for feedback are really necessary. Would the time not be better spent with the community itself? Those with no social science background find it difficult to take this side of their work seriously. For them it is the imperatives of the threat which are paramount, not the documentation of the research process.

The tension between reflection and analysis is present in all an-thropological work, but it is exacerbated in that which has a par-ticipatory and interventionist cast. In the case of AIDS research the magnitude of the perceived threat may all too easily come to domi-nate the achievement of good research. This chapter is an attempt at the reflection which may lead in this direction.

NOTES

1. As Brooke Schoepf and her colleagues (1992) point out, the critical anthropological message is not that local knowledge may have a value. Anthropologists have always argued this. Culture operates at more than this simplistic level, and anthropological techniques have more to offer than 'butterfly collecting' (Leach 1961).

2. Unlinked seroprevalence surveys carried out in a rural African com-munity of northern KwaZulu/Natal showed no evidence of infection in 1985, but by 1990 the prevalence stood at 1.2 per cent of the sur-veyed population, and by mid 1992 this had risen to 2.5 per cent (Ab-dool Karim, Preston-Whyte, and Abdool Karim 1992a; Q. Abdool Karim et al. 1992).

3. STDs are treated by both Western trained doctors and traditional healers, some of the latter claiming special expertise in illnesses of a sexual nature with some providing both preventative and curative medicine for sexual problems associated with physical symptoms believed to result from the attempts of others to control spouses and lovers who they suspect of having other partners. Medicine is correspondingly obtainable to attract the attention of the opposite sex. Since AIDS is explained in the media as being the result of sexual intercourse, some of these specialists claim the ability to cure it along with 'older' sexual problems. A pioneering study in KwaZulu/Natal showed that many women believed that, like other STDs, AIDS was also curable by a visit to the health clinic for 'an injection' (Abdool Karim, Abdool Karim, and Nkomokazi 1991).

4. This project forms part of the Women and AIDS programme conducted by the International Centre for Research on Women, Washington, DC, and was funded by the Office of Health of the US Agency for International Development. The team leader was Q. Abdool Karim and the researchers included E. Preston-Whyte, N. Zuma, Z.A. Stein, and I. Susser.

5. The major local research associates are Quarraisha Abdool Karim, Dr Salim S. Abdool Karim, and Dr N. Zuma, of the Medical Research Council, Durban, and overseas collaborators are Professor Z.A. Stein, Director, HIV Centre, Columbia University, and Professor I. Susser, Hunter College, New York.

6. Muriel Gcadinja, an anthropology graduate.

7. I am indebted to Adam Kuper for this insight. Indeed, it was his criticism of a research proposal for an AIDS intervention programme which alerted me to the problems discussed herein.

REFERENCES

Abdool Karim, Q., S.S. Abdool Karim, and J. Nkomokazi. 1991. Sexual Behaviour and Knowledge of AIDS Among Urban Black Mothers: Implications for AIDS Intervention Programmes. *South African Medical Journal* 80:340–343.

Abdool Karim, Q., E. Preston-Whyte, and S.S. Abdool Karim. 1992a. Teenagers Seeking Condoms at Family Planning Clinics: Part 1 — A User's Perspective. *South African Medical Journal* 82:356–359.

Abdool Karim, Q., E. Preston-Whyte, and S.S. Abdool Karim. 1992b. Teenagers Seeking Condoms at Family Planning Clinics: Part 2 — A Provider's Perspective. *South African Medical Journal* 82:360–362.

Abdool Karim, Q., S.S. Abdool Karim, B. Singh, R. Short, and S. Ngxongo. 1992. Seroprevalence of HIV Infection in Rural South Africa. *AIDS* 6:1535–1539.

Abdool Karim, S.S., Q. Abdool Karim, E. Preston-Whyte, and N. Sanker. 1992. Reasons for Lack of Condom Use Among High School Students. *South African Medical Journal* 82:107–110.

Ankrah, E.M., J.W. McGrath, D.A. Schumann, S. Nkumbi, and M. Lubega. 1991. The Impact of AIDS on Urban Families: An Assessment of Needs. Abstracts of VIth International Conference on AIDS in Africa. Dakar 1991, December 16–19.

Asad, T. 1973. *Anthropology and the Colonial Encounter*. London: Ithaca Press.

Barnett, T., and P. Blaikie. 1992. *Aids in Africa: Its Present and Future Impact*. London: Belhaven Press.

Bassett, M.T., and M. Mhloyi. 1991. Women and AIDS in Zimbabwe: The Making of an epidemic. *International Journal of Health Services* 21(1):143–156.

Bolton, R. 1989. *The AIDS Pandemic: A Global Emergency*. New York: Gordon and Breach.

Caldwell, S.C. 1982. *Theory of Fertility Decline*. London: Academic Press.

Caldwell, S.C., P. Caldwell, and I.O. Orubuloye. 1990. Changes in the Nature and Levels of Sexual Networking in an African Society: The Destabilisation of the Traditional Yoruba System. Health Transition Working Paper no. 4. Australian National University

Clatts, M.C. 1992. All the King's Horses and All the King's Men: Some Personal Reflections on Ten Years of AIDS Ethnography. Paper presented at a conference on 'Culture, Sexual Behavior, and AIDS', Department of Anthropology, University of Amsterdam, July 24–26. Forthcoming in *Human Organization*.

Coxon, A.P.M. 1988. Something Sensational ... The Sexual Diary as a Tool for Mapping Actual Sexual Behaviour. *Sociological Review* 362:353–367.

Dalrymple, L.A. 1991. A Drama Approach to AIDS Education. Unpublished report for the Department of National Health and Population Development, Pretoria.

Dalrymple, L.A., and E. Preston-Whyte. 1992. A Drama Approach to AIDS Education: An Experiment in 'Action' Research. *AIDS Bulletin* 1(1):9–11.

Dubb, A. 1974. The Impact of the City. In: *The Bantu-Speaking Peoples of Southern Africa*, edited by W.D. Hammond-Tooke. London: Routledge and Kegan Paul.

Frankenberg, R. 1992. What Identity's At Risk? Anthropologists and AIDS. *Anthropology in Action* 12:6–9.

Geertz, C. 1959. The Javanese Kijaji: The Changing Role of the Culture Broker. *Comparative Studies in Society and History* 2:228–249.

Geertz, C. 1983. *Local Knowledge*. New York: Basic Books.

Haas, M. de. 1987. Is There Anything More to Say About Lobolo? *African Studies* 46(1):33–35.

Herdt, G., and S. Lindenbaum, eds. 1992. *The Time of AIDS: Social Analysis, Theory and Method.* Newbury Park, CA: Sage Publications.

Illingworth, P. 1990. *AIDS and the Good Society.* London: Routledge.

Kark, S.L. 1949. The Social Pathology of Syphilis in Africans. *South African Medical Journal* 23:77–84.

Leach, E.R. 1961. *Rethinking Anthropology.* London: Athlone Press.

Ngugi, E.N., F.A. Plummer, R. Sajabi, P. Wambugu, E.K. Njeru, and J.O. Ndinya-Achola. 1992. Development of an Educational Booklet for STD/AIDS Control Among Female Commercial Sex Workers in Kenya. Paper presented at the VIIIth International Conference on AIDS. 19–24 July. Amsterdam.

PANOS. 1992. *The Hidden Cost of AIDS: The Challenge of HIV to Development.* London: The Panos Institute.

Patton, C. 1990. *Inventing AIDS.* New York: Routledge.

Preston-Whyte, E.M. 1978. Families Without Marriage. In: *Social System and Tradition in Southern Africa,* edited by W.J. Argyle and E.M. Preston-Whyte. Cape Town: Oxford University Press.

Preston-Whyte, E.M. 1981. Women Migrants and Marriage. In: *African Systems of Marriage in Southern Africa,* edited by E.J. Krige and J. Comaroff. Cape Town: Juta and Company.

Preston-Whyte, E.M., and C. Rogerson. 1991. *South Africa's Informal Economy.* Cape Town: Oxford University Press.

Preston-Whyte, E.M., and M. Zondi. 1991. Adolescent Sexuality and Its Implications for Teenage Pregnancy and AIDS. *Continuing Medical Education* 9(11):1389–1397.

Preston-Whyte, E.M., and M. Zondi. 1992. African Teenage Pregnancy: Whose Problem? In: *Questionable Issue: Illegitimacy in South Africa,* edited by S. Burman and E.M. Preston-Whyte. Cape Town: Oxford University Press.

Schoepf, B.G., Walu Engundu, Rukarangira wa Nkera, Payanzo Ntsomo, and C. Schoepf. 1992. Community-Based Risk-Reduction Support in Zaïre. In: *AIDS Prevention through Health Promotion: Changing Behaviour,* edited by R. Berkvens. Geneva: World Health Organization.

Whyte, W.F. 1991. *Participatory Action Research.* Newbury Park, CA: Sage Publications.

Wolf, E. 1956. Aspects of Group Relations in a Complex Society: Mexico. *American Anthropologist* 58:1005–1078.

Worth, D. 1989. Sexual Decision-Making and AIDS: Why Condom Promotion Among Vulnerable Women Is Likely to Fail. *Studies in Family Planning* 20(6):297–307.

INDEX

A

Abdool Karim, Q., 321
Abdool Karim, S.S., 320, 321, 324
Abramson, P.R., 258, 259, 261
Accion Familiar, 142
ACP, 81
Action-research
  and anthropology, iii, 38,
    316, 331, 333–334
  and performative
    ethnography, 38
  as empowerment strategy, 324
  informants in, 327
  limitations of, 332–333
  with adolescents, 102
  with mixed gender groups, 110
Adib, M.S., 185
Adler, P., 159
Adler, P.A., 159
Adolescents, 31, 89, 102–106, 324.
  See also Youth
Africa, xii, 29–45, 79–94, 265
African perception of AIDS, x–xi
  and the origin of HIV, 37
  sexuality, 32–35
Aggleton, P., 38
Ahlberg, B.M., 34
AIDS
  and anthropology, ii, vi, xiv, 54,
    289
  and cultural change, 31
  and economic development,
    30–32, 37
  and language use, 227
  and moralism, 173, 273
  and of anthropology, iii–v
  and the 'other', 98, 115, 147,
    269, 292
  and the public discourse, viii
  as a global crisis, v
  as a metaphor, 36, 229, 251
  as an industry, 80, 85
  coping with, 318
  natural history of, 42
  Northern and Southern, vii–ix
AIDS epidemic
  Western response, 317
AIDS prevalence
  in Haiti, 4
  in São Paulo, 98–99
  in Spain, 142
AIDS prevention. See also Drama
  and anthropology, 68
  and culture, 61
  and ethnographic research, 44
  and talking about sex, 41
  and the use of metaphors, 39
  in gay communities, 85
  perceived as a conspiracy, 67
AIDS research
  and anthropology, 295
  and applied anthropology, iv
  and cultural context, 277
  and ethnography, 252, 299–301,
    300
  and foreign researchers, ix–xi,
    84, 85
  and funding, 276
  and gay anthropologists, v, xiii
  and gender, xi
  and modes of commitment,
    iv–viii

and self-protection, 307
and Third World anthro-
    pologists, vi–viii
as a risk, 307
clients of sex workers, 140–141
community based, 325
ethics of, 85, 305–306, 330
foreign vs. local researchers, 85
in prisons, 304–305
local voices, 316
persons with HIV/AIDS,
    305, 330
present state of, 242
priorities in, 307
Western models in, 276
AIDSCAP, 265
AIDSCOM, 265
AIDSTECH, 265
Aina, T.A., 263
Akha, 55, 57, 58, 60, 61, 62, 63,
    64, 65, 66, 68
    women in commercial sex, 64
Albee, G.W., 186
Albert, J., 258, 259, 264
Aldwin, C., 187
Alexander, P., 139
Allman, J., 18
Alloway, R., 187
Allyn, E., 123
Alonso, A.M., 63, 69
Alting von Geusau, L., 55
Altman, L.K., 43
American Anthropological
    Association, 308
AMREF, 81
Anal intercourse, 157, 167, 169, 192
    active and passive, 218–219
    behavioural analysis of, 215–219
    condom use, 170
    incidence of, 215
    meaning of, 208, 234
    symbolic meaning of, 172

unprotected, 190
    in Belgium, 184
    in England and Wales, 184
    in Ireland, 185
    in Italy
    in San Francisco, 185
    in Switzerland, 184
    in The Netherlands, 184
    in the United States, 184
Anan Ganjanapan, 54
Ankrah, E.M., x, xi, 317
Anthropology
    and action-research, 44, 252, 289
    and AIDS research, 290, 291
    and biomedical research, 41–44
    and colonialism, 35, 318
    and creation of culture, 44–45
    and cultural relativism, 292
    and cultural sensitivity, 294–295
    and drama, 324
    and epidemiology, xv, 264
    and ethics, 68–70, 303, 304
    and HIV prevention, 316
    and responsibility, 292
    and sex research, 32, 274, 292
    and small goups, 139
    and subjectivity, iv
    and team work, iii, xi, 334
    and the AIDS epidemic, 288
    and the local context, iii
    as a dialogue, iv
    as cultural critique, 289
    creating culture, iii–iv, 302
    participant observation, 323
    response to AIDS, 317
    translation between
        cultures, 318
Antunes, M.C., 104
Archaeology of sexuality, 33
Ardener, E., 86, 141
Asad, T., 318
Atillasoy, A., 249

Attribution theory
  and unsafe sex, 190
Avison, W.R., 186

B

Bachrach, K.M., 187
Bangladesh
  migrants from, 57
Barbosa, R., 98, 101
Barnett, T., 317
Barrera, M., 187
Bassett, M.T., 31, 317
Baum, A., 186
Bayer, R., 289
Bebbington, P., 187
Beck, U., 136–137, 142, 151
Becker, M.H., 184
Bedoian, G., 103
Behavioural change
  and HIV testing, 291
  and peer groups, 276
  in gay communities, 301
Berkman, L.F., 187
Berkowitz, R., 157
Berridge, V., ix
Bibeau, G., 50
Billings, A.G., 187
Biomedical research
  and the representation of
    AIDS, 244
  dominance of, 34–35, 41–44, 45
Bjurström, E., 161
Blaikie, P., 317
Bolton, R., iii, v, vii, ix, xi, xiii, xiv,
    41, 62, 158, 172, 186, 188, 190,
    234, 242, 258, 259, 261, 262,
    289, 311, 317
Bone, G., 38
Border areas, xiii, 67, 69
Boxer, A., 262, 289

Brasil, V.V., 101
Brazil, xii, 97–112
  popular education in, 97
  private vs. public sphere,
    99–100
Brown, T., 263
Brox, O., 160
Bruyn, M. de, 21, 31
Bueno, R., 238
Burma (Myanmar), 55, 59, 60,
    64, 67

C

CAIDS (Community Acquired
    Immune Deficiency Syn-
    drome), 229
Caldwell, P., 321
Caldwell, S.C., 321
California Psychological
    Inventory, 277
Callen, M., 157
Calvez, M., 136
Camus, A., 289
Carballo, M., 213, 258, 259, 261,
    262, 289
Carrier, J.M., 242, 246, 262, 264
Cash, R., 123
Cass, V., 188
Cassel, J.C., 187
Casual encounters
  and love, 297
Catania, J.A., 184, 186
Catholic Church
  and condom use, 142
CDC, ix, 5, 291
Centro de Vigilancia
    Epidemiológica, 99
Chouinard, A., 258, 259, 264
Christianity, 80, 86–87, 86, 99
  Roman Catholicism and
    sexuality, 273
  split-level Christianity, 273

Chupinit Kesmanee, 59
Class
    and HIV transmission, 80
Clatts, M.C., v, ix, xiv, 229, 230,
    244, 246, 249, 251, 252, 318
Clients of sex workers. *See also*
    Sex workers
    HIV prevention strategies of,
        149
    perception of sex workers by,
        145–146
    self-image of, 144–146
Coates, T., 184, 185, 186, 234
Co-factors in HIV transmission
    economic inequity, 24
    poverty, 24
    STDs, 21–22
Cohen, E., 129
Coleman, E., 188
Collins, J.P., 123
Coming out
    and social support, 188
Commercial sex
    and cash economy, 58
    in Thailand, 64
Condom use
    and contraception, 322
    and culture, 34, 61, 81–82, 101
    and fertility, 40
    and gender relations, 31
    and gender roles, 93, 101
    and ignorance, 84
    and local culture, 322
    and pleasure, 92, 306
    and promiscuity, 81, 91
    and schools, 328
    and socioeconomic status, 121
    and STDs, 142
    and the Catholic Church, 142
    as scandalous, 84
    by sex tourists, 122
    in non-Western cultures, 318
    in sex work, 117, 121, 147–148
    in South Africa, 321

Condoms
    conceptions about, 321
    knowledge of, 92
    misconceptions about, 83
CONNAISSIDA, 36, 316
Control, perception of, 189, 190,
    192, 197
Cooper, R., 59
Corin, E., 33
Costa, P.T., 187
Coureau, S., 101
Coxon, A.P.M., xiv, 206, 208, 209,
    213, 215, 326
Coxon, N.H., xiv, 215
Coyne, J.C., 187
Crystal, S., 139
Cultural analysis
    in relation to social analysis,
        30, 68
Cultural construction
    in sex research, 260–261, 262
    of African sexuality, by
        Westerners, 37
    of AIDS, 29, 36, 98, 229
    of HIV, 66–67
    of homosexuality, 263
    of the 'other', 62
Cultural context
    and local voices, 317–319
Cultural influence model, 274
Cultural politics, 36–38
Cultural relativism, 274
    and homosexuality, 292
Cultural time-out
    and sex tourism, 125, 126
    sex workers in Thailand, 127
Culture
    and AIDS research, 309
    and anthropology, 318–319
    and blaming, 43
    and condom use, 83
    and disease conception, 66–67
    and gender roles, 242

and HIV prevention, 80
and language, 228
and political context, 139
and sexuality, 273–274
as an agent of change, 44–45
as a rationalization, 318
as mutable, 319
concept of, ii, 318
in relation to political
economy, 69
the limitations of, xi, xiv, 24
Cunningham, R., 189
Curran, W., 41

D

Dalrymple, L.A., 324, 325
Daniel, H., 263
Danielle Mitterrand Foundation, 82
Davies, P. M., 158, 173, 208
Day, S., 140
De Haas, M., 322
Delph, E.W., 158, 165, 166
Depression, 192
Derogatis, L.R., 192
Desvarieux, M., 5, 10, 19
Diaries. *See* Sexual diaries
Discourse
and linguistics, 228
biomedical, 228–230
colonial, 33
on AIDS, 138, 228
in Africa, 37
in Haiti, 20
in Sweden, 161
in Uganda, 84
on gender, 86–89, 104–106
on HIV prevention, 160
on sex, in AIDS research, 295
on sexuality, 32–35, 99, 272
on social hygiene, 99

Dore, P., 189
Douglas, M., 33, 136
Drama
and action-research, 327, 328
as HIV intervention, 38, 107,
324, 329
with adolescents, 329–330
Dubb, A., 332
Dubois-Arber, F., 184
Durrenberger, E.P., 67

E

Eibl-Eibesfeldt, I., 166, 168
Eiser, J.R., 190
Ekstrand, M., 157, 185
Elder, J.P., 186
Elias, C., 97
Ellis, H., 259
El sida, 143
EMPOWER, 116, 124
Empowerment, 317
and action-research, 333
and AIDS research, 308
and HIV prevention, 112,
131–132
and power, 250
of sex workers, 132
of women, 332
strategies of, 31, 38, 44, 107
English Collective of Prostitutes,
139
Ensel, W.M., 186
Epstein, P., 40
Eriksson, N., 174
Erotic oases
and HIV transmission, 161
in Sweden, 158
safer sex in, 171–173
Eroticization, 111
of minorities, 62
of prevention, xiii
of safe sex, 172, 174

Erotophobia
  and AIDS research, 295
Esparza, J., 43
Ethnographic method, 323
Ethnopornography, 35
Ewald, P.W., 30
Eysenck Personality Question-
  naire, 277

F

Fabian, J., 38
Family planning
  and condom promotion, 67
Farang, 115–131
Farmer, P., v, vii, viii, x, xi, 5, 7, 14,
  15, 20, 68, 69, 70, 289, 299
Fee, E., 80
Feilden, R., 16
Feldman, D., v
Feminism, and sexuality, 97–98
Fertility
  and contraception, 322
  and safe sex, 61
  and sex research, 34
  meaning of, 321–322
Finstad, L., 141
Flax, C.C., 220
Focus groups, 83, 91, 278, 280, 299
Folkman, S., 187
Foreign researchers. *See* AIDS
  research
Foucault, M., ix, 168, 241
Fox, D.M., 80
Franco (Luambo Makiadi), 36
Frankenberg, R., 289, 318
Freire, P., 38, 107

G

Gagnon, J.H., 63, 258, 260
Garcia, L., 263

Gay
  as a Western construct, 275
Gay Bowel Syndrome, 229
Gay men
  and social expectations, 188
  heterosexual behaviour, 213
  in the United Kingdom, 205–206
Gay saunas
  prohibition of, in Sweden, 160
Gay scene
  in Stockholm, 159–161
Geertz, C., 247, 318
Gelder, P. van, 71
Gender, xii
  and 'social skin', 243
  and AIDS discourse, 80
  and Christianity, 86, 99
  and conception of the body, 243
  and condom use, 19, 66, 100
  and control of female sexuality,
    34, 88
  and coping with stress, 189
  and empowerment, 332
  and HIV risk, 30, 68, 93, 324
  and HIV transmission, 80
  and identity, 243–244
  and multi-partner sex, 321
  and power, 31, 39, 58, 64, 66,
    68, 86, 88–89, 101, 296
  and risk perception, 245
  and stigma, 36
  culture of silence, 86
  male–female dichotomy, 243
Gender roles
  adolescents, 103, 105
  and kinship, 64
  and sexual behaviour, 280
  boys vs. girls, 108–110
  diversity of, 242
  female, in Thailand, 127
  motherhood, 101
  socialization into, 103
GESCAP, 13, 14, 21

GHESKIO, 5
Gibson, H., 126
Giddens, A., 136
Giele, J.Z., 189
Girault, C., 16
Glick-Schiller, N., 139
Global village, 275
Globalisation, v
   and medical discourse, x
Glory holes, 159
GMFA, 138
Goffman, E., 158, 159, 161, 167
Golding, D., 136
Gordon, G., 38
Gottlieb, A., 126
GRID (Gay Related Immune
   Deficiency), 229
GSRP, 190
Guimaraes, C.D., 101

H

Haff, J., 158, 165
HAIN, 272, 277
Health Action Information
   Network, 272
Haiti, xii, 3–24
   AIDS and the public health
      system, 22–23
   Carrefour, as an epicentre, 4
   heterosexual HIV transmission
      in, 5
   machismo in, 19
   origin of the HIV epidemic, 4–6
   position of women, 19
   prevalence of HIV, 4
   risk factors in, 11–12
   spread of HIV in urban areas, 4
   spread of HIV to the rural
      population, 11
   types of conjugal union, 17
Hanenberg, R., viii

Hanks, J.R., 60
Hanks, L., 60
Hart, A., xiii
Hart, D., 273
Hart, G.L., 184
Health behaviour, models of,
   186, 197
Health belief model, 276, 293
Henriksson, B., xiii, 160, 161,
   174, 326
Herdt, G., iii, v, ix, 164, 238, 258,
   259, 260, 261, 262, 265, 289,
   317, 334
Heroin trafficking, 57
Hilltribes
   in Thailand, 50–70
Hingson, R.W., 186
Hirdman, Y., 161
HIV prevalence
   among girls in Uganda, 83
   among sex workers, in
      Spain, 143
   in Haiti, 4–6
   in Northern Thailand, 56
   in São Paulo, 98–99
   in South Africa, 319–320
   in Sweden, 160
   in Thailand, 116
HIV prevention, 174
   among adolescents in São
      Paulo, 102
   among heterosexuals, in Spain,
      142
   among MSM, 304
   and anthropology, 279, 290–291,
      293
   and blame, 251
   and drama, 174
   and linguistic analysis, 228
   and partner reduction, 247
   and persons with HIV/AIDS,
      302–303
   and sex-positivity, 301–302

and sex tourism, 130
and sociocultural context, 280
and talking about sex, 80, 124
categories used in, 246
community based, 107
constraints of, 251
gay and bisexual men, 171–172
individual bias, 97, 138, 158, 294
in schools, 82
limitations of, 174
male dominance, 80
social context of, 81
Western models in, 318
workshops, 275
HIV risk
adolescents, 103, 324
and access to health care, 69
and political unrest, 20–21
and responsibility, 137
context of, 141
political and economic context
of, 68–69
HIV transmission
and economic disparity, 250
and economic pressure, 16–17,
57
and folklore rituals in Haiti, 19
and labour migration, 59
and political disruption, 20–21
and population pressure, 15–16
and poverty, 3, 6
and shame, 80
and sharing needles, 142
blaming women, 83
bridges in, 11–12
context of, 298
dynamics of, 15–17
in Spain, 143
knowledge of, 92, 102, 122
linking peripheral societies, 67
macro and micro context, 59–60
misconceptions about, 38
socioeconomic factors, 189
vertical, 320

HIV/AIDS, people living with,
and anthropology, 290–291
HIV-positive mothers, 83
Hmong, 55, 57, 59, 60, 61, 62, 63,
64, 65, 66, 67, 68
Hodzi, P., 38
Hoff, C., 184, 234
Hoigard, C., 141
Holahan, C.J., 187
Holanda, S., 100
Holmes, M.G., 273
Holmshaw, M., 44
Homosexuality
as a Western construct, 275
cultural construction of, 278
explanations of, 273
Hope, A., 38
Hopkins Symptom Check list, 192
Horwitz, A.V., 189
House, J.S., 187
Houweling, H., 184
Humphreys, L., 165
Hypersexuality, 62

I

IDRC, 265
Illicit economy, 57, 59, 60
Illingworth,P., 317
Individual autonomy and HIV
prevention, 97
Institute of Medicine, 186
Intervention
and action-research, 327
and anthropology, 316, 323, 324
and drama, 324
and interactive strategies, 108
and sex research, 261
consequences of, 111–112
in São Paulo, 107–108
in schools, 324
interactive strategies, 328
Islam, 80, 83

J

Jackson, P.A., 63
Janzen, J.M., 33
Jöhncke, S., 147
Johnson, R., 259
Johnson, W., 5, 6, 10
Jones, J.H., 41, 42
Joseph, J.G., 184, 185

K

Kahn, S., 197
Kammerer, C.A., xi, 31, 54, 59, 60, 61
Kane, S., 264
KAP surveys, 32, 35, 41, 242, 259, 278, 299
   in the Philippines, 272
Karen, 55, 58
Karimajong, 84
Kark, S.L., 321
Karma and sexual risk, 123
Kegeles, S.M., 186
Kelly, J.A., 184
Kempler, E., v
Keogh, P., 172
Kerkwijk, C. van, xii, xiii
Kessler, R.C., 186, 187
Kinsey, A., 259, 260, 261
Kisekka, M.N., 31
Kleiber, D., 121
Klein Hutheesing, O., xi, 57, 58, 59, 60, 64, 66
Klitzman, S., 187
Klouda, T., 38
Knutsson, S., 174
Kobasa, S.C., 197
Koreck, M.T., 63, 69
Krimsky, S., 136
Kunstadter, P., 57
Kunstadter, S., 57

L

Laguerre, M., 18
Lahu, 55, 62
Lazarus, R.S., 187
Leap, W.L., xiv, 229, 262, 265
Lee, J.A., 188
Leigh, B.C., 186
Levine, M., 234, 236, 237
Lewellen, D., 139
Liandis, K.R., 187
Liautaud, B., 4, 22
Lief, L., 23
Light, S.C., 187
Likert scale, 277
Lin Nan, 186, 187
Lindenbaum, S., iv, v, ix, xi, 32, 54, 258, 317, 334
Linguistic analysis
   and AIDS, xiv, 231–233
Linguistics
   and HIV prevention, 228, 237
Lisu, 55, 57, 58, 59, 60, 61, 63, 64, 65, 66, 67, 68
Local culture, v, x, xv, 69–70
   and homosexuality, 275
   and safe sex, 322
Local epidemics, 69
Local perceptions, xiv
Local researchers. *See* AIDS research
Local structures vs. larger structures, 68
Local voices, x, 318
Locher, U., 16
Locus of control, 247, 276
   and unsafe sex, 197
Lourea, D., 174
Love
   and unsafe sex, 185
Lynch, E., 38

M

MACS report, 184
Maddi, S.R., 197
Magaña, R., 262, 264
Mak, R., 184, 188, 190
Malinowski, B., 32
Mandel, J., 186
Mann, J.M., v, 55, 130, 262, 265
Månsson, S.A., xiii, 326
Mason, T., 264
Masters, W., 259
Materialist approach, xi, 68
Mattlin, J.A., 187
Mays, V., 186
McCall, P., 166
McCormick, D., 220
McCrae, R.R., 187
McCusker, J.J., 186
McGrath, J.E., 186
McKinnon, J., 59
McKirnan, D.J., 186
McLeod, J.D., 186
Mead, M., iv, ix
Meo, 55. *See* Hmong
Meyer, W., 118, 120, 125, 127
Mhloyi, M., 31, 317
Mien, 55
Migration
    and HIV transmission, 16, 59
Miller, H.G., 185, 190, 258, 259,
        260, 261, 264
Mintz, S., 19
Mirante, E.T., 59
Mirowsky, J., 186, 190
Misztal, B.A., 265
Molgaard, C.A., 186
Moos, R.H., 187
Moral, P., 17
Morgan Thomas, R., 186
Morin, S.F., 186

Moses, L.E., 185, 190, 258, 259,
        260, 261, 264
Moss, D., 265
MSM
    the concept, 275, 280–281
Muecke, M.A., 55
Mulder, N., 125
Multi-partner sex, 247
    and apartheid, 320–321
    and economic survival, 321
    and HIV transmission, 10
    and migration, 320–321
    in South Africa, 320
Murbach, R., 50
Murdock, G.P., 298
Murray, S.O., 19, 229
Mutchler, K.M., 229, 230, 244, 251

N

Nakamura, C.H., 186
National Resistance Council
    (Uganda), 82
Natural communication
    pathways, 69
Naturalistic paradigm
    in sex research, 259–260
Nature vs. nurture, 292
Neptune-Anglade, M., 16, 19
Nesselhof, S.E., 186
Netter, T.W., 55, 130, 262, 265
Newbury, C., 30
Ngugi, E, 317
Nicholls, D., 19
Nichols, E., 189
Nichols, M., 174
Nieri, G., 185
Niwat Tami, 62

O

Obbo, C., vii, viii, ix, x, xii, 31, 42, 79, 83, 88, 318
Orubuloye, I.O., 321
Ostrow, D.G., 185

P

Packard, R.M., 40
Paiva, V., iii, xv, 101, 102
Pan-American Health Organization, 4
PANOS, 333
Pape, J., 5, 6, 10, 19
Parker, R.G., iii, ix, x, xiv, 63, 99, 100, 112, 258, 259, 260, 261, 262, 263, 264, 289, 315–316
Participant observation
  in AIDS research, 299
  in sex research, 159
Passion
  different constructions of, 237
Patton, C., 161, 173, 174, 317
Payne, K., 229
Pearlin, L.I., 186, 197
Pellow, D., 35
Performative ethnography, 38, 44, 45. *See also* Role play
Peterson, P.L., 186
Philippines, xv, 269–281
Plant, M.A., 186
Plant, M.L., 186
Poisoned Blood, 274
Political economy
  and AIDS research, xi, 30
  and culture, 319
  in relation to culture, 69
  Thailand, 68
  vs. culture, 70
Polygyny, 87

Pomeroy, W.B., 220
Ponse, B., 188
Poverty, xiv
  and HIV risk, 3, 6, 7, 13, 59, 123, 249–250
  and HIV transmission, 10–12, 24, 30
  and sexual relations, 11
Preston-Whyte, E.M., iii, vi, xiv, 38, 320, 321, 322, 325, 332
Prevention
  and empowerment, 112, 131–132
  and gender relations, 66
  culturally inappropriate, in Haiti, 21
Price, R.H., 186
Proj Veye Sante, 7, 12, 13
Prostitution. *See* Sex work
  open ended, 129
Public vs. private sphere, 99–100

Q

Quinn, T.C., 35

R

Radley, H.M., 58
Ralana Maneeprasert, xi, 64
Rapid Assessment Procedures, 299
Relapse, concept of, 294
RFSL, 160
Richards, A., 32, 33, 38
Richardson, D., 173
Risk, in general, 111, 136, 294
Risk behaviour, 234
  rationality of, 294
Risk group
  the concept of, 6, 24, 69, 138–139
  vs. risk behaviour, 69, 138–139, 141, 150–151

Risk groups, construction of, 229
Risk society, 136
Riviere, P., 107
Robert, G.T., 186
Roberts, J.M., 295
Robertson, J.A., 186
Robinson, P., 259, 260
Rogerson, C., 332
Role play
    and condom use, 109–110
    and HIV prevention, 38, 39
Role reversal
    and sex tourism, 126, 127, 129,
        130
Rosenthal, R., 221
Rosnow, R.L., 221
Ross, C.E., 186, 190
Rotter's I-E Scale, 276
Rotter, J.B., 197, 276
Rubin, G., 260
Rukarangira, wa Nkera, 30

S

Sacanagem, 100, 111
Safe sex
    and culture, 61, 123
    and kinship system, 61
    and poverty, 31
    clients of sex workers, 145
    competence in, 93, 172, 173, 174
    in erotic oases, 171–173
    in video clubs, 169
    negotiations about, 124, 170,
        173, 326
    safer sex strategy, 160, 174
    workshops, 107, 280
Sairudee Vorakitphokatorn, 123
San Francisco Men's Health
    Study, 185
Sandfort, T., 184

Sandler, I.N., 186
Sasse, H., 184
Save the Children Fund
    Kampala, 88
Schafer, S., 188
Schmitt, A., 164
Schneider, S.F., 186
Schoepf, B.G., ii, iii, v, vi, xi, xii,
    xv, 29, 30, 31, 32, 34, 35, 36,
    39, 40, 41, 68, 69, 70, 250, 316
Seduction, and condom use, 100
Seidel, G., 33
Semiology of AIDS, 30
Serial monogamy, 18
Serostatus, and unsafe sex, 185
Sex
    and Christianity, 32–34, 320
    and colonialism, 32
    and fertility, 322
    and gender relations, 64
    and love, 104, 296
    and marriage, 322
    and modern science, 99
    and reproduction, 61
    as a commodity, 245, 248
    as survival strategy, 246, 332
    'natural sex', 147–149, 152
    talking about, 62, 71, 80, 90,
        111, 124, 325, 326
    vs. gender, 246
Sex education, among peers, 90
Sex modernism, 259
Sex-negativity, and HIV
    prevention, 301
Sex-positivity
    and culture, viii, xii
    and HIV prevention, 34,
        174, 301
    and middle classes, xiii
    and sex research, 295–298
    vs. sex-negativity, 301

Sex research. *See also* AIDS
  research, KAP surveys, and
  Sexual diaries
about Africa, 32–35
and anthropology, 265, 295
and behavioural change,
  242, 276
and culture, 278
and epidemiology, 261
and ethics, 41
and funding, 263
and health sciences, 260
and HIV prevention, 246, 247
and psychology, 196, 275–76
and the AIDS epidemic, 242
and the notion of pleasure, 295
and Western models, 276
approaches in, 197
assumptions in, 234
biomedical paradigm, 265, 274
categories used in, 243, 246
changing priorities, 264–265
clients of prostitutes, 140–141
contradictory findings, 157
different paradigms, 258–262,
  274, 292
individual bias, 186
interviewing, 234
methodological limitations,
  261–262
participant observation, 159,
  303–304
present state of, xv, 254–258,
  273, 297–298, 316
qualities of the researcher,
  297–298
quick models, 251
rational assumptions, 294
research agenda, 262–264
sociology and psychology, 186
stigma of, 297
theory in, 259–261, 274
Western models in, 278

Sex tourism, xiii, 274
and HIV prevention, 130
background of, 126
clients, 121
clients and condom use, 122
Sexual acts
  as described in diaries, 210
  behavioural analysis of, 208
  in video clubs, 168–169
Sexual alienation, 33
Sexual behaviour
  active and passive, 211–213
  and gender relations, 100
  and power, 208
  and psychology, 186
  and relationship type, 208, 215
  and social context, 186
  behavioural progression in, 217
  co-occurence of acts, 217–219
  encoding of, 209–210
  irrationality of, 294
  memory of, 206
  modality of, 209, 215
  of gay men, 213–215, 263
  outcome of, 209
  sequences in, 208
  sexual outlet, 214
  socialization, 280
  sociocultural context, 245–247,
    260, 274, 275, 277
  vs. sexual identity, 244, 246
Sexual culture
  and sex work, 102–106
  change of, 61, 63–66, 68
  creation of, 302
  in Brazil, 99
  of adolescents in São Paulo,
    102–106
  of gay men, 173
  of hilltribes in Thailand, 60–63
  Philippines, 272–274
  Thailand, 117

Sexual desire, sociocultural
context of, 259, 260–261
Sexual diaries
and anthropology, 220–221
as a method, xiv
collection of, 207–208
compared with interviews, 211
encoding of, 209
limitations of, 221
reliability of, 206–207
usefulness of, 219–221
Sexual encounters
and negotiation, 158
and the diary method, 209
anonymous, 304
Sexual identity, and risk
behaviour, 197
Sexuality
and culture, 280
and gender, 83
and marriage, 127
and reproduction, 33
as a social construct and
prevention, 173–174
conceptualization of, 274
in interethnic contact, 63
of gay men, 174
private and public expression
of, ix
symbolic value of, 172
the anti-social core of, xiii
Western preconceptions, 304
young gay men, 164
Sexual meaning, vs. sexual
behaviour, 266
Sexual negotiation, 80, 158, 159,
170, 172
avoidance strategies, 167
between strangers, 168
Sexual openness, and culture,
viii–ix
Sexual permissiveness, 274

Sexual relations
in Haiti, 17–19
types of, 213
Sexual risk, ii, v, xii, xiii
analysis of, 258
and gender, 245, 324
and HIV knowledge, 234
and perception of control,
195, 197
and political economy, 68–69
and poverty, 10–12, 123, 249–50
and social oppression, 188
and steady partnership, 196
and stress, 189
and traditional culture, 79
as suicide, 295
cultural construction of, 39
denial of, 136–137, 146
motives for, 234–235
perception of, 55, 143, 150–151,
244, 245, 281
risk factors, 5, 7
single women, 34
sociocultural context of, 158,
196, 294
Sexual session, 209–210
Sex work, 139–140
advantage of, 128–129
and cultural change, 65
and economic survival, 18
and love, 128, 129
and personal autonomy, 128
and poverty, 66
and stigma, 118, 137
in Spain, 142
in Thailand, 56
tolerance towards, 118
working conditions, 119
Sex workers
and drug use, 140
and HIV transmission, 140
as a group, 140, 144
attitudes of, 119

clients of, 136
  as a group, 140, 141
  mobility of, 120
  position of, 132
  research on, 297
Sex workers in Thailand. *See*
  Thailand
Shame
  and sexuality, 62
  and sexual relations, 66
Shedlin, M., 246
Shilts, R., 229
SIDA. *See* AIDS
Siegel, C., 234, 236, 237
SIGMA project, 205, 213
Silent community, 166
Simon, W., 63, 260
Singer, M., v, 41
Siraphone Virulak, 263
Social analysis, xi
  and ethnography, 23–24
  of HIV transmission in Haiti, 6,
    15, 23
Social constructionists, vs.
  essentialists, 292
Social Science Research
  Council, 308
Social support, 188
  and coping, 187
  and culture, xiii
  and unsafe sex, 185
Sofer, J., 164
Sophon Ratanakhon, 59
South Africa, 316–329
Sovine, M., 262, 265
Spain, 136–152
Speech events, and AIDS
  discourse, 228, 237
Stall, R., 184, 186, 234
Stavenhagen, R., 41
STDs
  among hilltribes in Northern
    Thailand, 66
  and lack of treatment, 18

co-factors in HIV transmission,
  21–22, 87
  discourse on, 229
  in South Africa, 321
  in Zaïre, 30
Stevens, J., 194
Stiffman, A.R.R., 189
Stigmatization, of sex work, 141
Stoller, R., iii, ix, 260
Stress
  and life events, 186
  and perception of control, 190
  chronic, 186
  coping with, 189
  definition of, 186–188
  sources of, 186
Structural Adjustment
  Programmes (SAPs), 30
Styles, J., 159
Sugar daddies, 82, 119
Sugar mummies, 82
Suicide, and rationality, 294
Sukanya Hantrakul, 127, 128
Sweden, 157–172
Symbolic economy, of sexuality,
  172, 174
Symonds, P.V., xi, 54, 59, 61, 64

T

Talkability, 54, 68, 71, 80
Tan, M.L., iii, x, xv, 318
Tarantola, D.J.M., v, 55, 130,
  262, 265
Tausig, M., 186
Taylor, C.C., 33
Taylor, C.L., 174
Temoshok, L., 186
Texts, analysis of, 228

Thailand, xii, xiii, 50–70, 115–132
  brothel circuit, 116
  commercial sex in, 56
  condom use by sex workers, 121
  condom use in, 123
  land shortage in (Northern), 59
  prevalence of HIV/AIDS in,
    55–56
  sex scene in, 116, 120
  sex workers, 118, 125
    perception of, by tourists, 127
    Western perception of, 125
  tribal minorities, 54. *See*
    Hilltribes
Third World
  and the impact of AIDS, viii
Thitsa Khin, 127
Tielman, R., 184
Timmel, S., 38
Traditional culture
  and HIV prevention, 40
Traditional healers
  as agents of change, 40
Training for transformation, 38
Transgression, 63, 88
Tribal minorities. *See* Hilltribes
Tribal people
  and prostitution, 65
Tribal Research Institute, 55, 64
Troiden, R.R., 188
Trouillot, M.R., 17
Tuberculosis
  and HIV infection in
    Haiti, 14–15
Turner, C.F., 185, 190, 258, 259,
    260, 261, 264
Turner, R.J., 186
Turner, T.A., 243
Turner, V., 295
Tuskegee Syphilis Study, 42

U

Uganda, 42, 43, 79–94
Umberson, D., 187
UNDP, 19
United Kingdom, 205–219
Unsafe sex
  adolescents, 102
  and age, 190
  and alcohol, 158, 185
  and attribution theory, 190
  and depression, 190
  and drugs, 185
  and knowledge, 190
  and love, 296–297
  and passion, 237
  and relapse, 158, 185
  and sexual desire, 234
  behavioural analysis of, 208
  causes of, 185–186
  clients of Thai sex workers, 124
  gay men, 157, 184–185
  theories about, 158

V

Vaccine testing, 42–43
  and ethics, 42
Vaccine trials, in Uganda, 85
Vance, C.S., ix, 274
Vanwesenbeeck, I., 121
Vaughan, M., 33
Vichai Poshyachinda, 56, 57, 69
Video clubs
  and safer sex, 165, 169
  as homo-social milieu, 164–165
  cruising scripts in, 166–167
  owners of, 165
  sexual interaction in, 162–170
  spatial organization, 162
  visitors of, 162, 164

Vincke, J., iii, xiii, 188, 190
Voices
  male, 80
  of elites, 80, 84
  of girls, 80
  of women, 80, 86
  of young men, 80
Vroome, E. de, 184
Vulnerability to HIV, xii, 54
  and poverty, 59–60
  as a concept, 67
  of marginalized groups, 69

W

Wallston, B.S., 276
Wallston, K.A., 276
Wanat Bhruksasri, 59
Weatherburn, P., 158, 173, 184, 208
Weeks, J., 260
Weinberg, T.S., 188
Weniger, B.G., 56
Werasit Sittitrai, 263
Western models, in Third World
  AIDS research, x
Wethinghton, E., 187
Wheaton, B., 187
Wheeler, C.C., 220
Whitam, F., 273
White, H.R., 189
WHO, 213, 301
  Global Program on AIDS, 205,
    264, 265

Whyte, W.F., 324
Wiley, J., 186
Woelfel, M.W., 187
Wolf, E.R., v, 318
Women
  and coping with AIDS, 317
  economic value of, 64–65
  self-protection, 325
World Health Organization, ix, 85
Worth, D., 317
Wortman, C.B., 186
Wyse, D., 185

Y

Yao, 55
Yates, B., 32
Yiannakis, A., 126
Young, A., 150
Youth. *See* also Adolescents
  and HIV risk, 89–93
Ytterberg, H., 160

Z

Zaïre, 30–44
  action-research in, 316
  HIV epidemic in, 30
Zalduondo, B.O. de, 261, 262, 264
Zautra, A.J., 187
Zero grazing, 80
Zondi, M., 320, 322